P9-EDE-118

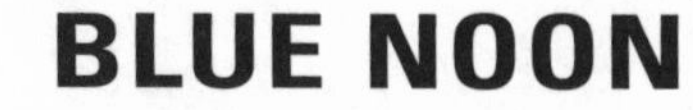

BLUE NOON

THE SLEEP REVOLUTION

THE SLEEP REVOLUTION

TRANSFORMING YOUR LIFE, ONE NIGHT AT A TIME

ARIANNA HUFFINGTON

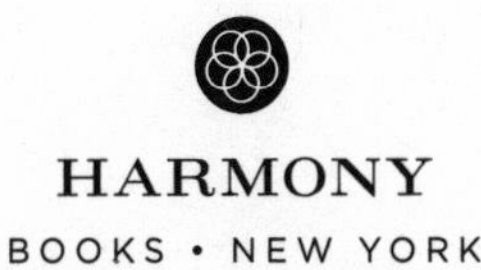

HARMONY
BOOKS • NEW YORK

Published in the United States by Harmony Books, an imprint of the Crown Publishing Group, a division of Penguin Random House LLC, New York.
crownpublishing.com

Harmony Books is a registered trademark, and the Circle colophon is a trademark of Penguin Random House LLC.

Library of Congress Cataloging-in-Publication Data
Names: Huffington, Arianna Stassinopoulos, 1950–, author.
Title: The sleep revolution : transforming your life, one night at a time / Arianna Huffington.
Description: New York : Harmony, [2016]
Identifiers: LCCN 2015039918 | ISBN 9781101904008
Subjects: LCSH: Sleep—Health aspects. | Sleep deprivation | BISAC: PSYCHOLOGY / Social Psychology.
Classification: LCC RA786 .H84 2016 | DDC 613.7/94—dc23
LC record available at http://lccn.loc.gov/2015039918

ISBN 978-1-101-90400-8
eBook ISBN 978-1-101-90401-5
International Edition ISBN 978-0-8041-8911-8

PRINTED IN THE UNITED STATES OF AMERICA

Jacket design by Christopher Brand
Jacket photograph by Peter Yang

10 9 8 7 6 5 4 3 2 1

First Edition

For all those who are sick and tired
of being sick and tired.

CONTENTS

INTRODUCTION

I GREW UP in a one-bedroom apartment in Athens where sleep was revered. After my parents separated when I was eleven, my mother, my sister, and I shared that one bedroom. But it was always understood that we should do everything in our power not to wake up anyone who was sleeping. If I had to study after my younger sister went to bed, I would study in the kitchen so the light wouldn't wake her. My mother was adamant about the importance of sleep for our health, our happiness, and our schoolwork. But despite this auspicious beginning, as soon as I left home—first to study at Cambridge and then to live and work in London—I bought into the prevalent cultural norm of sleep deprivation as essential to achievement and success. FOMO (fear of missing out) became part of my life long before the acronym was invented (probably by sleep-deprived millennials).

This new sleep-be-damned approach continued for years, until, as I wrote about in *Thrive*, I collapsed from sleep deprivation, exhaustion, and burnout in April 2007. I'd just returned home after taking my daughter Christina, then a junior in high school, on a tour of prospective colleges. The ground rules we'd agreed on—or, more accurately, that my daughter demanded—were that during the days I would not be on my BlackBerry. But that didn't mean I would stop working (sacrilege!). So each night we'd eat dinner late and get back to the hotel exhausted. Then, in some sort of role reversal, Christina would do the responsible thing and go to sleep while I acted the part of the sneaky teenager and stayed up late. After she'd fallen asleep, I'd fire up the computers and the BlackBerrys, responding to all the "urgent" emails and generally attempting to squeeze a full day's work into what should have been my sleep time. This would go on until about 3 a.m., when I couldn't keep my eyes open any longer. And after three or four hours of sleep, I'd be back up for the day shift. Work, after all, was much more important than sleep, at least to my 2007 self. Because, hey, I'm running a start-up—one that's got my name on it. Clearly I'm indispensable, so I must work all night, responding to a hundred emails and then writing a long blog post, while being the perfect mother during the day. This way of working and living seemed to serve me well—until it didn't.

The only part of that trip I seem to remember clearly is the cold, rainy morning at Brown, walking around in a daze as if it were finals week. About a third of the way into the tour, Christina leaned over to me and said, "I'm not going to apply here—how about we just drop out of the tour and go get coffee?" I felt like I'd just been given a get-out-of-jail-free card. Yes, yes! Where is the closest Starbucks? How quickly can we get there? I hope there's no line. Can't wait for my fourth infusion of caffeine of the day—just the pick-me-up I need to make it to the night shift.

So the college trip was over. But I didn't fly straight home. Instead I flew first to Portland for a speaking engagement that, in my scheduling hubris, I'd said yes to, and then on to L.A. that night. After getting home very late, I was up again four hours later for a CNN interview. I have no idea why I said yes, but there is that level of tiredness where you don't actually even notice you're tired because you no longer remember how not being tired feels. Like being drunk, being that tired not only causes you to make bad decisions, but it also makes you unaware that you're in no state to be making decisions at all. I was sleep-walking through my life.

Of course, being Greek, I should have known that hubris always gets punished. And mine was no exception. Once I got to my office after the interview, my body just couldn't take it anymore, and down I went, coming back to consciousness in a pool of blood. And that's how I painfully but powerfully rediscovered what my mother, with no formal education, and certainly no background in health or science, knew instinctively all those years ago in Athens: no matter the constraints, whether a tiny, crowded apartment or a crowded work schedule, sleep is a fundamental human need that must be respected.

It's one of humanity's great unifiers. It binds us to one another, to our ancestors, to our past, and to the future. No matter who we are or where we are in the world and in our lives, we share a common need for sleep. Though this need has been a constant throughout human history, our relationship to sleep has gone through dramatic ups and downs. And right now that relationship is in crisis.

The evidence is all around us. For instance, do you know what happens if you type the words "why am I" into Google? Before you can type the next word, Google's autocomplete function—based on the most common searches—helpfully offers to finish your thought. The first suggestion: "why am I so tired?" The global zeitgeist perfectly captured in five words. The existential cry of the modern age. And that's not just in New York but also in Toronto, Paris, Seoul, Madrid, New Delhi, Berlin, Cape Town, and London. Sleep deprivation is the new lingua franca.

Though we may not be getting much of it, we certainly talk (and post and tweet) about sleep a lot. There are nearly five thousand apps that come up when you search "sleep" in the Apple App Store, more than 15 million photos under #sleep on Instagram, another 14 million under #sleepy, and more than 24 million under #tired. A quick search for "sleep" on Google will bring up more than 800 million results. Sleep isn't just buried in our subconscious; it's on our minds, and in the news, as never before.

But even though we now know more about sleep than at any other time in history, and how important it is to every aspect of our physical, mental, emotional, and spiritual well-being, actually getting enough sleep is harder and harder to do. And here is a further paradox: advances in technology have allowed us to pull back the curtain on what's going on while we sleep, but technology is also one of the main reasons our relationship to this fundamental part of our existence has become so compromised.

Of course it's not just technology that's coming between us and a good night's sleep. It's also our collective delusion that overwork and burnout are the price we must pay in order to succeed. The method (or cheat code) we use isn't a mystery: feeling that there aren't enough hours in the day, we look for something to cut. And sleep is an easy target. In fact, up against this unforgiving definition of success, sleep doesn't stand a chance.

But this is a woefully incomplete vision of success. That's why I wrote *Thrive*—to explore the ways in which our lives can be much more fulfilling when we broaden our definition of success, moving beyond the modern metrics of money, status, and power to include well-being, wisdom, wonder, and the power of giving.

Sleep is a key element of our well-being and interacts profoundly with each of the other parts. Once I started getting seven or eight hours of sleep, it became easier to meditate and exercise, make wiser decisions, and connect more deeply with myself and others.

As I went around the country talking about *Thrive*, I found that the subject that came up the most—by far—was sleep: how difficult it is to get enough, how there are simply not enough hours in the day, how tough it is to wind down, how hard it is to fall asleep and stay asleep, even when we set aside enough time. Since my own transformation into a sleep evangelist, everywhere I go, someone will pull me aside and, often in hushed and conspiratorial tones, confess, "I'm just not getting enough sleep. I'm exhausted all the time." Or, as one young woman told me after a talk in San Francisco, "I don't remember the last time I wasn't tired." By the end of an evening, I'll have had that same conversation with any number of people in the room. And what everyone wants to know is, "What should I do to get more sleep?"

It's clear that if we're going to truly thrive, we must begin with sleep. It's the gateway through which a life of well-being must travel. From the moment we're born until the moment we die, we're in a relationship with sleep. It's the dominant subject for the parents of a newborn. "How's the baby sleeping?" people ask. Or "How are *you* sleeping?" Or, in an attempt to be helpful, "Here are twenty-five books to read in your spare time about how to get a newborn baby to sleep." To anyone who has a child, it's no surprise that Adam Mansbach's 2011 book *Go the F**k to Sleep* became a number-one best seller. And at the other end of the sleep spectrum, at the close of our lives, the phrase that's come to sum up what most people consider the best way to die is to "go peacefully in our sleep."

So we all have an intimate and unique relationship with sleep. Even when we fight against it, it's like an intense, on-again, off-again relationship with an ex who's never moved out. Sometimes it's healthy and supportive of everything we do while we're awake, and sometimes it's wildly dysfunctional and destructive. To paraphrase Tolstoy—who himself was fascinated with sleep—every unhappy relationship with sleep is unhappy in its own way. But whether we embrace it or resist it, one way or the other, we're all dealing with sleep every day, every night, all the time.

My own relationship with sleep has certainly been through ups and downs. For years, in one of our up periods, I chronicled my dreams every morning just after waking. In a small notebook I kept on my nightstand, I'd write as many details as I could remember before the day's demands intruded. It was like an intimate pen-pal relationship, only with someone—an elusive, timeless, and deeper version of myself—I had the chance to be with every night. And the effects of this habit, even though it was confined to the morning, echoed throughout my day.

But then, as so often happens, circumstances changed. In this case it was the arrival of my first daughter. My relationship to sleep didn't end—it can't, after all—but we certainly hit a rough patch. Gone was the enchanting experience of waking up naturally after a full night's sleep. In its place was a new reality, where sleep was perpetually just out of reach. Night-and-day transitions vanished, and sleep was something to be had only in tiny increments between other things—as if my entire diet was only what I was able to grab and scarf down on the way out the door. Sleep became an impediment, something to get past, a luxury I thought I could no longer afford. With the birth of my second daughter, it got only worse. In my mind, getting enough sleep would mean taking something away from my children—time spent with them or just time spent preparing everything for their next day. Of course, in reality what I was taking away from them was my ability to truly *be* with them.

Even after the immediate sleep demands of my children became less pressing, I never quite reentered that Garden of Eden of pre-child sleep. As so many of us do, I created a life in which I thought I no longer needed much sleep. And when my children stopped needing as much of my time, that space got filled with other things—columns and speeches and books that had to be written, and then a new baby, *The Huffington Post.* So that cycle of burnout and perpetual tiredness came to be my new normal—until my wake-up call.

The train is easy to board, hard to leave.

—Milan Kundera, *The Art of the Novel*

At the time, I didn't know the reason for my collapse (during which I hit my face on my desk as I toppled over and broke my cheekbone). But as I went from doctor to doctor and sat in waiting room after waiting room, trying to figure out the reason I'd blacked out, I began to think about how I'd been living my life. I had time to ask myself some big questions, such as the one at the heart of much of the work of Greek philosophers: What does it mean to lead "the good life"?

As it turned out, nothing was wrong with me. Except that, in fact, everything was wrong. The diagnosis was, essentially, an acute case of burnout, which Belgian philosopher Pascal Chabot has called "civilization's disease." And it all came back to sleep. If I was really going to make the sort of changes to my life I needed to, I was going to have to start with sleep. So I patiently set about repairing our strained relationship. And I'm happy to report that we are now solidly back together. But, as they say in recovery programs, it's one day (or night) at a time.

What I've learned is that in today's world, the path of least resistance is the path of insufficient sleep. And unless we take specific and deliberate steps to make it a priority in our lives, we won't get the sleep we need. Because today a full night's rest has never been more difficult to come by. With the demands of work and family and our ubiquitous and ever-growing arsenal of glowing screens and buzzing devices, we're hyperconnected with everyone in the world—often from the second we wake up to the second we finally fall asleep. But unless we're vigilant, we can become disconnected from ourselves.

What is more gentle than a wind in summer?
What is more soothing than the pretty hummer
That stays one moment in an open flower,
And buzzes cheerily from bower to bower?
What is more tranquil than a musk-rose blowing
In a green island, far from all men's knowing?

More healthful than the leafiness of dales?
More secret than a nest of nightingales?
. . . More full of visions than a high romance?
What, but thee, Sleep? Soft closer of our eyes!

—John Keats, "Sleep and Poetry"

If we look at our lives as a spiritual journey, sleep becomes a key paradox: when we completely identify with our persona in this world—with our job, our appearance, our bank account—we are asleep to life's deeper dimensions. In fairy tales such as *Sleeping Beauty* and *Snow White*, the heroines fall into a frozen sleep as the result of a dark spell and are awakened only through an act of grace personified in a savior-prince. In our daily lives, we are all in need of such a savior-prince, but we cannot afford to wait for Prince Charming. We have to be our *own* Prince Charming—to wake ourselves up by turning our gaze from the projects and distractions of the outside world to the many miracles within ourselves. That's the great sleep awakening. And as Carl Jung wrote, "Dreams give information about the secrets of the inner life and reveal to the dreamer hidden factors of his personality."

We are living in a golden age of sleep science—revealing all the ways in which sleep and dreams play a vital role in our decision making, emotional intelligence, cognitive function, and creativity. And how lack of sleep is often the culprit behind anxiety, stress, depression, and a myriad of health problems. It's only relatively recently that we've come to fully grasp the medical consequences of sleep deprivation. In the 1970s, there were only 3 centers in the United States devoted to sleep disorders. By the 1990s, that number had swelled to more than 300. Today there are more than 2,500 accredited sleep centers.

Even so, the delusion persists that we can do our jobs just as well on four or five or six hours of sleep as we can on seven or eight. It's a delusion that affects not only our personal health but our productivity and decision making. In other words, we may not have as many good ideas as we would have otherwise had, we may not be as able to come up with creative solutions to problems we're trying to address, or we may be short-tempered or waste a day (or day after day, or year after year) going through the motions. And in some occupations—in our hospitals, on our highways, or in the air—lack of sleep can be a life-or-death matter.

But even as we advance the science of sleep, we're also in desperate need of rediscovering its mystery. Every night can be a reminder that we are more than the sum of our successes and failures, that beyond all our struggling and our rushing there is a stillness that's available to us, that comes from a place deeper and more ancient than the unending noise that surrounds us. When we connect to that stillness through sleep, we can tap into it, even in the middle of the most action-packed day. "Learning to let go should be learned before learning to get," said Ray Bradbury. And surrendering to sleep every night is the ultimate letting-go.

I wrote *The Sleep Revolution* to examine this ancient, essential, and mysterious phenomenon from all angles, and to explore the ways we can use sleep to help regain control over our out-of-kilter lives. By the time you get to the chapter on tools and techniques, I hope you'll be convinced of the need to go from knowing what we must do to actually doing it, from awareness to action. In the first two chapters, I'll present the overwhelming evidence that we are indeed in a sleep crisis. More than 40 percent of Americans get less than the recommended minimum seven hours of sleep per night, with similar (or worse) statistics from around the world. We'll see how this is affecting various industries, from transportation and medicine to politics and law enforcement. In the third chapter, we'll take a look at the history of sleep. We're only now beginning to come out of a phase that started with the Industrial Revolution, in which sleep became just another obstacle to work. The veneration of sleep as a unique portal to the sacred was sacrificed to the idea of progress and productivity. The twentieth century saw the labor movement pushing back against the encroachment of work into our personal lives. And later, with the birth of the new science of sleep, we began to discover that sleep is in fact deeply connected to every aspect of our physical and mental health. But the end of the twentieth century also saw technological advances that allow our workdays to essentially never end, which is where we are today. Then I'll examine the science of sleep and what, exactly, is going on when we finally drift off. The short answer: a lot. Far from being a time of inactivity, sleep keeps many parts of the brain feverishly busy, and what they're doing—or not doing, if we neglect sleep—has huge consequences. We'll learn how sleep deprivation is linked with increased risks of diabetes, heart attack, stroke, cancer, obesity, and Alzheimer's disease. I'll then look at sleep disorders, from sleep apnea to insomnia to something called "exploding head syndrome" (yes, that's its scientific name!).

In "The Way Forward," Part Two of the book, I'll explore the innovations, reforms, inventions, and technology fueling the sleep revolution. People want more sleep, and the market is responding. Hotel rooms are being transformed into sleep temples, schools are modifying start times to suit the sleep needs of teenagers, an exploding market in wearable technology has emerged that tracks our sleep, and a range of smart products—from smart mattresses to smart headphones—has entered our lives. And yet there is a lot more to do. As I'll discuss in "The Way Forward," solving our sleep crisis requires not just practical changes to how we approach our days and our nights but also rethinking our priorities and what we really value. Sleep is, after all, at the center of our overall vitality. When we sleep well, we feel better, and vice versa. We may be what we eat, but also, to be sure, we are how we sleep.

I'm confident you will come away from this exploration with a newfound respect for sleep. But you may also find yourself beginning a love affair with it. We need to reclaim this special realm—not just because sleep makes us better at our jobs (though there's that) and not just because it makes us healthier in every way (there is that, too) but also because of the unique way it allows us to connect with a deeper part of ourselves. Because when we are asleep, the things that define our identity when we're awake—our jobs, our relationships, our hopes, our fears—recede. And that makes possible one of the least discussed benefits (or miracles, really) of sleep: the way it allows us, once we return from our night's journey, to see the world anew, with fresh eyes and a reinvigorated spirit, to step out of time and come back to our lives restored. These two threads that run through our life—one pulling us into the world to achieve and make things happen, the other pulling us back from the world to nourish and replenish ourselves—can seem at odds, but in fact they reinforce each other.

My hope is that by the end of this book you'll be inspired to renew your relationship with sleep—in all its mystery and all its fullness—and join the sleep revolution, transforming your life and our world one night at a time.

PART ONE

WAKE-UP CALL

1.

OUR CURRENT SLEEP CRISIS

SARVSHRESHTH GUPTA was a first-year analyst at Goldman Sachs in San Francisco in 2015. Overwhelmed by the hundred-hour workweeks, he decided to leave the bank in March. He soon returned, though whether this was a result of social or self-inflicted pressure is still unclear. A week later, he called his father at 2:40 a.m. saying he hadn't slept in two days. He said he had a presentation to complete and a morning meeting to prepare for, and was alone in the office. His father insisted he go home, and Gupta replied that he would stay at work just a bit longer. A few hours later, he was found dead on the street outside his home. He had jumped from his high-rise building.

DEATH FROM overwork has its own word in Japanese (*karoshi*), in Chinese (*guolaosi*), and in Korean (*gwarosa*). No such word exists in English, but the casualties are all around us. And though this is an extreme example of the consequences of not getting enough sleep, sleep deprivation has become an epidemic.

It is a specter haunting the industrialized world. Simply put: we don't get enough sleep. And it's a much bigger problem—with much higher stakes—than many of us realize. Both our daytime hours and our nighttime hours are under assault as never before. As the amount of things we need to cram into each day has increased, the value of our awake time has skyrocketed. Benjamin Franklin's "Time is money!" has become a corporate-world mantra. And this has come at the expense of our time asleep, which since the dawn of the Industrial Revolution we have treated like some dull, distant relative we visit only reluctantly and out of obligation, for as short a time as we can manage.

Scientists are resoundingly confirming what our ancestors knew instinctively: that our sleep is not empty time. Sleep is a time of intense neurological activity—a rich time of renewal, memory consolidation, brain and neurochemical cleansing, and cognitive maintenance. Properly appraised, our sleeping time is as valuable a commodity as the time we are awake. In fact, getting the right amount of sleep enhances the quality of every minute we spend with our eyes open.

But today much of our society is still operating under the collective delusion that sleep is simply time lost to other pursuits, that it can be endlessly appropriated at will to satisfy our increasingly busy lives and overstuffed to-do lists. We see this delusion reflected in the phrase "I'll sleep when I'm dead," which has flooded popular consciousness, including a hit Bon Jovi song, an album by the late rocker Warren Zevon, and a crime film starring Clive Owen. Everywhere you turn, sleep deprivation is glamorized and celebrated: "You snooze, you lose." The phrase "catch a few z's" is telling: the last letter of the alphabet used to represent that last thing on our culture's shared priority list. The combination of a deeply misguided definition of what it means to be successful in today's world—that it can come only through burnout and stress—along with the distractions and temptations of a 24/7 wired world, has imperiled our sleep as never before.

I experienced firsthand the high price we're paying for cheating sleep when I collapsed from exhaustion, and it pains me to see dear friends (and strangers) go through the same struggle. Rajiv Joshi is the managing director of the B Team—a nonprofit on whose board I serve, founded by Richard Branson and Jochen Zeitz to help move business beyond profit as the only metric of success. In June 2015, he had a seizure at age thirty-one during a B Team meeting in Bellagio, Italy, collapsing from exhaustion and sleep deprivation. Unable to walk, he spent eight days in a hospital in Bellagio and weeks after in physical therapy. In talking with medical experts, he learned that we all have a "seizure threshold," and when we don't take time to properly rest, we move closer and closer to it. Rajiv had crossed his threshold and fallen off the cliff. "The struggle for a more just and sustainable world," he told me when he was back at work, "is a marathon, not a sprint, and we can't forget that it starts at home with personal sustainability."

According to a recent Gallup poll, 40 percent of all American adults are sleep-deprived, clocking significantly less than the recommended minimum seven hours of sleep per night. Getting enough sleep, says Dr. Judith Owens, the director of the Center for Pediatric Sleep Disorders at Boston Children's Hospital, is "just as important as good nutrition, physical activity, and wearing your seat belt." But most people hugely underestimate their need for sleep. That's why sleep, says Dr. Michael Roizen, the chief wellness officer of the Cleveland Clinic, "is our most underrated health habit." A National Sleep Foundation report backs this up: two-thirds of us are not getting enough sleep on weeknights.

The crisis is global. In 2011, 32 percent of people surveyed in the United Kingdom said they had averaged less than seven hours of sleep a night in the previous six months. By 2014 that number had rocketed up to 60 percent. In 2013, more than a third of Germans and two-thirds of Japanese surveyed said they do not get sufficient sleep on weeknights. In fact, the Japanese have a term, *inemuri*, which roughly translates as "to be asleep while present"—that is, to be so exhausted that you fall asleep in the middle of a meeting. This has been praised as a sign of dedication and hard work—but it is actually another symptom of the sleep crisis we are finally confronting.

The wearable-device company Jawbone collects sleep data from thousands of people wearing its UP activity trackers. As a result, we now have a record of the cities that get the least amount of sleep. Tokyo residents sleep a dangerously low 5 hours and 45 minutes a night. Seoul clocks in at 6 hours and 3 minutes; Dubai, 6 hours and 13 minutes; Singapore, 6 hours and 27 minutes; Hong Kong, 6 hours and 29 minutes; and Las Vegas, 6 hours and 32 minutes. When you're getting less sleep than Las Vegas, you have a problem.

Of course, much of this can be laid at the feet of work—or, more broadly, how we define work, which is colored by how we define success and what's important in our lives. The unquestioning belief that work should always have the top claim on our time has been a costly one. And it has gotten worse as technology has allowed a growing number of us to carry our work with us—in our pockets and purses in the form of our phones—wherever we go.

Our houses, our bedrooms—even our beds—are littered with beeping, vibrating, flashing screens. It's the never-ending possibility of connecting—with friends, with strangers, with the entire world, with every TV show or movie ever made—with just the press of a button that is, not surprisingly, addictive. Humans are social creatures—we're hardwired to connect. Even when we're not actually connecting digitally, we're in a constant state of heightened anticipation. And always being in this state doesn't exactly put us in the right frame of mind to wind down when it's time to sleep. Though we don't give much thought to how we put ourselves to bed, we have little resting places and refueling shrines all over our houses, like little doll beds, where our technology can recharge, even if we can't.

Being perpetually wired is now considered a prerequisite for success, as Alan Derickson writes in *Dangerously Sleepy*: "Sleep deprivation now resides within a repertoire of practices deemed essential to survival in a globally competitive world. More so than in the time of Thomas Edison, depriving oneself of necessary rest or denying it to those under one's control is considered necessary to success in a 24/7/365 society. Americans have a stronger ideological rationale than ever to distrust any sort of dormancy."

And Americans are anything but dormant. From 1990 to 2000, American workers added the equivalent of another full workweek to their year. A 2014 survey by Skift, a travel website, showed that more than 40 percent of Americans had not taken a single vacation day that year. Much of that added work time has come at the expense of sleep. Dr. Charles Czeisler, the head of the Division of Sleep and Circadian Disorders at Brigham and Women's Hospital in Boston, estimates that in the past fifty years our sleep on work nights has dropped from eight and a half hours to just under seven. Thirty percent of employed Americans now report getting six hours of sleep or less per night, and nearly 70 percent describe their sleep as insufficient. Getting by on less than six hours of sleep is one of the biggest factors in job burnout.

And for far too many people in the world, the vicious cycle of financial deprivation also feeds into the vicious cycle of sleep deprivation. If you're working two or three jobs and struggling to make ends meet, "get more sleep" is probably not going to be near the top of your priorities list. As in the case of health care, access to sleep is not evenly—or fairly—distributed. Sleep is another casualty of inequality. A 2013 study from the University of Chicago found that "lower socio-economic position was associated with poorer subjective sleep quality, increased sleepiness and/or increased sleep complaints." But the paradox here is that the more challenging our circumstances, the more imperative it is to take whatever steps we can to tap into our resilience to help us withstand and overcome the challenges we face. There's a reason we're told on airplanes to "secure your own mask first."

Where we live can also affect our sleep. "I have never seen a study that hasn't shown a direct association between neighborhood quality and sleep quality," said Lauren Hale, a Stony Brook University professor of preventive medicine. If you're living in a neighborhood with gang warfare and random acts of violence, sleep will inevitably suffer—yet another example of sleep deprivation's connection with deeper social problems.

THE COST OF LOST SLEEP

It is industrialization, for all its benefits, that has exacerbated our flawed relationship with sleep on such a massive scale.

We sacrifice sleep in the name of productivity, but ironically, our loss of sleep, despite the extra hours we put in at work, adds up to more than eleven days of lost productivity per year per worker, or about $2,280. This results in a total annual cost of sleep deprivation to the US economy of more than $63 billion, in the form of absenteeism and presenteeism (when employees are present at work physically but not really mentally focused). "Americans are not missing work because of insomnia," said Harvard Medical School professor Ronald C. Kessler. "They are still going to their jobs, but they're accomplishing less because they're tired. In an information-based economy, it's difficult to find a condition that has a greater effect on productivity."

Sleep disorders cost Australia more than $5 billion a year in health care and indirect costs. And "reduction in life quality" added costs equivalent to a whopping $31.4 billion a year. A report, aptly titled "Re-Awakening Australia," linked lack of sleep with lost productivity and driving and workplace accidents. In the United Kingdom, a survey showed that one in five employees had recently missed work or come in late because of sleep deprivation. The researchers estimated that this is equivalent to a loss of more than 47 million hours of work per year, or a £453 million loss in productivity. And almost a third of all UK employees reported feeling tired every morning. Yet, though awareness is spreading, few companies have given sleep the priority it deserves, considering its effects on their bottom line. In Canada, 26 percent of the workforce reported having called in sick because of sleep deprivation. And nearly two-thirds of Canadian adults report feeling tired "most of the time."

It turns out that women need more sleep than men, so the lack of sleep has even more negative mental and physical effects on them. Duke Medical Center researchers found that women are at a greater risk for heart disease, Type 2 diabetes, and depression. "We found that for women, poor sleep is strongly associated with high levels of psychological distress, and greater feelings of hostility, depression and anger," said Edward Suarez, the lead author of the study. "In contrast, these feelings were not associated with the same degree of sleep disruption in men."

As women have entered the workplace—a workplace created in large measure by men, which uses our willingness to work long hours until we ultimately burn out as a proxy for commitment and dedication—they are still stuck with the heavy lifting when it comes to housework. The upshot is that women end up making even more withdrawals from their sleep bank. "They have so many commitments, and sleep starts to get low on the totem pole," says Michael Breus, the author of *Beauty Sleep*. "They may know that sleep should be a priority, but then, you know, they've just got to get that last thing done. And that's when it starts to get bad."

According to Dr. William Dement, the founder of the Stanford Sleep Disorders Clinic (the first of its kind), working mothers who have young children at home have seen an additional 241 hours of work and commuting time added to their lives annually since 1969.

Sarah Bunton, a mother and cognitive-skills trainer, described her experience on *The Huffington Post*: "Do you ever have one of those days where you want to hit pause? Let me rephrase: do you ever have a day where you don't want to hit pause? . . . There really isn't an end of the day for most moms, working or otherwise. There's usually not a beginning, either, just a continuation of whatever chaos preceded the momentary silence. . . . Mommy wants a nap."

"Let's face it, women today are tired. Done. Cooked. Fried," wrote Karen Brody, founder of the meditation program Bold Tranquility. "I coach busy women and this is what they tell me all the time: 'I spent years getting educated and now I don't have any energy to work.'"

Dr. Frank Lipman, the founder of the Eleven Eleven Wellness Center in New York, sees so many patients who are sleep-deprived and exhausted that he came up with his own term for them. "I started calling these patients 'spent,' because that was how they seemed to me," he writes. He compares this to his time working in rural South Africa: "There I saw many diseases arising from poverty and malnutrition but I didn't see anyone who was 'spent,' as I do today in New York."

The world is too much with us; late and soon,
Getting and spending, we lay waste our powers . . .
For this, for everything, we are out of tune.

—William Wordsworth, "The World Is Too Much with Us"

Just as sleep is universal, so is the belief that we don't have enough time to get the sleep we need. But we actually have far more discretionary time than we realize. The key is taking an honest look at how we spend it.

In her discretionary time, for example, Sherry Turkle, professor of the Social Studies of Science and Technology at MIT, has been using TV as a reward, letting herself watch shows such as *Mad Men*, *Homeland*, and *The Americans* after working on her book. "I felt like I earned these elegant treats," she told me. "I remember saying '*Orange Is the New Black* is mine' after I finished the 'Friendship' chapter of *Reclaiming Conversation*. As I worked on the 'Romance' chapter, it was *House of Cards*. I wouldn't have said, 'I'm prioritizing television drama,' but what strikes me is that I never said, 'I'm prioritizing sleep.' "

That's the case for millions of people around the world, despite how high the costs of sleep deprivation are. The incidence of death from all causes goes up by 15 percent when we sleep five hours or less per night. A 2015 CNN.com article based on the latest findings by the American Academy of Sleep Medicine, provocatively titled "Sleep or Die," discussed the connection between lack of sleep and an increased risk of heart attack, stroke, diabetes, and obesity. In other words, getting enough sleep really is a matter of life and death.

And even when it doesn't kill us, sleep deprivation makes us dangerously less healthy. Dr. Carol Ash, the director of sleep medicine at Meridian Health, points out that even losing an hour of sleep per week—which many of us do without a moment's thought—can lead to a higher risk of heart attack. Even the switch to daylight saving time can temporarily disturb our sleep patterns.

Looking for even more warning bells? A Russian study found that nearly 63 percent of men who suffered a heart attack also had a sleep disorder. Men who had a sleep disorder had a risk of heart attack that was 2 to 2.6 times higher and a risk of stroke that was 1.5 to 4 times higher. A Norwegian study determined that people who had trouble falling asleep were involved in 34 percent of fatal car accidents. And those with symptoms of insomnia are nearly three times more likely to die from a fatal injury. A lack of melatonin, the hormone that controls our sleep and wake cycles, is linked to higher rates of breast, ovarian, and prostate cancers.

By weakening our immune system, sleep deprivation also makes us more susceptible to garden-variety illnesses, like the common cold. It would actually be better for business if employees called in tired, got a little more sleep, and then came in a bit late, rather than call in sick a few days later or, worse, show up sick, dragging themselves through the day while infecting others.

A lack of sleep also has a major impact on our ability to regulate our weight. In a study by the Mayo Clinic, sleep-restricted subjects gained more weight than their well-rested counterparts over the course of a week, consuming an average of 559 extra calories a day. People who get six hours of sleep per night are 23 percent more likely to be overweight. Get less than four hours of sleep per night and the increased likelihood of being overweight climbs to a staggering 73 percent. That is due in part to the fact that people who get more sleep produce less of a hormone called ghrelin—the "hunger hormone," which increases our appetite. The sleep-deprived group also had lower levels of the hormone leptin, the "satiety hormone," which lowers our appetite. In other words, cutting back on sleep is a fantastic way to gain weight. Other research points to the role of sleep in the production of orexin, a neurotransmitter that normally stimulates physical activity and energy expenditure but is reduced when you are sleep-deprived.

The bottom line? When we're not well rested, we're not as healthy. And it shows. In a Swedish study, untrained participants were asked to look at photos of both sleep-deprived and well-rested people. Participants judged those in the sleep-deprived group as "less healthy, more tired, and less attractive." An experiment in the United Kingdom tested the effects of sleep deprivation on a group of thirty women. Their skin was analyzed and photographed after they slept for eight hours and then again after sleeping six hours for five nights in a row. Fine lines and wrinkles increased by 45 percent, blemishes went up by 13 percent, and redness increased by 8 percent. In other words, we wear our lack of sleep on our faces.

SLEEP: A KEY TO MENTAL HEALTH

As we go deeper under the hood, sleep becomes even more vital, playing a major role in brain maintenance. While we sleep, the brain is able to get rid of toxins, including proteins that are associated with Alzheimer's disease. Which is to say, if we don't allow the brain time to do this crucial work, the cost can be high.

Sleep affects our mental health every bit as profoundly as it does our physical health. Sleep deprivation has been found to have a strong connection with practically every mental health disorder we know of, especially depression and anxiety. "When you find depression, even when you find anxiety, when you scratch the surface 80 to 90 percent of the time you find a sleep problem as well," says University of Delaware psychologist Brad Wolgast. In the Great British Sleep Survey, researchers found that sleep-deprived people were seven times more likely to experience feelings of helplessness and five times more likely to feel lonely.

Nancy Fox, who runs the healthy-eating website Skinny Kitchen, wrote evocatively about the effects of sleep on her emotional health: "When I was short on sleep it felt like my 'cup of stress' was full and the least extra amount made it spill over. I remember sitting in my car in the parking lot of the restaurant and getting a call telling me that it was my day with the carpool, and I had forgotten to pick up the kids. . . . It literally blew me out! . . . The lack of sleep was making me more emotionally fragile . . . [and] making small problems feel like big ones."

Sleep deprivation also takes a toll on our mental abilities. "Your cognitive performance is reduced greatly," said Till Roenneberg, a professor at Ludwig-Maximilians University in Munich. "Memory capacity is reduced. Social competence is reduced. Your entire performance is going to suffer. The way you make decisions is changed."

Fact: When Golden State Warriors player Andre Iguodala improved his sleep habits, his playing time increased by 12 percent and his three-point shot percentage more than doubled. His points per minute went up by 29 percent, and his free-throw percentage increased by 8.9 percent. His turnovers decreased by 37 percent per game, and his fouls dropped by 45 percent.

In just two weeks of getting six hours of sleep per night, the performance drop-off is the same as in someone who has gone twenty-four hours without sleep. For those getting just four hours, the impairment is equivalent to that of going forty-eight hours without sleep. According to a *Today* show survey, the side effects of not getting enough sleep include difficulty concentrating (29 percent), losing interest in hobbies and leisure activities (19 percent), falling asleep at inappropriate times throughout the day (16 percent), losing your temper or behaving inappropriately with children or partners (16 percent), and behaving inappropriately at work (13 percent).

If a friend described chronic behavior like this to you, you might reasonably worry that he or she was having a drug or alcohol problem and stage an intervention. But we still have a long way to go toward treating sleep deprivation with the same seriousness and urgency.

Sometimes these side effects hit hard. Nalini Mani, a consultant living in Washington, D.C., averaged 2.5 to 3 hours a night throughout her thirties. Mani described the moment her body couldn't take it anymore: "I walked into my home at 10 p.m. after having gotten off the shuttle from La Guardia Airport. I walked in, took my shoes off and sat for a moment on my couch. I don't remember much of what happened. The next thing I knew was that I was still sitting there, on my couch, in the same position, at 9:30 the next morning, completely dressed. My body shut down, and I could not physically move."

DRIVING WHILE DROWSY

An Australian study found that after being awake for seventeen to nineteen hours (a normal day for many of us!), we can experience levels of cognitive impairment equal to having a blood alcohol level of .05 percent (just under the legal limit in many US states). And if we're awake just a few hours more, we're up to the equivalent of 0.1 percent—legally drunk. While there is of course a roadside test for drunk driving, there is no equivalent test for sleep-deprived driving. But if we truly want to address all the ways in which drivers become impaired, police officers should consider asking "Have you gotten enough sleep?" when they pull over people who are driving erratically. Building awareness of the impact of sleep deprivation on driving can't come too soon. Nearly 60 percent of train operators, 50 percent of pilots, 44 percent of truck drivers, and 29 percent of bus and taxi drivers admit that they never or rarely get a good night's sleep on work nights.

And that has predictable consequences. "Every aspect of who you are as a human, every capability is degraded, impaired, when you lose sleep," says Mark Rosekind, the Administrator of the National Highway Traffic Safety Administration. "What does that mean? Your decision making, reaction time, situational awareness, memory, communication, and those things go down by twenty to fifty percent."

So why do we tolerate, much less venerate and applaud, sleep deprivation? In much of our culture, especially in the workplace, going without sleep is considered a badge of honor. Yet since the effects of sleeplessness are largely the same as those of being drunk, when we get behind the wheel of a car without enough sleep, we are engaging in behavior that's dangerous to both ourselves and others.

In 1982, there were 21,113 deaths due to drunk driving. By 2013, that number had plummeted to just more than 10,000. A key factor was a change in thinking and a desire on the part of citizens, law enforcement, and society to take the problem seriously. The crisis of drowsy driving deserves that same attention. According to researchers at the University of Pennsylvania, "Sleepiness-related motor vehicle crashes have a fatality rate and injury severity level similar to alcohol-related crashes."

A report from the Centers for Disease Control and Prevention found that 4.5 percent of drivers aged eighteen to twenty-four had fallen asleep behind the wheel in the previous month. For those twenty-five to thirty-four years old, the number was 7.2 percent. And in a National Sleep Foundation poll, 60 percent of adults admitted to driving while drowsy within the past year. That translates into 168 *million* people—and those are just the ones who admit to it. More than a third of those, or 56 million people, have actually nodded off behind the wheel.

Carin Kilby Clark, founder of the Mommyhood Mentor, described how sleep deprivation nearly caused her to drive into an active intersection. "Dazed and confused, I thought I was pressing the brakes—but apparently not hard enough. Thanks to the loud horn of a driver passing by, I was jolted out of my trance. . . . I was driving half asleep. To be brutally honest, I was living life half asleep."

And if that isn't sobering enough, drowsy drivers are involved in 328,000 accidents each year, 6,400 of which result in deaths.

Sleep experts have a name for this phenomenon of nodding off: "microsleep." Microsleep occurs when we unknowingly fall asleep for anywhere from a few seconds to a minute or so. It is a terrifying phenomenon when you are behind the wheel of a car. Imagine commuting home from work, driving down the highway at 60 mph; at that speed, your car is traveling at 88 feet per second. If your eyes close for only four seconds, your car has traveled roughly the length of a football field before you jerk awake—and the consequences can be deadly.

Men are 11 percent more likely than women to climb behind the wheel knowing they're drowsy. Worse, they are nearly twice as likely to fall asleep at the wheel. That's not surprising, given the macho status we give to the willingness to forgo sleep.

And nowhere is this more true than in the trucking industry. "The men engaged in long-haul trucking have always been a different breed of blue-collar worker," writes Alan Derickson. "At the core of that identity is a rugged version of masculinity. . . . On the stage settings offered by highways, rest areas, and truck stops, men who pilot big rigs have been putting on very public performances of masculine endurance for almost a century."

There are now an estimated 2 million truckers on our highways, and accidents involving trucks and buses are responsible for 4,000 deaths and more than 100,000 injuries in the United States each year. More than 60 percent of the drowsy drivers involved in fatal crashes in 2013 were driving trucks, and nearly half of all truckers said in a government survey that they'd fallen asleep behind the wheel in the previous year. In 2014 alone, 725 truckers died behind the wheel.

That same year, the danger posed by drowsy drivers was made tragically clear with the news that a Walmart truck on the New Jersey Turnpike had slammed into a limousine carrying, among others, the comedians Tracy Morgan and James McNair, killing McNair and seriously injuring Morgan and two others. A report by the National Transportation Safety Board confirmed that the driver had not slept for twenty-eight hours leading up to the crash. He had driven overnight eight hundred miles from his home in Georgia to a Walmart in Delaware, where his shift then began at 11 a.m. He was on his last delivery when the accident occurred, nearly fourteen hours later, at 12:54 a.m. The crash made national headlines because it involved a celebrity, but thousands of crashes take place each year under the media radar.

Playwright Ron Wood became an advocate for stricter rules on trucking companies when his mother, sister, and three nephews were killed by a truck driver who'd been on the road for thirty-five consecutive hours. "My response to the Tracy Morgan truck crash is that it's been ten years since my family was obliterated, and we're not any safer," he said. "It makes me angry." Several states are considering measures that would make driving while sleep-deprived a criminal offense. But only two states—Arkansas and New Jersey—have such laws on the books.

Just days before Tracy Morgan's crash, Senator Susan Collins (R-Maine) had added an amendment to a bill that would loosen rules mandating driver rest. "With one amendment, we're doing away with rules we worked years to develop," said Daphne Izer, whose son was killed by a truck driver—also from Walmart—who fell asleep behind the wheel in 1993. To spare other parents the same anguish, Izer founded Parents Against Tired Truckers, which lobbies on transportation safety. Current regulations allow drivers to be on the road for eleven hours within a fourteen-hour workday. Since drivers, for the most part, are paid by the mile, and their employers are not required to pay overtime, it's a system set up to incentivize sleep-deprived driving—and on that score, it's working.

Airlines have much stricter standards, with rules mandating specific rest periods for pilots between flights and dictating how many hours they're allowed to fly in a given period of time. And in the airline industry, there are usually many levels of safety redundancy: copilots in the cockpit on commercial flights, autopilot technology, and air-traffic controllers tracking a plane's progress. But tragedies still occur. A study by the National Transportation Safety Board showed that fatigue was a factor in 23 percent of all major aviation accidents between 2000 and 2012.

In 2010, a report by investigators of an Air India crash that resulted in 158 fatalities noted that "heavy breathing and snoring" could be heard coming from the cockpit. And then there are the near misses, which we don't hear about. As the captain of a Boeing 747 said on the PBS documentary *Sleep Alert*, "It is not unusual for me to fall asleep in the cockpit, wake up twenty minutes later, and find the other two crew members totally asleep."

Even when the consequences are not tragic, sleep deprivation can lead to some bizarre incidents. In April 2014, flight attendants on an Alaskan Airlines jet were startled when they heard banging sounds from the cargo hold, prompting an emergency landing. The culprit? A sleep-deprived baggage handler who fell asleep as he loaded luggage onto the plane and awoke to find himself thirty thousand feet in the air. More seriously, this problem extends to luggage screeners, whose effectiveness, according to a study by the University of Pennsylvania and the Department of Homeland Security, deteriorates rapidly when they are sleep-deprived, and to federal air marshals, 75 percent of whom were found by a Harvard study to be sleep-deprived.

And a study by NASA and the Federal Aviation Administration found that US air-traffic controllers averaged only 5.8 hours of sleep per night, dropping to 3.25 hours of sleep when they worked overnight shifts. Of the controllers who made safety errors on the job, 56 percent attributed the mistake to fatigue.

In 2014, five years after a plane crashed in Buffalo, New York, killing fifty people—with pilot fatigue cited as a factor in the crash—new rules went into effect that require pilots to have ten hours of rest, eight of which must be uninterrupted sleep, between shifts. The maximum that pilots are allowed to fly is eight to nine hours, and they must have thirty consecutive hours off each week.

Train accidents resulting from sleep deprivation have made headlines recently as well. William Rockefeller, an engineer with more than a decade of experience, momentarily dozed off one December morning in 2013 as his Metro-North train sped at 82 mph through a 30-mph curve in the Bronx. Rockefeller awoke and hit the brakes, but the train derailed, killing four people and injuring dozens of others.

Sleep deprivation may have been a factor in another crash that same year, this one involving an Amtrak train in Philadelphia that killed eight people. The Brotherhood of Locomotive Engineers and Trainmen union believes that engineer Brandon Bostian suffered from exhaustion due to demanding new train schedules. "We feel 100 percent confident that the issue of the new schedule, the reduced rest period and layover period for this young man, was an immediate and direct contribution to this incident," union member Karl "Fritz" Edler said.

DOCTORS WITHOUT BEDTIMES

Also infamous for sleep deprivation are doctors and nurses, who make life-or-death decisions while dealing with long overnight shifts and the demands of on-call hours. "Health is deeply intertwined with culture: what we eat, how active we are, how much we sleep," said US Surgeon General Dr. Vivek Murthy. "When I was training in medicine, . . . there was a culture that strong people didn't need sleep. . . . It is not helpful to have a culture that supports unhealthy practices like that."

The medical community has a "part martyr and part hero" culture, as Dr. Brian Goldman, an emergency physician at Mount Sinai Hospital in Toronto, described it. " 'Jack Bauer' [after the lead character in the TV show *24*] is British hospital slang for a physician who is awake and taking care of patients despite being up for more than 24 hours," wrote Goldman. "That we invent slang for a sleep-deprived colleague rather than tackle the problem is strong evidence that we doctors are so inured to its impact, that we don't even recognize it."

Researchers from Harvard Medical School and Brigham and Women's Hospital examined the effects of sleep deprivation on nearly three thousand first-year residents. The number of hours an intern may work per week is capped at eighty hours, but individual shifts can run more than twenty-four hours. They found that in months when interns worked five or more shifts longer than twenty-four hours, "fatigue-related adverse events" increased by 700 percent and "fatigue-related adverse events" resulting in patient death increased by 300 percent. In a Pennsylvania hospital in 2015, a nurse fell asleep while feeding a newborn baby and dropped him on his head. The baby survived but suffered a fractured skull.

Sleep-deprived health-care workers also show less empathy, which, in turn, can lead to more adverse outcomes. James Reason, a professor of psychology at the University of Manchester, compared the medical community's defense system against errors to a stack of Swiss cheese slices: There are holes at every level, but they usually do not align—a nurse realizes an intern's mistake and corrects it, for example. But when the holes do overlap, it can result in injury or death for the patient. And the metaphorical holes are more likely to overlap when those involved haven't gotten a good night's sleep.

NOT KIDDING AROUND: CHILDREN AND SLEEP

Sleep disruptions are particularly dangerous for infants, toddlers, and children. The brains of young children go through a critical period of plasticity as they scramble to absorb as much information as possible and pick up a whole array of language, motor, visual, and cognitive skills—which is why babies and toddlers learn so quickly. All this is not possible without sufficient quality sleep. Researchers at the University of Pennsylvania found that "REM sleep . . . makes traces of experience more permanent and focused in the brain. . . . Experience is fragile. . . . These traces tend to vanish without REM sleep and the brain basically forgets what it saw."

Sleep deprivation affects behavioral development as well. Dr. Aneesa Das, the assistant director of the Sleep Medicine Program at The Ohio State University, says that it's not always obvious when young children are sleep-deprived. When adults don't get enough sleep, they feel and look tired. For kids, the opposite is true—sleep deprivation can actually make them hyperactive and can lead to a diagnosis of ADHD.

In 2012, researchers from the Albert Einstein College of Medicine and the University of Michigan observed more than eleven thousand British children from infancy to seven years old. They found that those who snored, had sleep apnea, or were mouth breathers—all potential sleep disruptors—at age four were 20 to 60 percent more likely to develop behavioral issues. By age seven, that likelihood jumped to 40 to 100 percent. Hyperactivity was the most common symptom.

As children hit school age, the external challenges become stronger still, and sleep difficulties increase. Researchers from the University of Hong Kong found that nearly 20 percent of adolescents studied experienced difficulty falling asleep, waking up during the night, and waking up too early in the morning for school. One of the reasons behind their difficulty in getting enough sleep is that school starts too early for many students. And as children get older, the structure of the school day becomes even more out of sync with the natural rhythms of children and adolescents.

Mary Carskadon, a professor of psychiatry and human behavior at Brown University, conducted a study that looked into the ways circadian rhythms change as children get older and how school start times can affect their sleep. What she found was that as children age, they begin to resist the sleep signals—in the form of sleep hormones—their bodies are giving them. So even though older kids need the same amount of sleep as those a few years younger, they stay up later—often many hours past the time when their brains are ready for sleep. The pattern, Carskadon told me, emerges in the early teen years and is connected to secretions of melatonin, the "Dracula hormone" that calibrates our circadian rhythms. Melatonin is released later in the evening in teens than in adults, which manifests itself in their wanting to stay up later—a challenge when teens face early school start times. As Steven Lockley of Harvard Medical School put it, "Asking a teenager to get up at 7 a.m. is like asking me to get up at 4 a.m."

The problem is exacerbated by how technology affects teenagers. Teens sleeping with their iPhones and staying up all night texting are staples of our brave new digital world. As Dr. Rakesh Bhattacharjee, a pediatric sleep expert at the University of Chicago, told me, "Television, video games, smartphones, tablets have all been recently identified as agents that frequently disrupt a child's sleep, including leading to total sleep deprivation." The light from those devices, while bad for all of us before bedtime, is even worse for adolescents.

The consequences of ignoring these facts are profound. Most immediately, students are not learning much. As researchers from Uppsala University in Sweden showed, adolescents getting less than seven hours of sleep per night were at a higher risk of failing. This relationship among poor sleep, grades, and dropout rates applies to college students, too.

A 2014 study by the University of Sydney and the Mount Sinai School of Medicine in New York found that among teens and young adults, short sleep duration was directly associated with higher levels of stress and anxiety. For every hour of lost sleep, the risk of psychological distress went up 14 percent. A 2015 survey by the Sleep Council in the United Kingdom found that 83 percent of British teenagers said their sleep was compromised by anxiety and stress over exams.

Of course, beyond grades and stress are the deadly consequences of sleep deprivation that every parent dreads. Which is why it was so shocking to read in May 2012 of the death of Marina Keegan, a talented writer who was in college with my daughters, killed in a car crash when her boyfriend fell asleep at the wheel just days after their graduation.

SLEEP DEPRIVATION AND PUBLIC SERVICE: FROM POLITICS TO POLICE

Our political campaigns constantly feature candidates bragging about how little they sleep and all the long hours they put in. What they're actually proclaiming with their burnout machismo is "Hey, vote for me—I structure my life so badly that my decision making is chronically compromised. If you want a leader who's effectively drunk—all the time—I'm your man (or woman)!" It's an under-the-radar double standard. "No politician would smoke in front of a camera," says Till Roenneberg, "but all politicians clearly declare—and show it in their faces—how little they have slept. We know how important sleep is, but they convey to the world that sleep deprivation is good."

A 2015 *New York Times* piece on Wisconsin governor Scott Walker's presidential campaign ran the headline "A Sleep-Deprived Scott Walker Barnstorms Through South Carolina." Walker was quoted as saying, "I tried to sneak in a few z's, but it's hard when your head is up against an armrest." The article went on to claim that "the lack of sleep doesn't seem to have fazed him." No reporter would ever write that drinking didn't "faze" a candidate. Nor would you vote for a candidate who boasted about being drunk. As former President Bill Clinton once said, "Every important mistake I've made in my life, I've made because I was too tired."

In his book, *Eyewitness to Power*, David Gergen went

deeper on Clinton's sleep habits. In the weeks after his election, Gergen wrote, "Clinton was still celebrating the victory and loved staying up half the night to laugh and talk with old friends. The next morning, he would be up at the crack of dawn to hit the beach for an early run or perhaps a game of touch football." This had a visible impact on him. "He seemed worn out, puffy, and hyper," Gergen continued. "His attention span was so brief that it was difficult to have a serious conversation of more than a few minutes. . . . In a short encounter with Clinton, I tried to say gently that the presidency is a marathon, not a hundred-yard dash, and I hoped he would have a chance for some downtime in the three weeks still remaining. I don't think I registered. . . . Those who saw him in his first weeks at the White House often found him out of sorts, easily distracted, and impatient." Citing the work of Clinton biographer David Maraniss, Gergen noted that "Clinton had been sleeping only four to five hours a night since a professor said in college that many great leaders of the past had gotten by that way." This aversion to sleep may well have played a part in several early lapses in presidential judgment, including his inept handling of the issue of gays in the military—now widely considered to be one of the low points of his two-term presidency. As Gergen dramatically summed it up, this "planted seeds that almost destroyed his presidency."

The daily email newsletter *theSkimm*, in its coverage of the 2016 presidential election, asked the candidates, "How many times do you hit snooze in the AM?" (Ted Cruz hits it twice, Carly Fiorina "doesn't have time to hit snooze these days," and for Hillary Clinton it "depends on the morning.") Now, of course, hitting the snooze button isn't a sin, but if you need to do it—because you can't get up when your alarm goes off—that's a strong message that you're not getting enough sleep (and the decision-making benefits that come with it). One of the persistent clichés of the presidential campaigns is the question "Would you want this person to have his or her finger on the nuclear button?" Well, when it comes to having a president operating on all cylinders, we should also ask whether we want someone with one finger on the snooze button and the other on the nuclear button.

Yet another sign our leaders aren't getting enough sleep at night is that they're dozing off at inappropriate times during the day, in meetings, interviews, public events, and even during sessions of Congress—you know, the place where they make laws that govern the rest of us. Supreme Court Justice Ruth Bader Ginsburg dozed off during President Obama's 2013 and 2015 State of the Union addresses. Secretary of Homeland Security Janet Napolitano fell asleep during the 2010 State of the Union speech. Vice President Joe Biden nodded off in 2011 during a speech on the national debt. Former President Bill Clinton struggled to stay awake during a Martin Luther King Day event in Harlem in 2008; the *New York Post* headline read, "Bill Has a 'Dream.'" The head of the National Economic Council, Larry Summers, fell asleep in (at least) two White House meetings in the midst of the financial crisis in 2009.

And it's not just American leaders who are asleep on the job. Former British prime minister Gordon Brown snoozed in public just before he took the stage to speak to the UN Security Council in 2008. Members of Parliament in Japan have been caught on camera nodding off during sessions. In Uganda, it's become something of a national pastime to look for snoozing ministers and members of Parliament during televised sessions—even President Yoweri Museveni was caught sleeping during a budget meeting. In fact, if you Google "politicians sleeping," you'd think that some mass sleep sickness has broken out.

In the middle of the Greek economic crisis in 2015, meetings dragged on through the night, with one marathon session running for seventeen hours. European Commission President Jean-Claude Juncker commented on the exhausting proceedings. "I don't like this way of working, which leaves me sleepless," he said. "We can't make the right decisions when we are tired."

"Clearly it is a very suboptimal way to make these very important decisions which affect millions of people," says Michael Chee, a professor at Duke-NUS Graduate Medical School in Singapore. "But this pattern of late-night meetings has been going on for years. . . . The way they operate is essentially the torture method to break people's will by keeping them up so they are physically and mentally drained. . . . All the fundamental elements of having to process information rapidly are diminished. . . . People take riskier bets and they become more insensitive to losses when they are deprived of sleep." Not a good idea when you're deciding on military actions or a Eurozone-wide financial crisis.

Political campaigns are also notorious breeding grounds for sleep deprivation, with a direct correlation to damaging decisions. During the 2012 US presidential election, for example, after senior adviser Eric Fehrnstrom caused a media firestorm with his unfortunate quote that Mitt Romney was an Etch-A-Sketch candidate, it was reported that Fehrnstrom routinely slept only three or four hours a night, with his cell phone beside him. He would wake up and check his email, send out replies, and then get another hour of sleep. You'd think with the high stakes of a campaign, political professionals would begin to correlate this kind of sleep deprivation with the bad decisions we know it results in.

When it comes to our military personnel, a 2015 report by the RAND Corporation showed that a third of servicepeople sleep only five hours a night or less. More than 18 percent of the survey participants said they use sleeping pills. Lieutenant Colonel Kate Van Arman, the medical director of the Traumatic Brain Injury Clinic at Fort Drum, New York, describes sleep problems as "the absolute number-one military disorder when people come back from deployments," pointing to the vicious cycle of sleeplessness that many soldiers endure. The rigorous demands of duty, alongside the stresses of the battlefield, have fueled what Van Arman calls a "culture of caffeine," which only exacerbates the sleep problems our soldiers struggle with. Reflecting on soldiers' cognitive impairment from sleep deprivation, Surgeon General of the Army Lieutenant General Patricia Horoho said, "We never will allow a soldier in our formation with a .08-percent alcohol level, but we allow every day [sleep-deprived soldiers] to make those complex decisions."

The same problems exist in law enforcement. In a study of almost five thousand police officers, nearly 30 percent reported "excessive sleepiness." A follow-up survey showed that officers who exhibited more uncontrolled anger toward suspects were more likely to fall asleep while driving and more likely to commit a safety violation. Given the recent controversies surrounding police behavior, sleep deprivation and its effects must become part of the conversation.

2.

THE SLEEP INDUSTRY

IF BURNOUT is civilization's disease, sleep deprivation is one of its chief symptoms. It's a paradox of modern life that we live in a state of continuous exhaustion and yet we're unable to sleep—which leaves us even more exhausted the next day, and the day after that. In fact, alarm clocks, which are so ingrained in our culture, are work-arounds to get us up when we're not able to wake up naturally.

Most of us force our reluctant brains—indeed, our reluctant selves—to wake up with multiple alarms, often set five minutes apart on our phones, insistently nudging us toward what passes for consciousness. Lifehacker even published an article detailing how to wire your alarm clock to a car horn—for those of us who *really* can't get out of bed in the morning. Just think about the definition of the word "alarm": "a sudden fear or distressing suspense caused by an awareness of danger; apprehension; fright," or "any sound, outcry, or information intended to warn of approaching danger." So an alarm, in most situations, is a signal that something is not right. Yet most of us rely on some kind of alarm clock—a knee-jerk call to arms—to start the day, ensuring that we emerge from sleep in full fight-or-flight mode, flooded with stress hormones and adrenaline as our body readies itself for danger. That adrenaline is needed because our sleep-deprived bodies want to—are begging to—continue sleeping, because we didn't get enough sleep in the first place. The American Academy of Sleep Medicine reports that 70 million Americans have trouble getting a good night's sleep.

SLEEPLESSNESS AND SLEEPING PILLS: A MATCH MADE IN BURNOUT HEAVEN

An entire industry has arisen to facilitate our attempts to get more sleep. In the United States, more than 55 million prescriptions for sleeping pills were written just in 2014, with sales topping $1 billion. A 2013 Centers for Disease Control report stated that 9 million Americans—4 percent of all adults—use prescription sleeping pills. It also found that women are bigger users of sleeping pills than men; that sleeping-pill consumption increases with age and education; and that white adults consume more than any other racial group.

I asked several sleep experts what they thought of the 4 percent number from the CDC, and the general conclusion was that the survey number involved significant underreporting. A National Sleep Foundation poll found startlingly high rates of sleep-aid usage among women, with 29 percent reporting that they use a sleep aid of some kind at least a few nights each week. A survey by *Parade* magazine of more than fifteen thousand people found that 23 percent of respondents took sleeping pills once a week and 14 percent took them every night. The problem is global: in 2014, people around the world spent a staggering $58 billion on sleep-aid products, a figure projected to rise to $76.7 billion by 2019. Not surprisingly, the use of sleeping pills is highest among those who regularly get less than five hours of sleep a night.

For the drug industry that stands to profit from today's sleep crisis, business is good and the future looks bright. But the strength of this market is just a reflection of the depth of the problem. And although marketers use the soothing term "sleep aids," burnout is the necessary condition that feeds the sleep-aid market.

"In twenty years, people will look back on the sleeping-pill era as we now look back on the acceptance of cigarette smoking," Jerome Siegel, director of UCLA's Center for Sleep Research, told me. "Movies and TV glamorized smoking. Advertisements, often with doctors or actors posing as doctors, were used to sell cigarettes." Only after many years and many studies linking cigarettes to lung cancer and other diseases did the government step in to regulate tobacco advertising. So we may have moved beyond the era of Joe Camel and advertisements proclaiming "More doctors smoke Camels than any other cigarette!" and "Give your throat a vacation . . . Smoke a fresh cigarette," but as Siegel put it, "history appears to be repeating itself. The chronic use of sleeping pills is an ongoing public health disaster."

Sleep difficulties can turn into serious medical problems, as I discuss in the Sleep Disorders chapter. For the vast majority of us, however, sleep difficulties are a lifestyle problem. Yet we tend to treat all our sleep-related woes the same way: with a pill. This is hubris on the scale of Greek mythology. We expect, as if by magic, to wrestle sleep into submission. This isn't accidental. Combine the marketing power of the modern pharmaceutical industry with a client market that includes, potentially, every fatigued and burned-out worker—which is to say nearly every worker—and you've got the makings of the juggernaut that is the modern sleep-aid industry. As Matthew Wolf-Meyer put it in *The Slumbering*

Masses, by "empowering medical practitioners, pharmaceuticals, and caffeine as mediators in individuals' relationships with sleep," we have created a world where "rather than a gentle sovereign, sleep has become demonized and rendered an object of medical and scientific control."

As so many of us burn out in our efforts to keep up in today's high-pressure, always-on world, we've made it easier and easier for the pharmaceutical industry to tighten its grip on us and expand its reach. Instead of questioning how we live our lives, we fall prey to sophisticated marketing that promises us health, happiness, sleep, and energy. And who wants to be the naysayer, the Luddite who rejects such progress? A great deal of ingenious and insidious brainpower, along with billions of dollars, goes into selling us a solution that doesn't actually solve our problems but only disguises and prolongs them.

The most common pharmaceutical weapon we use to knock ourselves out is the drug zolpidem, which you probably know as Ambien. It accounts for more than two-thirds of the sleeping pills sold in the United States. It is also sold under the soothing names Intermezzo, Sublinox, Zolfresh, and Hypnogen. That last one is especially apt, since zolpidem is part of a class of drugs known as hypnotics, which work to induce and lengthen the duration of sleep. Of the 55 million prescriptions written for sleeping pills in the United States in 2014, 38 million were for zolpidem, accounting for sales of more than $320 million. Lunesta, another hypnotic, marketed with a seductive green butterfly logo, had more than $350 million in sales in the United States in 2014, and that figure does not include the generic version, eszopiclone, which generated another $43 million.

When you hear the stories of people who have become

dependent on sleeping pills, you realize that they actually shouldn't be called sleeping pills at all. Because we now know that simply not being awake doesn't necessarily mean you're actually asleep. It's not the clean, binary, zero-sum game the drug manufacturers would have us believe. Which is why sleeping pills aren't the solution to our sleep-deprivation crisis—they're another crisis masquerading as a solution, offering a false promise that takes us further from the benefits of real, restorative sleep.

Mohamed El-Erian, the chief economic adviser at Allianz and former PIMCO CEO, told me about his experience at a sleep clinic that a friend suggested he visit because he was having trouble sleeping. "At the end of the test, the doctor said to me, 'There is good news and bad news. The good news is that there is no sleep apnea or other issue. The bad news is that your brain doesn't stop, and it keeps you up at night. But I have a solution for you—I can put you on medication.'" El-Erian refused. "It is really unfortunate," he told me, "that drugs are most often the only alternative offered to millions of people who have trouble sleeping." Instead, he made some significant changes to his nightly routine, the most important being removing electronics from his bedroom.

Harvard Medical School professor Patrick Fuller explained to me the difference between natural sleep and drug-induced sleep. Sleeping pills typically target only one of the many different chemical systems used by the brain as part of the sleep process, which "necessarily produces an imbalance in the chemical signaling by which the brain achieves normal sleep and may limit restorative slow-wave sleep. The newer drugs like Ambien produce more naturalistic sleep but can have side effects, albeit rarely, like sleep eating and sleepwalking, which by definition are not a part of normal sleep behavior."

This limbo state, when we are not really awake but not really asleep, can result in behaviors ranging from the harmless and humorous to the disturbing and dangerous. And part of the danger is that you will more than likely have no memory of whatever you do.

In a November 2014 appearance on *The Late Show*, actress Anna Kendrick regaled David Letterman with stories of taking Ambien while flying. "It's a hell of a drug," she told Letterman. "I just sort of black out the second that I take it, and it's like, I wake up, and I wake up to a surprise every time—like all my DVDs are in my fridge or something. Surprise! . . . This last time I took it as soon as we took off, and I remember thinking, 'Ah, I should put on something comfy to sleep in.' . . . And then nothing. And when I woke up, I was wearing everything that was in my carry-on bag, and I had a ninety-second video of my salad."

"And then nothing" refers to the fact that Kendrick had no memory after that point. It's kind of a funny story—until you realize that she's describing doing things such as putting on clothes and videotaping her food after having completely blacked out.

The *Today* show's Julia Sommerfeld was a regular user of Ambien until what she describes as her "wake-up call." Her credit card company called to report suspicious activity on her account—nearly $3,000 charged to the store Anthropologie at 2 a.m. Her initial reaction—fraud!—was quickly disproven, in the form of an e-receipt at the top of her in-box: she had been the perpetrator of an Ambien-induced online shopping spree. On other occasions, while on Ambien, she had also consumed large quantities of brown sugar right out of the bag, devoured two of her sons' decorated Easter eggs, and written an embarrassing email to her boss. What finally got her to kick the hypnotic habit was her husband invoking their toddler son. "How can you be sure you'd never hurt Jude?" he asked. "What if you decided to put him in the car?"

Former representative Patrick Kennedy (D-Rhode Island), after taking Ambien and a drug for a stomach disorder, smashed his car into a barrier on Capitol Hill at 3 a.m. He later had no memory of the incident. He had left his headlights off and swerved into the wrong lane; police officers described him as appearing intoxicated, unable to maintain his balance, with slurred speech and watery eyes. The next day he publicly admitted to an addiction to prescription medications: "I simply do not remember getting out of bed, being pulled over by the police, or being cited for three driving infractions. That's not how I want to live my life." In fact, in a University of Washington study, people who took generics of Ambien, Desyrel, or Restoril were nearly two times more at risk of being involved in a driving accident.

In response to growing concerns, the FDA in 2013 cut the recommended dose of zolpidem in half—in half!—for women and began requiring stronger warning labels highlighting the dangers of driving a motor vehicle after taking extended-release versions of the drug. It was a significant step forward—as well as a dramatic, unequivocal acknowledgment of how the drug manufacturers have been allowed to profit from a sleep-deprived public for so long.

Ambien has also been used as a defense in criminal trials—a pharmaceutical version of the "Twinkie defense." On The Fix, a site about recovery and addiction, Allison McCabe told the story of Lindsey Schweigert, a thirty-one-year-old working for a defense contractor. Returning from a business trip exhausted, she took one dose of generic Ambien. Several hours later, when she emerged from her zombie state, she was in police custody. She'd gotten out of bed, filled the bathtub and left the water running, taken her dog out, climbed into her car, and, while driving, collided with another car. She failed a sobriety test after falling three times when asked to walk a straight line. The police charged her with driving under the influence. Prosecutors sought a sentence of six months, but Schweigert's lawyer pointed to the warning label on the Ambien she took and argued that she belonged in the hospital, not jail. The label read:

> After taking Ambien, you may get up out of bed while not being fully awake and do an activity that you do not know you are doing. The next morning, you may not remember that you did anything during the night. . . . Reported activities include: driving a car ("sleep-driving"), making and eating food, talking on the phone, having sex, sleep-walking.

Put aside for a moment the absurdity of this label and the fact that it exists. Or file it under: Warning Labels Apparently Written by *The Onion*. The charges were dropped, though Schweigert was left with a suspended license and nearly $10,000 in lawyers' fees. The more of these stories I hear, the more shocked I am at the number of people who walk away from such incidents with similar consequences—a suspended license, a financial burden, but ultimately nothing more. Because of the FDA warning, the consequences of Ambien use are treated as a side effect, not as a crime. I asked Ted Olson, a former US solicitor general, to explain why something that would be a crime in one context is not in another. "Criminal laws are not well-suited for prosecutions in these kinds of cases," he explained, "because of the difficulty in articulating standards for impairment from various types of medication and, for that matter, for driving while tired, sleep-deprived, emotionally distracted, et cetera. And there are probably not adequate tests or articulated standards as there are with alcohol impairment. One drug might affect one person quite differently than another. On the other hand, civil cases might be easier and present less insurmountable obstacles of proof and standards for liability."

There are, of course, times in our lives—a traumatic experience, the death of a loved one—when we might need some temporary help getting to sleep. But it's important to make a distinction between turning to sleep aids at such moments and turning to them—as ads suggest we should—as an everyday, long-term cure for sleeplessness.

In 2009, Julie Ann Bronson, a flight attendant based in Texas, took Ambien after drinking wine earlier in the day. When she woke up, she was in jail in her pajamas. To her horror, she learned that she had gotten behind the wheel of her car and run over three people. One of them was an eighteen-month-old baby, who survived but suffered severe brain damage. She could have gotten ten years behind bars, but the fact that she was on Ambien reduced her sentence to six months with ten years of probation—despite the fact that she had violated the warning not to drink while taking the drug.

There's no shortage of such stories, of lives derailed or destroyed in ways that could never be contained in the pharmaceutical-industry parlance of "side effects." And in many instances the people involved took the drug exactly as directed.

Human-rights activist Kerry Kennedy was arrested for erratic driving, after swerving and hitting a truck in 2012. Kennedy said that her memories of the incident were "really jumbled" and that she hadn't realized how impaired she was. Claiming she'd taken the generic version of Ambien by mistake, thinking it was her thyroid medication, she was acquitted by a jury.

Shortly before her death, my friend Nora Ephron told me about taking Ambien one night in Paris. She woke up in the morning disoriented, with wet hair. It turned out that she'd gotten up during the night, filled the bathtub with water, and gotten in. She recounted it to her friends as a funny anecdote—Nora could make anything funny—but it's a story that easily could have had a very different ending.

Another friend of mine who regularly takes Ambien told me of receiving a large UPS package she didn't remember ordering. When she opened it, she discovered a large amount of, as she put it, "hooker clothes," which it turned out she—or perhaps her subconscious—had purchased in the middle of the night while on Ambien. (Though Ambien's FDA warning covers a wide range of side effects, there is no mention of how to properly dispose of unwanted hooker clothes. Perhaps online retail sites should start to list their return policies for Ambien-fueled purchases.)

Lunesta has many of the same dangers as Ambien. As a result, in May 2014 the FDA required a lower starting dose for the drug, citing "the risk of next-morning impairment." The bottom line is that consumers are taking drugs that even the FDA admits are not fully researched or understood. They promise to "update the public as new information becomes available." The risks, though, are outlined clearly in the drug warning to users: "The morning after you take

Lunesta your ability to drive safely and think clearly may be decreased. . . . Lunesta may cause serious side effects that you may not know are happening to you including daytime sleepiness, not thinking clearly, acting strangely, confused or upset, or walking, eating, driving or engaging in other activities while asleep. Other abnormal behaviors include aggressiveness, agitation, hallucinations and confusion. In depressed patients, worsening of depression including risk of suicide may occur." Most concerning is the fact that these are effects "you may not know are happening to you."

But even as it continues to evaluate the safety of sleep drugs, the FDA continues to approve new ones, such as Belsomra, the brand name of suvorexant, distributed by Merck. When it was approved in 2014, it was hailed in the press as "groundbreaking" because it's supposedly more targeted than previous prescription sleeping pills. But the list of side effects cataloged in a 2015 commercial for the drug are almost identical to those of Ambien and Lunesta: "Walking, eating, driving or engaging in other activities while asleep, without remembering it the next day . . . Aggressiveness, confusion, agitation, or hallucinations . . . In depressed patients, worsening depression including risk of suicide may occur." If this is groundbreaking, what do the drugs that *don't* get approved look like?

The potential dangers of sleeping pills don't stop at your being turned into a mindless zombie. There are also longer-term health hazards to go along with *Night of the Living Dead*–like misadventures. Researchers from the University of Montreal and the University of Bordeaux discovered that the use of benzodiazepines (such as Xanax and Restoril), usually taken for anxiety or as a sleep aid, increases the risk of developing Alzheimer's by 32 percent after being used for three to six months. Taking these drugs for more than six months raises the risk by 84 percent.

Sleeping pills carry major health risks even for occasional users. One study from the Scripps Research Institute led by Dr. Daniel Kripke compared data from a sample group of more than 10,000 people taking sleeping pills, including zolpidem (Ambien) and temazepam (Restoril), with a control group of more than 23,000 not taking sleeping pills. Researchers found that those prescribed as few as 18 doses of sleeping pills a year had a three-times-higher risk of death during the study's two-and-a-half-year follow-up period than their counterparts in the control group, "with greater mortality associated with greater dosage prescribed." Furthermore, those taking the highest dosage of sleeping pills (more than 132 doses per year) had a 35 percent increased risk of cancer—including lung, lymphoma, prostate, and colon cancers. This association between sleeping pills, cancer rates, and death remained strong even after controlling for health conditions such as obesity, heart disease, and diabetes.

Yet we hear little about these increased risks, even as other, much smaller risks get tons of airtime. I have many friends, for example, who obsess about organic produce, organic diapers, organic dish soap, and organic shampoo but pop sleeping pills as though they're candy. It's sort of like taking great care to eat a nutritious breakfast and then think nothing of smoking a pack a day.

In 2015, Kripke, in an effort to protect consumers and hold the sleeping-pill industry more accountable, submitted a citizen petition to the FDA requesting a complete overhaul to the distribution, labeling, and regulation of sleeping pills. His proposals included requiring drug manufacturers to perform more studies on the risks of taking sleeping pills, helping doctors educate their patients about those risks, and requiring drug labels to include the mortality hazards.

Given these major dangers, what do sleeping pills actually do for us? In 2015, *Consumer Reports* found that Ambien and Lunesta put people to sleep only about twenty minutes faster on average than a placebo and added only three to thirty-four minutes of total sleep time: "Their effectiveness is so limited that as of late 2014 they were no longer considered a first-choice treatment for chronic insomnia by the American Academy of Sleep Medicine."

What about over-the-counter sleeping pills? Procter & Gamble, the maker of ZzzQuil, estimates the over-the-counter sleep-aid market at more than $500 million and growing fast. What helps a ZzzQuil user fall asleep is the active ingredient diphenhydramine, which is also found in Benadryl, the allergy drug often taken for its drowsiness effect, especially on long flights. Dr. Shalini Paruthi, from the Cardinal Glennon Children's Medical Center in St. Louis, Missouri, explained "that when we use something like diphenhydramine to help us sleep at night, we're actually using it for its side effect—not its treatment, which is to fight allergies." Aside from the primary side effects of drowsiness and fatigue, ZzzQuil may also cause headaches, tremors, and a fast, irregular heartbeat. That's even more of a problem because 41 percent of people take over-the-counter sleeping pills for a year or longer—hardly a short-term solution—according to a 2016 *Consumer Reports* survey. Also, a 2015 study from the University of Washington discovered a link between higher risks of developing dementia, including Alzheimer's disease, and the use of anticholinergic medications such as Benadryl.

Perhaps most disturbing is how many adolescents and

young people are finding their way to sleeping pills. Researchers at the University of Michigan determined that teenagers who have been prescribed medication for sleep difficulty or anxiety were up to twelve times more likely to abuse the medications than those who had never been prescribed them. And the longer teens have had a prescription, the more likely they are at some point to abuse the drug. Are they just mimicking the values and practices of the adults they see around them—learning that being sleep-deprived and burned out is the inevitable price of success, and the way to deal with that in the modern world is with a pill?

I have personally never taken a sleeping pill. That doesn't mean that I've never had trouble sleeping. There were many times when either because of jet lag or because I was worried about something and couldn't switch my mind off, I had trouble falling asleep or woke up in the middle of the night. Wanting to avoid the sleeping-pill trap, I experimented instead with every possible alternative, starting with listening to soothing guided meditations. I must have listened to hundreds until I found a couple that clicked with me. My best endorsement for them is that I have no idea how they end—because I always fall asleep before they finish! I have also tried magnesium powder and herbal remedies such as valerian root. But I've found that my mind-set is just as important as my methods, as I discuss at length in Part Two, "The Way Forward."

CAFFEINE: A COMPLICATED LOVE AFFAIR

With the creation of the world's massive market for sleeping pills—pills that often leave us groggy or zombified the next day—has come the need for a force to counteract it: the creation of an equally massive market for stimulants, including all sorts of hypercaffeinated drinks. It's a perfect circle of commodified burnout.

Because we don't get enough sleep to feel refreshed and awake, we jack ourselves up with a vitality substitute instead—increasingly, from a variety of "energy" drinks. And when we falter later in the day, we grab another Red Bull, sugary soda, or shot of 5-hour Energy. We're constantly forcing our bodies into a state we're unable to achieve naturally, because we don't allow ourselves enough sleep. So we're tired during the day and wired during the night.

Of course, coffee and tea have been around for centuries. We prize them for their power to make us more alert, but many cultures have other traditions around coffee and tea—traditions that encourage us to slow down, be in the moment, take a break (hence, the "coffee break"), or enjoy the legendary Japanese tea ceremony. They are rituals associated with a cessation of work, a pause, a time-out to socialize, read, or, as Oprah puts it, "steep your soul," before heading back to work recharged—and not just by the caffeine they've delivered to us. Compare this to the way so many of us drink our coffee—on the run, refueling rather than actually recharging ourselves, just to speed up, without any semblance of ritual.

I could lay my head on a piece of lead
And imagine it was a springy bed
'Cause I'm sleepy, sleepy

—Cat Stevens, "I'm So Sleepy"

Today caffeine has become a key component of our sleep-deprived culture. But when taken too late in the day—when we are trying to fight off that afternoon slump—caffeine hinders our ability to fall asleep at night. As a result, we are even more tired the next day. So we reach for another caffeinated drink in an endless sleep-deprived cycle.

In *A History of the World in 6 Glasses*, Tom Standage explained that in the eighteenth century "factory workers had to function like parts in a well-oiled machine and tea was the lubricant that kept the factories running smoothly." Also, in *Uncommon Grounds*, Mark Pendergrast traced increasing coffee consumption to the Industrial Revolution. In short, we're using the same methods that factory owners used two hundred years ago to maximize employee productivity. We would think it cruel to use this method on somebody else, so why do we think it's okay or even noble when we do it to ourselves? I write this as someone who absolutely loves coffee and drinks it every morning (although I try not to drink it after 2 p.m., which is roughly the time sleep experts recommend we stop consuming caffeinated drinks).

Coffee consumption in the United States has actually fallen by half since the 1940s. We're instead guzzling super-caffeinated and sugar-packed sodas. Annual US sales of carbonated sodas, at $77 billion, are six times the annual sales of coffee, at $13 billion. And eight out of the top ten best-selling soft drinks in the United States contain caffeine. As Murray Carpenter explained in *Caffeinated*, at the turn of the twentieth century the U.S. Department of Agriculture's Bureau of Chemistry viewed the caffeine in Coca-Cola as harmful and addictive. "Why should the people of this country be subjected to this awful drugging?" asked bureau chairman Harvey Washington Wiley. "Fatigue is nature's signal that there is danger ahead. Will you make a railroad more safe if you go along and take all the red lights away from the open switches? They are the marks of danger. What is fatigue? It is nature's notice that you have done enough."

A century later, caffeine has spilled out of beverages and into products such as topical sprays, soap and toothbrushes (why wait for that morning coffee?), stockings, beer, candy, oatmeal, sunflower seeds, breath fresheners, popcorn, hot sauce, lip balm, and water! There was even a report that a Swedish condom company was going to produce caffeine-laced condoms (supply your own punch line).

The most recent rage in caffeinated drinks is energy drinks mixing caffeine with other substances, such as the amino acid taurine—Red Bull, anyone? Mintel Group, a global-market research agency, estimates that US energy-drink sales will grow by 40 percent from 2014 to 2019. Red Bull sold more than 5.6 billion cans worldwide in 2014, and its major competitor, Monster Beverage, saw its sales grow by more than 9 percent to $2.8 billion in 2014, which included increased consumption in developing markets such as India, South Africa, and Turkey.

Our addiction to energy drinks is making us sick. Consuming too many, too fast can result in a laundry list of side effects, including nausea, vomiting, tremors, nervousness, delirium, seizures, altered heart rhythms, mood changes, diarrhea, increased blood pressure, and kidney problems. Emergency-room visits involving energy drinks in the United States doubled from 10,068 in 2007 to 20,783 in 2011. And one in ten of these was serious enough to require hospitalization.

THE STUPIDITY OF "SMART DRUGS"

Some of us looking for an afternoon or late-night boost are increasingly looking beyond a fourth cup of coffee or can of Red Bull. Among the modern pick-me-ups of choice are drugs such as Provigil (originally created to treat people with narcolepsy and other severe sleep disorders, it's become popular with shift workers and exhausted execs) and so-called smart drugs—stimulants such as Adderall, Ritalin, and other drugs claiming to enhance cognitive function, such as piracetam.

Though the efficacy of these drugs is still being debated, a 2014 study found that long-term use may lower brain plasticity, especially in young people. "In other words," wrote Betsy Isaacson in *Newsweek*, "the cost of short-term productivity may be long-term creativity, adaptability and intelligence."

According to the Partnership for Drug-Free Kids, one-fifth of students have abused prescription stimulants during their college years. "The profile that emerges," says Sean Clarkin of the Partnership, "is less that of an academic 'goof-off' who abuses prescription stimulants to make up for lost study time, than a stressed-out multitasker who is burning the candle at both ends and trying to keep up." Among Ivy League students, 18 percent have used such "cognitive enhancers." With so many stressed-out parents taking prescription drugs, clearly the burned-out apples haven't fallen far from the success-at-any-price trees. In fact, a 2014 report by the American Psychological Association found that millennials were the most stressed generation, almost a third saying they can't sleep because they are "thinking of all the things they need to do or did not get done" and because "they have too many things to do and do not have enough time." For an alarming number of students, college has been turned into one long training ground for burnout. And the deeply ingrained association of college with sleep deprivation is one the sleep industry is only too happy to exploit. As one ad for Red Bull put it, "Nobody ever wishes they'd slept more during college."

BURNOUT U

Talk to college students, and they'll tell you they feel as if they're in a no-win situation, forced to choose between sleep and life. As an advertisement for Spotify says, "College is about making decisions—big ones—like to sleep . . . or not to sleep?" Sarah Hedgecock, in a piece titled "The Ivy League's Insomnia Problem," gave a firsthand account. "Sleep, it seemed, was discouraged the moment I moved into the dorms at Princeton," she writes. "I began hearing the same axiom uttered over and over again from all corners: 'Sleep, grades, social life: pick two.' Consensus on which two should be prioritized was clear: we could sleep when we were dead (or graduated)."

Angela Della Croce observed the same problem in an article she wrote for Vassar College's *Miscellany News*:

> When we were young, we had naptime, recess, and lunch break. As we got older, naptime was omitted and recess soon followed suit. A time dedicated to eating lunch was also taken from us as we entered college—now we hardly even have time to breathe, let alone sleep or relax. Since when has sleep—something so crucial that it was incor-

> porated into our school day—become such a luxury that many people sacrifice it? . . . As a social norm, we simply don't emphasize the need to sleep. . . . Fun is focused around late-night activities; studying reaches its epitome with pulling all-nighters; and people from around the world flock to "the city that never sleeps." . . . The bottom line is that we DO have the time to sleep, we just choose not to.

Here is how some of our HuffPost college editors-at-large have described the sleep culture on their respective campuses:

> "I get this notion that sleep deprivation is a huge badge of honor. People sometimes refer to Leavey Library as 'Hotel Leavey' because a lot of students pull all-nighters there." —Fernando Hurtado, USC

> "Catching up on sleep is what the summer is for." —Hannah Tattersall, University of Delaware

> "People don't really prioritize sleep here. It's very common to see entire dorm and apartment buildings with nearly every room lit up." —Luis Ruuska, University of Tennessee

> "Who needs sleep when you have coffee?" —Kenza Kamal, Ohio State University

> "I'll get Snapchats during finals week of people advertising how late they stayed in the library, and it's like a competition." —Madeline Diamond, Bucknell University

In recent years, there's been a lot of attention given to the problems of binge drinking and drug use among high school and college students. But a 2014 study by the University of St. Thomas in Minnesota showed that the effect of sleep deprivation on grades is roughly equivalent to binge drinking and drug use. "I don't think sleep problems are often included on the questionnaire intake forms for health services," says Roxanne Prichard, a psychology professor at the University of St. Thomas, "and that could be explaining a lot of the other problems that you see showing up, including recurrent illnesses."

What makes getting sleep in college much harder is the fear of missing out, which leads to smartphone addiction, obsessively checking for texts, messages, updates, notifications, and alerts, at all hours. Researchers at California State University, Dominguez Hills, looked at more than seven hundred college students and found that those who felt anxious when separated from their phones were more likely to stare at their electronic screens right until the moment they went to sleep. They also woke up more frequently throughout the night to check their phones.

Not only is too little sleep as bad for students' grades as too much alcohol, but the two are actually connected. A 2015 study from Idaho State University found that teens with sleep problems were 47 percent more likely to binge-drink than their classmates who slept well. They were also more likely to experience alcohol problems a year later and to drive under the influence. Even five years later, the sleep-deprived high-schoolers were more likely to get behind the wheel drunk. Each hour of extra sleep in high school is associated with a 10 percent drop in binge drinking—a remarkable statistic given the focus on curbing excessive drinking.

And sleep-deprived students turn to stimulants. We don't yet know all the long-term consequences for young adults and teens (and children) who take prescription stimulants. But we do know some of them. "Sporadic use can lead to severe sleep deprivation and cause stimulant-induced psychosis, when a student gets paranoid and may hallucinate," says Miami University psychiatrist Dr. Josh Hersh.

The University of Florida found that almost 15 percent of ten- to eighteen-year-olds reported that they'd used a prescription stimulant at some point, and just as they like to share photos and music, they also like to share their prescription medications. The Partnership for Drug-Free Kids study found that nearly a third of eighteen- to twenty-five-year-olds said they'd shared their medication with friends and about the same number said they had exaggerated their symptoms in order to be prescribed a larger dose. More than half said the drugs were not hard to get. In other words, students are artificially jacking themselves up during the day and artificially bringing themselves down at night.

The good news is that there's a solution: get enough sleep without sleeping aids, and there's no need for all the Red Bulls and Adderalls in the daytime. It's hard to quit only one half of the perfect circle of burnout without quitting the other. Admittedly, getting out of the vicious cycle isn't easy. There are endless flashing lights and signposts telling us we have a medical problem—after all, there are billions of dollars to be made by getting us to believe that sleeping pills are the answer to our sleep deprivation. Yet what we really have is not a medical problem but a lifestyle problem. It's just that there's much less of a market for telling us how to solve that.

3.

SLEEP THROUGHOUT HISTORY

SLEEP IS one of the great recurring themes in the long narrative of humanity. But how we think about it, and how much we value it, has changed through the centuries. In the last four decades, science has validated much of the ancient wisdom about the importance of sleep. We've made incredible discoveries about all the things going on in our brains and our bodies while we're sleeping, and these findings have fueled a sleep renaissance. While science continues to make the case for sleep in terms of our physical health, cognitive functions, athletic performance, and general productivity, it's worth looking back at what the ancients valued about the mysteries of sleep: the rhythm it brings to our daily lives and the gateway it provides to something greater than ourselves, beyond the realm of our daily activities, beyond our achievements and our failures.

A PATHWAY TO THE SACRED: SLEEP IN THE ANCIENT WORLD

From the beginning of recorded time, sleep and dreams have played a singular role in virtually every religion and spiritual tradition. Sleep was revered—so much so that good sleep was considered something of a luxury, reserved for the rich and those favored by the gods, or something that could be earned by living the proper kind of life. "People sought peaceful sleep the way hunters pursued prey and gatherers searched for nuts and roots to carry them through lean times," writes Kat Duff in *The Secret Life of Sleep*. "Sleep was like food, a cherished and necessary—though not always available—source of physical and spiritual sustenance."

In both ancient Egypt and ancient Greece, people would often spend the night in "sleep temples" to have their dreams interpreted, asking the gods for answers to life's questions and the healing of diseases. But sleep and dreams were not just shortcuts to solutions for earthly problems. They were a sacred bridge to the divine, a means of transcendence. The Upanishads, among the oldest sacred Hindu texts, dating back to 700 BC, include a reference to dreams, full of poetic metaphors:

> *The Golden God, the Self, the immortal Swan*
> *leaves the small nest of the body, goes where He wants.*
> *He moves through the realm of dreams; makes numberless*
> *forms;*
> *delights in sex; eats, drinks, laughs with His friends;*
> *frightens Himself with scenes of heart-chilling terror.*
> *But He is not attached to anything that He sees;*
> *and after He has wandered in the realms of dream and*
> *awakeness,*
> *has tasted pleasures and experienced good and evil,*
> *He returns to the blissful state from which He began.*

In Genesis we see the status accorded to dreams as Joseph, son of Jacob and Rachel, impresses the pharaoh with his unique gift of interpreting dreams. "Since God has shown you all this," the pharaoh tells him, "there is none so discerning and wise as you are. You shall be over my house, and all my people shall order themselves as you command. Only as regards the throne will I be greater than you."

Even a soul submerged in sleep
is hard at work and helps
make something of the world.

—HERACLITUS, *Fragments*

The Greeks and the Romans each had their gods of sleep: Hypnos for the Greeks, Somnus for the Romans. As David Randall writes in his book, *Dreamland*, the Greeks considered sleep to be a kind of middle state between life and death. And indeed the twin brother of Hypnos was Thanatos, god of death. Lethe, the river of forgetfulness, flowed through Hypnos's cave, helping people sleep by forgetting their worldly identities and their worldly problems. I love that the name Lethe is also related to (and contained within) the ancient Greek word for philosophical truth, *aletheia.* As Heraclitus, the fifth-century BC Greek philosopher, wrote, "The waking have one common world, but the sleeping turn aside each into a world of his own."

Around the same time, the Greek doctor and philosopher Alcmaeon of Croton came up with the first known theory of sleep. He suggested that sleep comes about as the result of blood on the surface of the body withdrawing into the body's interior. One hundred years later, Aristotle defined sleep in his treatise *On Sleep and Sleeplessness* as "a seizure of the primary sense-organ, rendering it unable to actualize its powers; arising of necessity . . . for the sake of its conservation." He was wrong on the seizure, but the conservation part was amazingly prescient, given what science has now revealed about the restorative powers of sleep.

Ancient Chinese literature, as Kat Duff writes, referencing the fourth-century Taoist text *Liezi*, "regards sleeping and waking worlds as equal counterparts in a greater whole, akin to night and day, winter and summer, and yin and yang." In Islam, the existence of sleep is enumerated among the signs of Allah's greatness. Muhammad stressed the importance of a clear transition between daytime and bedtime: "Whenever you go to bed, perform ablution like that for the prayer." Muhammad was also an advocate of naps: "Take a short nap, for Devils do not take naps."

In the seventeenth century, René Descartes, like Aristotle, focused on the restorative function of sleep. "During sleep," he wrote in his *Treatise of Man*, "the substance of the brain, being in repose, has leisure to be nourished and repaired, being moistened by the blood contained in the little veins or arteries that are apparent on its external surface." Again, a little off on the mechanism, but otherwise spot-on.

PRE-MODERN AND EARLY MODERN SLEEP

Pre-industrial sleep differed from our own not just in the reverence attached to it but in the nature of sleep itself. In most cultures, sleep wasn't the uninterrupted stretch of time it is now. Throughout most of human history, night was divided into two separate periods of sleep, known as segmented sleep. One of the earliest references to this practice of segmented sleep is in *The Odyssey*, where Homer wrote about a "first sleep." Between the two sleep stages was a period of wakefulness, which would last up to several hours. But this wakeful interlude wasn't the same as being awake during the day. It was a prized and valuable time. "This non-continuous sleep pattern is characteristic of virtually all mammals and is also the pattern we experience early and late in life," Dr. Gregg Jacobs, an insomnia specialist at the University of Massachusetts, told me.

Roger Ekirch, the author of *At Day's Close*, described this special time between sleep: "Fires needed to be tended or perhaps a tub of ale brewed. Still, most persons never left their beds, preferring instead to ponder dreams from which they awakened. No other period afforded such a secluded interval of darkness in which to absorb fresh visions of solace, spirituality, and self-revelation." It was also a time of prayer. Indeed, "When you awake in the night" was a special section in prayer books of the time. And, Ekirch noted, this was also considered the best time for sex if a couple was trying to conceive a child: "A sixteenth-century French physician ascribed the fecundity of rural peasants to early morning intercourse 'after the first sleep' when, he claimed, they 'have more enjoyment' and 'do it better.'" Whether these frisky rural peasants enjoyed sex after brewing some ale or after reciting prayers and contemplating their souls, we can't be sure.

So sex, prayers, reading, and writing occupied at least some of the hours before falling asleep again. But nothing was more important than using that time that blurred the frontiers "between the waking and invisible worlds"—as Ekirch put it—to make sense of dreams: "The influence dreams had upon individuals and their personal relationships is difficult to imagine. Reverberations could last from fleeting minutes to, in rare instances, entire lifetimes."

The quiet relaxation of these special hours, without the distractions of daily activities, allowed people to become aware of subtler things and digest the unique insights that so often occur in that transition state between waking and sleeping. Edgar Allan Poe called them "a class of fancies, of exquisite delicacy, which are not thoughts, and to which, as yet, I have found it absolutely impossible to adapt language. . . . They arise in the soul . . . only at its epochs of most intense tranquillity . . . and at those mere points of time where the confines of the waking world blend with those of the world of dreams. I am aware of these 'fancies' only when I am upon the very brink of sleep." These "fancies" have inspired many writers, including Robert Louis Stevenson, who wrote about the special magic of that time: "It seemed to me as if life had begun again afresh, and I knew no one in all the universe but the almighty maker."

Our ancestors' reverence for sleep and for dreams is particularly remarkable when you consider how difficult it was to actually get any sleep! Today we may feel besieged by technology, by overwork, by the clamor and chaos of modern life. But our ancestors were besieged by more down-to-earth disruptions, by rustlings, smells, and movements—including from the farm animals that were often sleeping in the same room (and you think your partner is annoying at night?). There were definitely no blackout curtains, white-noise machines, high-thread-count sheets, and lavender sachets. "Within some homes . . . such was the tumult created by rats and mice that walls and rafters seemed on the verge of collapse," wrote Ekirch of the conditions in the late seventeenth and early eighteenth centuries. "Ill-constructed houses generated their own cacophony, owing to shrinking timber, loose boards, drafty doors, broken windows, and open chimneys."

And though it's not on the recommendations list of today's sleep consultants, communal sleeping served an important social purpose. Sleeping was, in many ways, a social activity and a means of family cohesion. "Sleeping with others," Carol Worthman, a professor of anthropology at Emory University, told me, "was virtually universal from infancy onward, providing security, safety, and the most intimate context that can be shared by all ages."

Sometimes co-sleeping may be simply a necessity, like if you're a college student trying to make ends meet. Or just a couple of guys trying to found a country: a few months after the American colonies declared their independence from England, Benjamin Franklin and John Adams had to share a bed at an inn in New Brunswick. They quarreled over whether they should keep the tiny window open or not, and Adams fell asleep to Franklin's disquisition on his "theory of colds"—proving once again that great men do not necessarily make great roommates.

And while there are many reasons that segmented sleep went out of fashion in the modern world, there's some evidence it might be our natural state. In a National Institute of Mental Health study, when subjects were put into a setting with no artificial light for fourteen-hour blocks, they reverted back to segmented sleep like our pre-industrial ancestors. According to Dr. Thomas A. Wehr, the study's author, "consolidated sleep in human beings may be an artifact of modern lighting technology."

So some sleep disorders may be the natural expression of our pre-modern sleep wiring coming to the surface: "It's the seamless sleep that we aspire to that's the anomaly, the creation of the modern world," Ekirch says. Yet people who wake up in the middle of the night "regard themselves as abnormal, which only heightens their anxiety, thereby accentuating their inability to sleep."

What ultimately killed off segmented sleep—and changed our relationship with sleep forever—was the spread of artificial light. The first public lamp, a candlelit lantern, was hung at the Grand Châtelet in Paris in 1318. In 1667, under the reign of Louis XIV, the "Sun King," Paris became the world's first city to install artificial lights on a large scale. Other cities soon followed.

This early movement to light up the night used candles and sometimes oil—materials that had been available for hundreds of years. So why did the illumination of cities only begin in the seventeenth century? History professor Craig Koslofsky at the University of Illinois says it was because of changes in the way people began thinking of nighttime: "The night was closely associated with danger, both natural and supernatural. But in the 17th century, Europeans were beginning to see opportunities to expand their authority throughout the world. . . . We go from seeing darkness as something dangerous and best to be avoided to something that could be used selectively." The night was yet another frontier to be conquered in an age of expansion.

By the end of the seventeenth century, more than fifty cities across Europe were illuminated at night. In 1807, London's Pall Mall became the first city street to be lit with gas lamps. By the dawn of the twentieth century, Paris had more than fifty thousand gas streetlamps. Across the pond,

Baltimore established the first gas company in the United States in 1816 and lit its streets with gas lamps a year later. In Southeast Asia, Singapore installed gas lamps in 1864. When it comes to our modern society's relationship with sleep, all this is still prehistory. Our modern sleep narrative really begins with the Industrial Revolution.

FROM SACRED TO A WASTE OF TIME: THE INDUSTRIAL REVOLUTION AND SLEEP

The Industrial Revolution is what truly fueled the sea change in our relationship to sleep. Artificial light allowed the night to be colonized, but mechanization allowed it to be monetized, and capitalism had no use for sleep. Through the nineteenth century, as was the case with factories, machines, and workers, sleep became just another commodity to be exploited as much as possible. Indeed, sleep became not just devalued but actively scorned. After all, every hour spent sleeping was another hour spent not working—therefore another wasted hour. "Increasingly," write Kevin Hillstrom and Laurie Collier Hillstrom in *The Industrial Revolution in America*, "owners and managers treated human labor as a commodity in the production cycle—one that they tried to obtain cheaply and use as efficiently as possible."

To support this new way of working and compel workers to go along with it, going without sleep was cast as an act of masculinity, a sign of strength—what Alan Derickson in his book *Dangerously Sleepy* called "heroic wakefulness" and "manly stamina." Sleep became a sign of "unmanly weakness," and this macho notion of sleep persists to this day—a way of measuring masculinity without a ruler. "Extreme hours become a way men compete to establish whose is bigger," Joan Williams, a law professor at the University of California Hastings College of the Law, told me. "Are we really just talking about schedules?"

To ensure maximum efficiency, factories began to be run throughout the night, adding shifts around the clock. Women particularly suffered, since even as their working days became longer, their responsibilities to maintain the home and care for the family remained. As awareness of inhumane conditions increased, states began to pass laws to protect women. What followed was a period of mounting consensus from courts, legislatures, and public officials around the need to reform working conditions. Sleep was often cited as a key consideration. In fact, Louis Brandeis, who was later appointed to the Supreme Court, submitted a brief showing the latest social science data on the health effects of sleep deprivation, especially on women: "Sleep is so important from the health standpoint that there is perhaps no function which should be so conscientiously exercised." One effect of the ensuing court battles over the legislation was a pushback against this new idea of human beings—and their sleep—as a product to be monetized as exhaustively as possible.

Despite the efforts of labor activists, these piecemeal legal reforms were overshadowed by the growing popular sentiment that sleep was for the weak. "Places that clung to their traditional sleeping schedules were quickly derided as backwaters filled with people who weren't fit for the industrialized world," writes David Randall.

"EIGHT HOURS FOR WORK, EIGHT HOURS FOR REST, EIGHT HOURS FOR WHAT WE WILL"

One of the worst industries when it came to sleep was the steel industry. Steelworkers across America went on strike in 1919, demanding a reduction of their working hours, but their efforts failed and conditions remained dismal. Throughout the early 1920s, steelworkers endured double shifts every other week, allowing companies to avoid employing an additional shift of workers. The scourge of sleep deprivation from such long days affected entire communities. Charles Rumford Walker, the author of *Steel: The Diary of a Furnace Worker*, described the impact in 1922. "The twelve-hour day, as I observed it," he wrote, "tended to either destroy, or to make unreasonably difficult, that normal recreation and participation in the doings of the family group, the church, or the community, which we ordinarily suppose is reasonable and part of the American inheritance."

Plus there was the matter of very sleepy people operating very dangerous machines. "Workers regularly crawled off to sleep wherever and whenever they could and were sometimes horribly killed," write John Hinshaw and Peter N. Stearns in *Industrialization in the Modern World*. "Accidents peaked when workers ended a long turn, or when they shifted from days to nights." Alan Derickson quotes Alfred Kiefer, a steelworker, lamenting, "I often grieved when I saw the men lined up at the Steel Plant gates waiting for relatives to bring their meals for another twelve hours. What a shame! Work a horse twenty-four hours and you go behind the bars." Kiefer himself was fired for falling asleep—*twenty-one hours* into a shift!

Demand for an eight-hour workday had been building in the labor movement. Trade unionists had marched through Worcester, Massachusetts, in 1889 with a banner held high reading "Eight Hours for Work, Eight Hours for Rest, Eight Hours for What We Will." But it was not until 1926 that one of the major American companies, Ford, introduced the forty-hour workweek.

The idea of sleep as a labor issue was famously raised in the case of the Pullman porters, the workers who manned the railroad sleeping cars of the Pullman Company. Their fight over working conditions led to the formation of the first all–African American union, the Brotherhood of Sleeping Car Porters. A 1935 article described the horrible conditions they were forced to endure: "The Pullman porter . . . must sleep at night in the smoking compartment of his car unless a certain upper berth near that compartment happens to be vacant. He does not retire until the occupants of the smoking compartment go to bed. He is subject to call at every moment of the day or night while on service. . . . Hours of service are barbarously long."

The consequences of too many hours of work and too little sleep—not just for Pullman porters but for engineers, signal operators, and all railroad personnel—were predictable: crashes, derailments, and fatalities. At the turn of the century, Edward Moseley, the secretary of the Interstate Commerce Commission, wrote that "it is undeniable that many of the accidents which occur are largely contributed to, if not directly caused by, the long hours of duty to which trainmen are subjected." He then noted a train wreck that had happened in Illinois, quoting a Chicago newspaper account which concluded that "the officials of the company might as well fill their engineers and firemen with whiskey or drug them with opium as to send them out for fifteen and seventeen hours of continuous work expecting them to keep their heads, and apply intelligently the general rules of the road." The same could be written about many companies today.

THE AMERICAN WAR ON SLEEP

Though this shift in thinking about sleep took place across the industrialized world, there was also something uniquely American in this modern attitude toward work and sleep. Our up-by-the-bootstraps national narrative, combined with a deeply ingrained Puritan work ethic, made the New World fertile ground for a culture that equated sleep with laziness. "The truly moral man," writes Daniel Rodgers in *The Work Ethic in Industrial America, 1850–1920*, "was at once a person of strength and a *perpetuum mobile*," whose days, as Bishop Henry Potter put it at the time, "are so crowded full of honest and healthy tasks that he has no room for dreaming." It's a sentiment espoused in colonial times by none other than the enterprising young Benjamin Franklin, in *Poor Richard's Almanack*: "Up, Sluggard, and waste not life; in the grave will be sleeping enough."

It was certainly a way of thinking embraced by an American business class in the thrall of Charles Darwin, whose theory of "the survival of the fittest" was extended from the jungle to the boardroom. Rodgers notes the popularity of connecting relentless work, status, and success and quotes Horace G. Burt, the president of the Union Pacific Railroad, summing up the secret of success: "Application. Work, work, work, work, work, work."

Considering this heritage and history, it's no surprise that maximizing work and minimizing sleep are still firmly embedded in our national consciousness. It's one of America's foundational creation myths. If you were to pinpoint one man who most embodied this delusion, it would be Thomas Edison, who was convinced that sleep was unnecessary. He bragged that he never needed more than four or five hours a night, and believed that America should follow his example on the brightly lit path of progress and self-improvement.

In fact, it's hard to find an account of Edison that doesn't mention his heroic dedication to hard work and sleepless nights, as he tried and failed and tried again to perfect the lightbulb. The implication was, of course, that his willingness to forgo sleep was strongly connected with his genius, commitment, and eventual success. The *Chicago Tribune* lauded his "willingness to work at all hours, night or day," even during his honeymoon. (Other than that, Mrs. Edison, how did you enjoy the honeymoon?)

On the thirty-fifth anniversary of the invention of the incandescent lightbulb in October 1914, Edison was interviewed by *The New York Times.* The prescient headline, displayed in large letters across the page, quoted Edison: "THE FUTURE MAN WILL SPEND LESS TIME IN BED." "In the old days man went up and down with the sun," Edison explained. "A million years from now he won't go to bed at all. Really, sleep is an absurdity, a bad habit. We can't suddenly throw off the thralldom of the habit, but we shall throw it off. . . . Nothing in this world is more dangerous to the efficiency of humanity than too much sleep." Helpfully, he even did the math: "Suppose a crusade which would educate the people might be started which would keep the 90,000,000 people of the United States out of bed one hour each night.

That would add 365 hours a year to each individual's life, or much more than a month of working days of ten hours each. To the 90,000,000 it would give about 3,500,000,000 hours every year. I can think of no way in which a vast addition to the wealth of the world could be made so certainly as by this method." He concluded that "everything which decreases the sum total of man's sleep increases the sum total of man's capabilities. There really is no reason why men should go to bed at all." And you thought *your* parents gave you a hard time when you slept in as a teenager. Imagine being Thomas Edison's kid (he had six) on Saturday mornings.

> *Seeing everybody so up all the time made me think that sleep was becoming pretty obsolete, so I decided I'd better quickly do a movie of a person sleeping.*
>
> —Andy Warhol, *POPism*

So Edison believed he had rendered sleep obsolete by giving us the ability to be productive at night. And heroically forgoing sleep became even more woven into the triumphal American narrative of progress. When another quintessential American hero, Charles Lindbergh, became the first man to fly across the Atlantic Ocean solo in 1927, sleep was once again cast as an obstacle to overcome. Lindbergh remembered his battle with sleep this way in his autobiography, *The Spirit of St. Louis*:

> I simply can't think of sleep. I have an ocean yet to cross, and Paris to find. Sleep is a trivial thing. . . . It has no

> business bothering me now. It will interfere with my judgment, my navigation, my accuracy of flying. . . . The worst part about fighting sleep is that the harder you fight the more you strengthen your enemy, and the more you weaken your resistance to him.

And conquer "the enemy" he did. Lindbergh went on to be praised by President Calvin Coolidge in a welcome-home address as a man of "valiant character, driven by an unconquerable will and inspired by the imagination and the spirit of his Viking ancestors." In other words, the recipe for becoming a great man involved not just valiant character and the Viking spirit, but also heaping portions of exhaustion and sleep deprivation (bake until baked).

We see these same sleep-be-damned themes reflected throughout our culture and our literature. In "Rip Van Winkle," Washington Irving writes about a man who daydreams, tells stories, and likes to take walks by himself in the woods—suspect actions that are cast as the opposite of hard work and are appropriately punished. After going into the mountains one day with some strange explorers, he gets drunk and, fatefully, goes to sleep. He wakes up twenty years later, having missed his wife's death and the American Revolution. Talk about sleep as something deeply un-American: by falling asleep, Van Winkle missed out not just on his own life but also on the birth of his country. His story is a cautionary tale for a new country defining itself and what it values. Daydreaming and sleeping are seen as anathema to participation in modern life.

And of course that new country was made possible in part by Paul Revere, the American Revolutionary hero who stayed awake through the night and, while others slumbered, alerted the militia to the approach of British forces.

The problem is that these kinds of heroic and necessary instances of overcoming sleep—Paul Revere alerting the militia, Charles Lindbergh crossing the Atlantic, and, more commonly, a mother staying up with a sick child—are the exceptions we legitimately celebrate. Clearly, Lindbergh would not have been able to cross the Atlantic if he had dozed off. And Paul Revere could not have warned the militia if he had been tucked in bed. And someone's got to stay up with the baby. But in popular culture, these achievements were used to amplify a narrative that conquering sleep should be what we aspire to as an everyday virtue.

SLEEP IN RETREAT AROUND THE GLOBE

The desire to triumph over sleep isn't limited to America. One of the most eloquent denunciations comes courtesy of the novelist Vladimir Nabokov, who in his memoir called sleep "the most moronic fraternity in the world, with the heaviest dues and the crudest rituals. It is a mental torture I find debasing. . . . I simply cannot get used to the nightly betrayal of reason, humanity, genius. No matter how great my weariness, the wrench of parting with consciousness is unspeakably repulsive to me. I loathe Somnus, that black-masked headsman binding me to the block."

When Napoleon was asked how much sleep is good, it is said he replied, "Six for a man, seven for a woman, eight for a fool." To Napoleon, sleep was just another enemy to be vanquished. As William Henry Hudson explains in *The Man*

Napoleon, "Even bodily fatigue had no effect upon the vigour and flexibility of his mind. Sleep itself had been made a slave, and came and went at the word of command."

And he extended the idea to his troops. "Napoleon always talked about fatigue as the fundamental limitation," says David Dinges, the chief of the Division of Sleep and Chronobiology at the University of Pennsylvania. "If you could keep your troops active for longer periods of time with less sleep, you had a greater tactical advantage, assuming they would remain behaviorally effective."

That, of course, is the big assumption. Maybe if Napoleon had increased his nightly total to the fool level, things might have gone differently at Waterloo. But, as Dinges said, Napoleon's sleep regimen is the "perfect description of the way high-performing people with a great degree of prefrontal cortex control imagine they can extend that to sleep." This may be the original "Napoleon complex." In fact, Dinges has put this to the test in large-scale experiments and found that sustained sleep deprivation results in "cumulative deficits in cognitive performance." In other words, whether you're a brilliant general, a great inventor, or a "30 Under 30" CEO, cheating sleep isn't an act of courage or a test of will. According to the latest science, it's hubris and folly.

Yet this new Industrial Revolution view of sleep could be seen everywhere in society. During the nineteenth century, the idea of sleep as a reminder of human frailty and something to be ashamed of was expressed in how people thought of their bedrooms. Until that time, in much of the world the bedroom had been a social and public part of the house, reflecting the communal reverence that sleep enjoyed. King Louis XIV was known to hold court and receive official visitors from his bed. But by the Victorian era, as sleep began its downward slide into shame, the bedroom retreated from public view.

A SCIENTIFIC AWAKENING

As the nineteenth century progressed, doctors and scientists began to devote more energy and resources to the study of sleep. Harvard's Division of Sleep Medicine chronicles many of these advancements in its online sleep history hub "Healthy Sleep." In 1827, Scottish doctor Robert Macnish published *The Philosophy of Sleep*, the first known sleep study of the modern age. In 1869, William Hammond, a military physician and neurologist who had been the US surgeon general before the Civil War, published *Sleep and Its Derangements*. In 1885, Henry Lyman published his book *Insomnia, and Other Disorders of Sleep*, and as scientists tried to understand what sleep was, the idea of the "sleep disorder" as something to be cured medicinally began to gain traction. In 1903, the first sleeping pill, barbital (a synthesized barbiturate sold under the brand name Veronal), was developed. Its popularity grew quickly—as did reports of abuse and fatal overdoses. Other sleeping pills hit the market, and by 1930 the number of doses of barbiturates being taken annually in the United States was estimated to top a billion.

An important milestone occurred in 1913, when the French researcher Henri Piéron published *The Physiological Problem of Sleep*, widely considered the first work to take an entirely physiological approach to sleep. In Germany, a psychiatrist, Hans Berger, created the first electroencephalograph (EEG), a machine that measures electrical brain activity, and in 1929 published his studies, which revealed that human brain waves were different in waking than in sleeping states. In 1935, the German biologist and botanist Erwin Bünning came up with the term "biological clock" to describe the principle of circadian rhythms.

As universities began to embrace sleep science, the field gained legitimacy—and momentum. In 1925, the famed sleep researcher Nathaniel Kleitman opened the world's first laboratory dedicated to the study of sleep at the University of Chicago, exploring the physiology of sleep and human consciousness. He published his seminal work *Sleep and Wakefulness* in 1939. And in 1953, Eugene Aserinsky, Kleitman's graduate student, discovered rapid eye moment (REM) sleep (discussed in greater length in the Science chapter).

The Association of Sleep Disorders Centers (now the American Academy of Sleep Medicine), the first accrediting organization of sleep professionals, was founded in 1975 (as mentioned in the Introduction, today more than 2,500 sleep centers have been accredited). Three years later, the first issue of the peer-reviewed medical journal *SLEEP* was released, with Stanford sleep researchers Christian Guilleminault and William Dement at the helm.

In 1982, the cognitive scientist Carlyle Smith discovered the connection among sleep, learning, and memory consolidation. And the next year, the University of Chicago sleep researcher Allan Rechtschaffen demonstrated the fatal consequences of prolonged sleep deprivation.

So centuries after Aristotle, Heraclitus, and their ancient brethren, we're once again beginning to give sleep its due—only now with the scientific and technological ability to collect groundbreaking data. Enter a search for the word "sleep" today in PubMed, the online science database overseen by the U.S. National Library of Medicine, and you will get more than 150,000 results. At *The Huffington Post*, we launched a section devoted to sleep in 2007.

OVERWORK: POSTWAR AMERICA'S MOST DANGEROUS STATUS SYMBOL

The onset of the Cold War, together with the slowing of the postwar growth of the middle class and heightened global competition, added to a sense of unease and self-doubt, as Americans perceived themselves falling behind the Soviet Union in the arms race and the space race. That led to an unrelenting focus on economic growth. Shorter working hours were linked to Communist ideas, and labor unions were increasingly hindered by the wave of anti-Communist sentiment. As Juliet Schor notes in *The Overworked American: The Unexpected Decline of Leisure*, people were working 163 hours more per year in 1987 than in 1969. Sleep was dispensable. Sam Walton, the founder of Walmart, described in his autobiography the way his relentless work schedule extended to the weekends: "I come in every Saturday morning usually around two or three, and go through all the weekly numbers. I steal a march on everybody else for the Saturday morning meeting. . . . I do this with each store every Saturday morning."

The rise of the finance industry dealt sleep another blow; the industry's attitude toward sleep was summed up by the slogan Citibank chose in 1978: "The Citi Never Sleeps." The campaign was revived in 2008, with this commercial: "Opportunities never sleep; the world never sleeps. . . .

That's why we work around the clock, to turn dreams into reality. That's why Citi never sleeps." Perhaps if they had, they wouldn't have needed more than $300 billion in bailouts and guarantees from the federal government later that year. (And given what we know about decision making, you definitely don't ever want to hear your financial adviser brag about "working around the clock.") The iconic embodiment of this mind-set was the suspender-wearing, greed-endorsing Gordon Gekko of the movie *Wall Street*, a fictional blend of real-life financial tycoons and junk-bond kings, who told us that "money never sleeps." And though Gekko remains a widely recognized symbol of everything wrong with our corporate culture, many modern executives around the world continue to live—and sometimes die—by such tired (literally) slogans.

One of the tragic examples of this attitude toward sleep and success is the rise of the Japanese "salaryman," the white-collar office worker characterized by an unfailing dedication to the company, often at the expense of life outside of work. He's at his desk until his supervisor leaves, even if there's nothing left to be done, and entertaining clients late into the night before rising at dawn for the morning commute. The reward for his unwavering loyalty was built into the paternalistic relationship with the company, with cultural approval and generous bonuses handed down after decades of employment.

The culture of the salaryman, however, has proven increasingly unstable. Employee stress and burnout have become national epidemics, as globalization has severed the lifelong bonds between employee and company. But while there may not be as many young Japanese workers today sacrificing their lives for their company, the concept of the salaryman persists. In 2015, the popular YouTube vlogger Stu in Tokyo, who works at a financial-services firm, documented a typical week during the company's busy season (seventy-eight hours of work and thirty-five hours of sleep) in a video that has now been viewed more than a million times.

According to Joan Williams, burnout is so associated with success, it's become a cultural symbol. "Overwork has also become a way to signal class status: 'I am slammed' is a way of saying 'I am important,'" she told me. "This represents a sharp shift from a prior era when having leisure was a 'class act.' . . . We have this weird reversal in the US where the elite work very long hours, while the poor typically can't get even forty hours a week of work."

Women stand at a particular disadvantage in this culture of overwork. When women work harder to climb the ladder and shatter the glass ceiling, sleep is often the first thing to go. "Women typically have a fragile hold in these kinds of workplaces," Williams said, "and often get the message that the only way they can succeed is by being 'one of the guys,' including proving themselves by working even harder than the men."

So although the science of sleep has evolved dramatically over the last century, our cultural attitudes have a lot of catching up to do, and everyday practices even more. They are, however, changing even as I write this. We are now at a crossroads. New findings about the science of sleep and its impact on performance and decision making, which I explore in depth in the Science chapter, are published every week. And there is an increasing awareness that sleep helps us to perform better both physically and cognitively, to learn faster, to consolidate memories, and, generally, to be healthier. Sleep deprivation undermines all these things. But this growing awareness clashes with our daily lives, tethered as we are to our devices and endlessly distracted by our 24/7 connection to the world. This clash has created a cultural tension that we are still trying to resolve. In a world in which silence and stillness are becoming increasingly rare, sleep for some has become almost a form of cultural resistance, as Jonathan Crary describes in his book *24/7: Late Capitalism and the Ends of Sleep*: "Sleep poses the idea of a human need and interval of time that cannot be colonized and harnessed to a massive engine of profitability, and thus remains an incongruous anomaly and site of crisis in the global present."

In response to the crisis of sleep, there is a new and growing sleep consciousness. Everywhere I look, I see articles about the benefits of sleep. And they're appearing not just in health publications but on sports and business pages—*The Wall Street Journal*, *The Financial Times*, *The Economist*, *Forbes*, *Business Insider*, *Fast Company*, etc. They describe the downsides to sleep deprivation, share practical tips on how to get more and better-quality sleep, and announce the latest gadgets and devices to help us. From sleep trackers to smart beds to apps on our tablets and smartphones, they all claim to help us sleep by disconnecting us from the very technology that has helped rob us of our sleep. Paradoxically, some of the most promising devices are made by the same companies that hyperconnected us in the first place.

That's why I say we are in the midst of a sleep revolution. Among those who are paying attention to the latest science, sleep is no longer belittled or denigrated as a waste of time. Indeed, increasingly, getting enough sleep is all about performance—job performance, physical performance, mental performance, athletic performance. And though it's much more than that, this is a big step in the right direction.

The good news is that despite our distractions and time pressures, our glowing screens and vibrating phones—our hyperconnectivity, often from the moment we wake up until the instant we drift off—we now have the knowledge and the tools to create a golden age of sleep. We have the ability to safeguard and savor the realm of sleep—not just for the benefits it confers in terms of performance and decision making but for the way it forces us to disconnect from the world and to connect with our deeper selves.

4.

THE SCIENCE OF SLEEP

Physics says: *go to sleep. Of course*
you're tired. Every atom in you
has been dancing the shimmy in silver shoes
nonstop from mitosis to now.
Quit tapping your feet. They'll dance
inside themselves without you. Go to sleep.

Geology says: *it will be all right. Slow inch*
by inch America is giving itself
to the ocean. Go to sleep. Let darkness
lap at your sides. Give darkness an inch.
You aren't alone. All of the continents used to be
one body. You aren't alone. Go to sleep.

Astronomy says: *the sun will rise tomorrow,*
Zoology says: *on rainbow-fish and lithe gazelle,*
Psychology says: *but first it has to be night, so*
Biology says: *the body-clocks are stopped all over town*
and
History says: *here are the blankets, layer on layer, down and down.*

—Albert Goldbarth, "The Sciences Sing a Lullabye"

WHY WE SLEEP

The science of sleep has exploded in recent years, revolutionizing our understanding about a need that has stayed constant through the centuries. New findings come out every day, and though their subject matter is varied, they all point toward the same conclusion: the notion that our brains and bodies are inactive during sleep—the nighttime "off" switch to our daytime "on" switch—couldn't be further from the truth.

Though much about sleep remains a mystery, scientists have made fascinating discoveries about what, exactly, is going on while we sleep—and as a result they've put to bed, if you will, our most misconceived and harmful views. Knowing all that's going on in our brains while we're sleeping, it's hard to believe that a body seemingly at rest can be so busy.

The first question most of us have is: Why do we sleep at all? What's the purpose of spending a third of our lives in a state that is seemingly at best unproductive and at worst a complete waste of time? When we think of fundamental human needs and urges, we usually think of food and sex. But the need to sleep is just as critical to our survival. In fact, as Erin Hanlon, an assistant professor at the University of Chicago's Sleep, Metabolism and Health Center, points out, it can take precedence: "The drive to sleep is so strong it will supersede the drive to eat. Your brain will just go to sleep, despite all of your conscious efforts to keep it at bay."

There are many studies that show what happens to us if we don't sleep, but here is one extreme real-life story: In

1959, New York disc jockey Peter Tripp stayed awake for 201 hours (just over eight days) to benefit the March of Dimes, continuing his daily radio broadcasts from a glass booth in Times Square throughout the "wakeathon," as the stunt was billed. After three days, Tripp became mean and abusive, and two days later he began to suffer intense hallucinations, leading to paranoia. His body temperature dropped, and, although he appeared to be awake, brain scans showed him to be asleep. And on the final day of the wakeathon, he thought his doctor was an undertaker planning to cart off his corpse.

We've all experienced—though hopefully not to that degree—the burnout that comes when we deny ourselves the sleep we need. (And is there anything that feels more welcome, more right, than crawling into bed when you're exhausted?) But where does this urge to sleep come from? There are a number of hypotheses about why we need sleep. Here are four of the leading theories. First, there's the inactivity theory, which holds that sleep is a product of natural selection; our inactivity during sleep allowed our ancestors to hide quietly and go unnoticed by predators. The obvious problem with this theory is that although stillness can be a helpful defense mechanism, stillness coupled with a lack of awareness of your surroundings doesn't seem like a particularly strong predator-avoidance strategy (nor a plus in making sure your genes get passed on). Then there's the energy conservation theory, in which sleep, by putting our bodies into a slower metabolic state, developed as a way to reduce the number of calories, or energy, we need to consume and expend each day. Think of it as lowering your monthly expenses to make you financially healthier in the long term. The third theory is the restorative theory, in which sleep is seen as a way of restoring the resources we use during the day. And last is the brain plasticity theory, which holds that sleep is a function of the development and ongoing maintenance of the brain itself. In many ways, these theories are interconnected, particularly the last two, highlighting that, as Harvard's Patrick Fuller told me, "sleep is for the benefit of wake." Or, as Harvard's Allan Hobson once said, "Sleep is of the brain, by the brain and for the brain."

Now, blessings light on him that first invented sleep! It covers a man all over, thoughts and all, like a cloak; it is meat for the hungry, drink for the thirsty, heat for the cold, and cold for the hot. It is the current coin that purchases all the pleasures of the world cheap, and the balance that sets the king and the shepherd, the fool and the wise man, even.

—Miguel de Cervantes, *Don Quixote*

We may never be certain about how sleep evolved, but, as the University of Chicago sleep researcher Allan Rechtschaffen said, "If sleep does not serve an absolutely vital function, then it is the biggest mistake the evolutionary process has ever made." And science is now showing just how vital it is. Sleep involves a range of complex functions associated with memory, our ability to learn, brain development and cleaning, appetite, immune function, and aging. And that doesn't even begin to scratch the surface of what it does for our mood, our well-being, our creativity, and our relationships.

So what puts us to sleep at night, and what wakes us up in the morning? Sleep and wakefulness are regulated by two complementary systems: our sleep/wake homeostasis, which responds to the body's internal cues, and our circadian rhythm, which responds to external cues, especially daylight. Sleep/wake homeostasis has a complex name but describes an intuitive process: the longer we stay awake, the sleepier we get; the longer we sleep, the more likely we are to wake up. Scientists call this "sleep pressure," which builds up as you stay awake and releases when you go to bed.

The second system, our circadian rhythm, comes from the Latin *circa* (around) and *dies* (day), and is a cycle that roughly corresponds to one day. In humans, circadian rhythm is governed by a small group of brain cells located in the hypothalamus (just above the optic nerves). Another way to think of it is as a master clock set to a schedule of approximately twenty-four hours, the exact time varying for each of us. Our circadian rhythm cycle, dipping and rising at different times of the day, needs constant input in the form of natural light to be calibrated properly and interacts with the buildup of sleep pressure from being awake to regulate our sleepiness and wakefulness throughout the day.

Our sleep rhythms are in many ways fluid; factors such as how much we sleep and when are likely to change over time. For newborn babies, this rhythm takes several months to become circadian—as sleep-deprived parents know all too well. New phases of life bring new patterns of sleep as our rhythms continue to shift and adjust.

Though it may feel mundane to us, the onset of sleep is highly choreographed and even beautiful in its complexity. The circadian rhythm cycles downward in the late evening, dovetailing with the high sleep pressure built up throughout the day. Scientists sometimes refer to this transition as the "primary sleepiness zone" or the opening of the "sleep gate," which Peretz Lavie, president of the Technion-Israel Institute of Technology, defines as "the sudden change from a high level of alertness to one of extreme sleepiness." And if we go to bed while our sleep gate is open, then we hit the sleep bull's-eye or the sleep sweet spot.

Fact: 60 percent of people around the world have slept holding their mobile phone.

Before I saw the light about the importance of sleep, I treated it like an enemy, something that needed to be fended off or even ignored entirely. The "primary sleepiness zone" was to be avoided, like a heavily mined border crossing. I even had my go-to methods of powering right through that zone: playing workout music to pump me up, eating (even if I wasn't hungry), splashing cold water on my face (though stopping short of prying my eyelids open with toothpicks!). Essentially, each night the sleep train would pass through my life, headed for the sleep gate, and I would do whatever I could to make sure I wasn't on it.

THE FOUR STAGES OF SLEEP

Once we do finally make it through the sleep gate, there are four stages of sleep. Each is characterized by different types of brain waves, which reflect the level of the brain's electrical activity. Stage one is light sleep, a transitional stage between wakefulness and sleep. In this state we can wake up easily and our eyes and muscles are still moving. Stage two is slightly deeper and characterized by the slowing and stopping of eye movement and a decrease in core body temperature. In stage three, slow-wave deep sleep (also known as delta sleep) begins. In this stage the brain creates slow, high-amplitude delta waves—a departure from the higher-frequency beta waves of our waking hours. This is our deepest phase of sleep, during which eye and muscle movements have nearly ceased and it's very difficult to wake us up. If we *are* woken up, we'll likely be disoriented and groggy. The depths of this third stage contain some of sleep's most fascinating mysteries and oddities, like sleepwalking and sleep talking.

Once, when we were living in Washington, D.C., and Isabella was four years old, I put her to sleep and then went out to dinner with her dad, leaving her with my mother, who was staying with us. When we got back, I went to check on her and her bed was empty! You can imagine the fear that gripped us as we frantically searched the whole house. Finally, in desperation, we went back to her bedroom and started looking under the furniture. We found her peacefully asleep on the floor under a little daybed for friends to sleep in during sleepovers.

Sleepwalking occurs in approximately 17 percent of children and 4 percent of adults. The symptoms can be more complex than the name might suggest. According to the National Sleep Foundation, the behavior can range from "simply sitting up in bed and looking around, to walking around the room or house, to leaving the house and even driving long distances." It's commonly believed that sleepwalkers should not be awakened, but given the unpredictability of what people might do while sleepwalking (um, are those your car keys?), the best thing you can do is gently wake them and guide them back to bed.

Then there's sleep talking, which occurs in about half of young children and 5 percent of adults. There is a genetic component to it, but sleep deprivation and stress can also increase instances of sleep talking. What we say in our sleep can range from gibberish to complex monologues. And although sleep talking presents no health hazard, spilling your darkest secrets while asleep can prove problematic, as Lady Macbeth discovered:

> *Gentlewoman: This is her very guise, and upon my life fast asleep; observe her; stand close . . .*
> *Doctor: You see her eyes are open.*
> *Gentlewoman: Ay but their sense are shut . . .*
> *Lady Macbeth: Yet here's a spot . . . Out damned spot—out I say.*
> *. . . Who would have thought the old man to have had so much blood in him.*
> *. . . Here's the smell of the blood still—all the perfumes of Arabia will not sweeten this little hand. O, O, O. What's done, cannot be undone.*

Or, to quote a more recent musical example from the Romantics: "I hear the secrets that you keep / When you're talking in your sleep."

The fourth and final phase of sleep is REM sleep, characterized by rapid eye movement. In REM sleep, which starts about an hour and a half after we fall asleep, our breathing becomes shallower and quicker, our blood pressure and heart rate—which have been slowing in the earlier stages—go back up, and our brain waves become faster in frequency, resembling those of our awake brain. Our muscles are essentially in a state of paralysis. It's in REM sleep that we do most of our dreaming, and if we wake up during this phase, we are more likely to remember our dreams.

The connection between REM sleep and dreaming is part of what led to the discovery of REM sleep in 1953. Dr. William Dement—who went on to open the first sleep-disorders clinic in 1970 at Stanford University—was a graduate student at the time working with Nathaniel Kleitman and Eugene Aserinsky. He told me that their team had one of the very first electroencephalograph (EEG) machines and that while using it to monitor sleeping patients, they noticed electrical activity that was not coming from the brain. "My job, which was extraordinarily tedious," he explained, "was to sit by the bed of someone who was sleeping and to see if the subject was making any movement when these artifacts appeared. At some point, I looked at the face and noticed the eyes were twitching. I thought it was a wink!" But the EEG indicated that the subject was asleep. So when he saw activity on the EEG, Dement held a flashlight to the eyes to see if they were moving—and they were. (Almost as impressive as the discovery itself is the fact that people can sleep with a researcher sitting by the bed watching them!)

Kleitman hypothesized a connection between the eye movements and dreaming. So the researchers began to wake the subjects immediately after eye movements were observed and ask them if they were dreaming. They discovered that dream recall was much higher when eye movement was present; instead of the vague morning dream recall, subjects could remember multiple dreams in vivid detail. "My favorite analogy," Dement told me, "is that before REM was discovered, sleep was thought to be like putting the car in the garage and turning off the ignition—no activity, no energy. I like the analogy that sleep is more like you park the car, put it in neutral, and the motor keeps running." I love that metaphor, and to perhaps even update it, going to sleep is like the car becoming a self-driving car and running all sorts of essential errands for us.

Further study has deepened our knowledge of the link between eye movement and dreams. These eye movements may be the result of a "change of scene" in our dreams—as if we are "moving on to the next dream frame." Throughout the night, we cycle through the four stages of sleep, the REM stage getting longer with each of the three to five cycles we experience during a normal night's sleep. The first cycle of REM sleep may be as little as ten minutes; subsequent cycles may last as long as an hour. Adults tend to spend 20 percent of their time in REM sleep; for infants, it is closer to 50 percent.

We're only beginning to discover what's going on in our brains during REM sleep, besides dreaming. A study from the University of California, Berkeley, found that REM sleep can help us process emotional stress. Participants were shown images designed to elicit an emotional response. Twelve hours later they were shown the images again. The brain scans of the group that was allowed to sleep during that interval showed a less stressful response to the second viewing, with less activity in the amygdala, the emotional center of the brain. That allowed the calmer, more rational part of the brain to process the images. "This research shows that sleep plays a crucial role in emotional processing and opens up doors for therapeutic avenues," wrote lead author Els van der Helm.

The relationship between sleep deprivation and stress is also profound. Sleep deprivation results in higher levels of the stress hormone cortisol the next day. And many of the genes affected by lack of sleep are involved in processing stress and regulating our immune system. Researchers from the University of Surrey in the United Kingdom found that lack of sleep actually changes the gene expression of more than seven hundred genes and increases the activity of genes linked to inflammation. This shift takes place after just one week of getting too little sleep. Our ancestors' bodies readied themselves for potential injury (such as animal attacks) by triggering inflammation genes as protection. And that's very similar to what happens when we don't sleep. Sleep deprivation "puts the body on alert for a wound but no wound happens," said Malcolm von Schantz, a researcher on the study. "This could easily help explain the links between sleep deprivation and negative health outcomes such as heart disease and stroke."

IF YOU VALUE YOUR BRAIN, GET MORE SLEEP

One of the most important recent findings is that sleep is essentially like bringing in the overnight cleaning crew to clear the toxic waste proteins that accumulate between brain cells during the day. Dr. Maiken Nedergaard, a codirector of the Center for Translational Neuromedicine at the University of Rochester, has studied the mechanism underlying these cleaning functions. "It's like a dishwasher," she said. Just as we wouldn't eat off dirty dishes, why should we settle for going through the day with anything less than the full power and potential of our brains?

What Nedergaard's research on mice revealed is that the glymphatic system, essentially the brain's plumbing system, functions at a much higher rate during sleep and plays a critical role in brain maintenance. As the mice slept, their brain cells actually shrank in size, creating more space for the spinal cord and brain fluid to flow throughout the brain and literally sweep away the toxic buildup associated with Alzheimer's. Initial studies have shown that a similar process may occur in the human brain, a fact that could provide a major step forward in the prevention and treatment of dementia. This washing-away of waste chemicals and toxins happens only when we sleep—when we're awake, the brain is too busy handling our body's many functions. As Nedergaard put it, "The brain only has limited energy at its disposal, and it appears that it must choose between two different functional states—awake and aware or asleep and cleaning up. You can think of it like having a house party. You can either entertain the guests or clean up the house, but you can't really do both at the same time."

The consequences of not giving your brain this needed time to wash away toxins and waste chemicals go far beyond simple maintenance. According to Claire Sexton at the Oxford Centre for Functional Magnetic Resonance Imaging of the Brain, a lack of sleep over time is associated with a decline in the size of the brain itself. "We found," she told me, "that poor sleep quality was associated with an increased rate of decline in brain volumes over three to five years. The question is whether poor sleep quality is a cause or an effect of changes in brain structure, or if the relationship is bidirectional."

Never waste any time you could spend sleeping.

—Frank Knight, Cofounder of the Chicago School of Economics

One thing is clear: sleep is profoundly intertwined with virtually every aspect of brain health. Lack of sleep over time can lead to an irreversible loss of brain cells—yet another debunking of the myth that sleep debt can be made up. Researchers from the University of Pennsylvania and Peking University found in a joint study that sleep-deprived mice lost 25 percent of their LC neurons, which are involved in mental alertness, cognitive function, and attention span. "In general, we've always assumed full recovery of cognition following short- and long-term sleep loss," Dr. Sigrid Veasey, one of the study authors, said. "But some of the research in humans has shown that attention span and several other aspects of cognition may not normalize even with three days of recovery sleep, raising the question of lasting injury in the brain." Up until recently, she added, "no one really thought that the brain could be irreversibly injured from sleep loss."

A 2014 study from Duke-NUS Graduate Medical School found that the less we sleep as we grow older, the faster our brains age. In Alzheimer's patients, the brain ventricles—chambers that hold cerebrospinal fluid—widen as the brain shrinks, and the grooves and folds of the brain become more pronounced, creating gaps. Researchers found that lack of sleep in older adults increased the pace of brain-ventricle enlargement and decreased cognitive performance, the very markers of brain aging associated with the onset of Alzheimer's.

Two studies from Uppsala University in Sweden highlighted this further. One study showed that men who self-reported a sleep problem were one and a half times more likely to contract Alzheimer's. The other revealed that just one night of sleep deprivation leads to an increase in two rare molecules in the brain (NSE and S-100B) that are signs of brain damage. (If you want to go to sleep now, feel free to put the book down!)

Fact: In the United States we lose $63 billion of productivity every year due to sleep deprivation.

Sleep is also intricately connected with our general mental health. Researchers from Canada and France found that consistent early bedtimes may reduce the risk of mental illness. The underlying mechanism involves our ultradian rhythms—cycles within our body's twenty-four-hour circadian day—which govern body temperature, hormone regulation, and appetite. These rhythms are regulated by dopamine, a neurotransmitter associated with the reward and pleasure parts of our brain. Sleep disturbances interfere with our dopamine levels, leading to an imbalance associated with bipolar and schizophrenic disorders.

Then there's the matter of longevity. As of this writing, "Miss Susie," Susannah Mushatt Jones of Brooklyn, New York, is the world's oldest person at 116 years old. When asked for her secret by a reporter from the New York *Daily News*, she replied, "I sleep." She then proceeded to demonstrate her nap style.

UNFORGETTABLE: SLEEP, MEMORY, AND COGNITIVE FUNCTION

Scientists are also starting to unravel the connection between sleep and memory. A recent study from the University of California, Berkeley, found that there is a circular relationship between poor sleep and poor memory, based on the protein beta-amyloid, believed to be the cause of Alzheimer's. "The more beta-amyloid you have in certain parts of your brain, the less deep sleep you get and, consequently, the worse your memory," said lead author, neuroscientist Matthew Walker. "Additionally, the less deep sleep you have, the less effective you are at clearing out this bad protein. It's a vicious cycle."

It's not just that sleep deprivation impairs our ability to remember, it also makes us remember things that didn't happen. A study from the University of California, Irvine, found that sleep deprivation can actually create false memories. Participants who slept five hours or less per night were much more likely to report remembering having seen a news video they hadn't seen. This same group was much more likely to incorporate false information that researchers had given them into their own personal stories. "We already know that sleep deprivation wreaks havoc on your health and cognitive functioning," said lead researcher Steven Frenda. "It seems another consequence may be that it makes our memories more easily manipulated and more pliable."

In 2015, researchers at Washington State University showed just how severe our cognitive impairment can be after sleep deprivation. For the two-day study, participants were divided into two groups: one slept normally, while the other didn't sleep at all for sixty-two hours. Then they were asked to press a button when shown specific numbers and to refrain from pressing a button when shown other numbers. Once this pattern was learned by both groups, the instructions were reversed. Not a single individual from the sleep-deprived group was able to complete the task correctly even after forty attempts. "It wasn't just that sleep-deprived people were slower to recover," said lead author Paul Whitney. "Their ability to take in new information and adjust was completely devastated."

Fact: Twenty-four hours without sleep is the equivalent of a blood alcohol level of 0.1 percent—at which point you are more than legally drunk.

Matthew Walker of the University of California, Berkeley, and Dr. Robert Stickgold of Harvard's Division of Sleep Medicine studied the role sleep plays in how we learn motor skills and create memories. Participants were taught a series of finger-tapping sequences. After a night's sleep, they showed a 17 to 20 percent improvement in speed in all the sequences. But in the most challenging tasks, their improvement was 28.9 percent, showing that the more difficult the task, the more sleep prepares us to meet the challenge.

As Stickgold said in a TEDx Talk, "Sleep, Memory and Dreams: Fitting the Pieces Together," by helping us make sense of the world around us, sleep is also helping us make sense of ourselves. He tells the story of a shoemaker who cut the leather for a pair of shoes and left them out before retiring to bed. To the shoemaker's surprise, when he awoke, he found the pair of shoes finished, with no sign that anyone had been there. "This is not a fairy tale," Stickgold explains. "This is what happens for us each and every night. Like a nocturnal elf, our sleep sews those pieces together, leaving us in the morning with something better than a pair of shoes." What it leaves us with, he says, is a higher level of understanding of our lives: "When we talk about the meaning of events in our lives, what we're really talking about is how this event fits in with everything else."

The complex workings of the sleeping brain aren't just keeping sleep scientists busy—they're also inspiring and informing the work of innovators like Demis Hassabis, whose artificial-intelligence company, DeepMind, was purchased by Google in 2014. The company's mission is to use artificial intelligence and insights from neuroscience to help solve some of the world's biggest problems.

As they are making advances in artificial intelligence, Hassabis and his team are being driven by a key insight summarized by artificial-intelligence expert Stuart Russell: "Basically a machine that sleeps and dreams learns more and performs better in the long run than one that is always awake. What it means for a machine to sleep is to essentially switch off its direct connection to perception and action, while to dream means to repeatedly replay experiences in order to extract the maximum learning signal from them." As Hassabis told me, "It is a paradox. We think of sleep as an inefficient use of time, and in fact it is the most efficient use of time in terms of learning and memory." Yet again we see that in the most scientifically advanced, futuristic fields, our brightest minds increasingly grasp the link between sleep and results.

> *It is a common experience that a problem difficult at night is resolved in the morning after the committee of sleep has worked on it.*
>
> —John Steinbeck, *Sweet Thursday*

Science continues to prove that "sleeping on it" when grappling with a problem is a real thing. A study by the University of Exeter in the United Kingdom found that "sleep almost doubles our chances of remembering previously unrecalled material. The postsleep boost in memory accessibility may indicate that some memories are sharpened overnight. This supports the notion that, while asleep, we actively rehearse information flagged as important." Students, take note: next time you feel the need to pull an all-nighter to cram for an exam, remember that you'd be better off just going to bed.

Neuroscientists Russell Foster, of Oxford, and Steven Lockley, of Harvard, further underscore the link between sleep and memory consolidation by tracing it back to evolution. It was while sleeping that the earliest life-forms learned new processes that increased their likelihood of surviving. Their brains had sufficient energy to learn but registered less "noise" from the outside—the ideal conditions to efficiently consolidate new experiences. "There is considerable support for the notion that sleep is required for the processing of recently acquired short-term memories (converting some to long-term memory) and the strengthening of long-term memory." Sleep doesn't just preserve our memories; it can transform them in a process linked to creativity, according to a study out of Brazil, which found that during REM sleep neural processes not only strengthen connections between neurons but also reorganize them.

SLEEP AND OUR HEALTH

Sleep is as important for our bodies as it is for our minds. For instance, we may not have a cure for the common cold yet, but we do know how to increase the likelihood of getting one: don't sleep. Researchers from Carnegie Mellon University monitored the sleep of participants for fourteen days. Test subjects were then given nasal drops containing rhinovirus (which causes the common cold). Those who had averaged less than seven hours of sleep per night were nearly three times more likely to come down with a cold than those who had slept eight hours or more. Sleep efficiency, the percentage of time the participant was actually asleep, was an even stronger predictor. Those with an efficiency score of only 92 percent were 5.5 times more likely to develop a cold than those at 98 percent.

So cure that cold before you get it. But if you do get it, sleep is also essential for recovery—or, as an Italian proverb goes, "Bed is a medicine." And as Dr. Axel Steiger at Munich's Max Planck Institute of Psychiatry says, nature works for us: "With an infection, patients often become sleepy, and . . . sleep helps them recover." But only if we let it. The fact that sleepiness is one of the symptoms of illness is a further reminder of what our bodies instinctively know about the power of sleep.

Sleep can also amplify the effectiveness of other treatments. A 2012 study from the University of Pittsburgh showed that getting more sleep greatly increased antibody levels of those who had just received the hepatitis B vaccine, and that averaging less than six hours of sleep could render the vaccine ineffective.

Sleep deprivation may even allow cancer to spread faster. Researchers from the University of Chicago and the University of Louisville found that in mice injected with cancer cells, sleep disturbances and poor sleep quality resulted in more aggressive tumors, quicker cancer growth, and a reduced ability of the immune system to root out the early stages of cancer. "It's not the tumor, it's the immune system," explained study director Dr. David Gozal, chairman of pediatrics at the University of Chicago Comer Children's Hospital. "Fragmented sleep changes how the immune system deals with cancer in ways that make the disease more aggressive."

A 2015 study from the Fred Hutchinson Cancer Research Center in Seattle found a correlation between a pattern of poor sleep before a diagnosis of breast cancer and the likelihood of dying of the disease. Women who reported getting five hours or less sleep per night before they were diagnosed were one and a half times more likely to die of the disease than women who reported getting seven or eight hours per night. Also, when we're sleep-deprived, our pain tolerance is decreased, so normally tolerable levels of pain can feel much more intense.

Fact: One American falls asleep at the wheel every second.

Another sign of sleep as a biological imperative is the fact that it's also associated with our ability to, well, make more of us. Sleep deprivation has been linked to infertility in both men and women, as disruption of our circadian rhythms affects hormone production and sperm count. A 2013 Danish study found that men who slept less than six hours or reported high levels of sleep disturbance saw a reduction in sperm count of more than 25 percent. Sleep deprivation has also been associated with erectile dysfunction. "Testosterone is produced during the night," wrote Dr. Lisa Shives, the founder of Northshore Sleep Medicine in Evanston, Illinois. "There are studies showing not only that a decrease in the total amount of sleep can lower a man's testosterone, but also that REM sleep is important to the production and release of testosterone."

Once a new baby is on the way, sleep continues to be vital. The phrase "eating for two" is commonplace, but pregnant women should remember they're also "sleeping for two." Coming up with a birth plan of how the mother wants her labor experience to go is becoming common, but it's less well known that sleep makes it a lot more likely for that plan to succeed. Researchers at the University of California, San Francisco, found that women who slept less than six hours a night in their ninth month of pregnancy had longer labors and were 4.5 times more likely to require cesarean deliveries.

Appetite and metabolism are also profoundly affected by sleep. In a 2012 Harvard Medical School study, healthy adults who slept an average of 5.6 hours a night for three weeks had a decreased resting metabolic rate and increased glucose levels after meals, increasing the risk of obesity and diabetes.

In fact, diabetes and sleep deprivation are intricately linked. Sleep deprivation sets the stage for diabetes by increasing the risk of resistance to insulin, a hormone that's essential for absorbing blood sugar and either converting it to energy or storing it. And insulin resistance is a precursor of diabetes. Once diabetes is diagnosed, sleep is as crucial as diet for managing it. (As it happens, Thomas Edison, who claimed to have triumphed over sleep, also developed diabetes.)

The connection between sleep and weight problems has been well documented, but what we're finding out is just how strong that link is. It takes only one night of poor sleep to leave us wanting to eat more fat the next day. In a University of Pennsylvania study, one group of participants was kept awake all night, while the other was allowed to sleep. (Maybe there needs to be a study on the effects of all these sleep studies!) The people who stayed up ate nearly a thousand extra calories during the night. And the next day, even though their caloric consumption was roughly equal to that of the well-rested group, more of the calories in the sleep-deprived group came from fats. The reason why, said study author Hengyi Rao, is that even one night of no sleep is enough to alter what is called the brain's "salience network," the region associated with decision making—in this case, what participants decided to eat.

This is thy hour O Soul, thy free flight into the wordless,
Away from books, away from art, the day erased, the lesson done . . .

—Walt Whitman, "A Clear Midnight"

Self-control requires mental energy, and each of us has a limited reservoir. When we're tired, these energy reserves run low, and our self-control suffers. This is why, warns a 2015 review from Clemson University, sleep deprivation puts us at greater risk of "succumbing to impulsive desires, poor attentional capacity, and compromised decision making." Indeed, a study on smokers found that sleep deprivation made it much harder to quit.

"BUT I'M STILL TIRED": PERCEPTION VERSUS REALITY

Sometimes while we're fretting about not getting enough sleep, we're really getting more than we realize. Researchers from Chicago, Missouri, and Stanford universities found that how we *think* we sleep at night doesn't always match up with how we *actually* sleep at night. Participants wore small wrist monitors that recorded their sleep. In the morning, they were asked how much sleep they had gotten. Thirteen percent said they never or rarely felt rested when they woke up. Yet that group logged only four minutes less sleep than the two-thirds who said they felt rested most of the time. Those who said they had woken up during the night had in fact woken up, but they had also gotten nineteen minutes more sleep than those who said they had slept through the night. "That time you're awake [at night], if you're full of anxiety, may feel much more important than if you can pass the time calmly," study coauthor Diane Lauderdale said.

But there are reasons, despite getting a full night's sleep, that we still wake up tired. Michael Decker and Elizabeth Damato of Case Western Reserve University call this "sleep inertia." They explained to me that we usually wake up during light non-REM sleep or REM sleep, when our brains are active, which eases the transition from sleep to consciousness. But if we're in slow-wave sleep when we wake up, as they put it, "the leap to an alert and vigilant state of consciousness is comparable to jumping over a canyon." The reason is that during non-REM, slow-wave sleep "our brain undergoes a metabolic slowdown. During that time our cortex, the part of our brain that senses and reacts to the environment and is the essence of 'us,' becomes 'disconnected' from activity in other brain areas." Usually this type of slow-wave sleep happens early in the night, but if our sleep sequence is disrupted by things such as jet lag, drinking, or a crying baby, our slow-wave sleep might not kick in until the early morning—right when our alarm starts sounding.

YAWNING

It's contagious, but you can't do it on command. Maybe you're even doing it now (and that's okay, because even reading about yawning can make you yawn). Another fun fact: yawning starts early. According to Robert Provine, a neuroscientist at the University of Maryland, Baltimore County, and an expert on yawning, we begin yawning even before we're born.

We think of yawning as a sign of being sleepy, but it's also a signal for our bodies and brains to wake up, be alert, or come back to the moment—a kind of gentle course correction. And yes, we yawn when we're bored, but we also yawn when we anticipate something happening. "Olympic athletes sometimes yawn before their events; concert violinists may yawn before playing a concerto," Provine said.

Provine has broadened his theory to include the idea of yawning as a way of bridging mental states: "wakefulness to sleep, sleep to wakefulness, alertness to boredom, threshold of attack, sexual arousal, switching from one kind of activity to another." As for the contagiousness of yawning, new research shows it may be a primitive form of empathy. So remember to point that out to your boss the next time you're caught yawning in a meeting.

SHORT SLEEPERS

A lot of people in our culture—especially hard-charging men—like to think they don't need much sleep and even brag about it. It usually goes something like this: "Sure, other people need a full night's sleep in order to function and be healthy and alert. But I'm different." The truth, however, is that less than 1 percent of the population actually qualifies as "short sleepers"—those rare few able to get by on little sleep without experiencing negative consequences. Though many people would like to believe they can train themselves to gain admission to the short-sleeping 1 percent, the trait is actually the result of a genetic mutation. If you would like a recondite genetic-mutation dinner-party talking point, you can explain that according to researchers at the University of California, San Francisco, "a single DNA sequence change causes a switch from proline to arginine in the 385th amino acid of the DEC2 protein." For those of us without advanced degrees in genetics, let me offer a rough translation: you either have it or you don't, so it's not something you can develop over time or something you magically acquire because of your dedication to your job. While we cannot turn ourselves into short sleepers by force of will, we may be able, via gene editing, to implant a short sleep gene in embryos and thus shorten the sleep needs of our unborn children. But as Till Roenneberg put it, "I have the suspicion that once we really understand what sleep does, we will not choose to shorten it."

Even with all the new science about the critical importance of sleep, many still cling to the belief that they've somehow found a loophole. Or they grab onto any new morsel of information that tells them they can get by just fine on only a few hours of sleep a night (as I did for years).

That's exactly what some in the press did with a 2015 study published in the journal *Current Biology*, led by Jerome Siegel at UCLA. The study focused on three hunter-gatherer communities in South America and Africa that reportedly sleep between 5.7 and 7.1 hours a night. Many in the media, and even some in the science community, seized on this, resulting in a series of overblown headlines implying that sleep isn't all that important after all.

Granted, it's much easier to believe a study that reaffirms our current habits than one that tells us we need to change them. And as Siegel put it when I reached out, "Some media may have emphasized the lower sleep-duration numbers because it made for a more striking story." But the real story is much bigger: as our scientific sleep awareness grows, we also need to be on guard against wishful thinking and overblown headlines masquerading as sound science.

If one conclusion can be gleaned from all the scientific studies on sleep, it is that, as Dr. David Gozal put it, "At all ages and across all cultures and professions, the public needs to acquire the deep understanding that similar to other healthy behaviors, sleep is not a tradable commodity but rather is a life-sustaining physiological function." Only when we grasp this fundamental truth can we truly live the lives we want and not the lives we settle for.

5.

SLEEP DISORDERS

THOUGH MOST of the reasons people have trouble sleeping are self-inflicted, originating from the low priority we put on sleep, there are a number of sleep disorders that stem from medical problems and are less under our control.

SLEEP APNEA

More than 25 million American adults suffer from sleep apnea. These apneas, or interruptions, can last from a few seconds up to several minutes and can occur hundreds of times per night, making it impossible to fall into a deep sleep. In obstructive sleep apnea, the most common type, the soft tissue in the back of the throat can briefly block the airway—often the reason a person is a chronic snorer. A second kind of sleep apnea, known as central sleep apnea, results from a failure of the brain to correctly communicate with the muscles that control breathing. Though you may not remember waking up throughout the night, you will likely feel tired, have trouble concentrating during the day, and be at risk for a host of illnesses caused or exacerbated by the sleep deprivation.

Research on sleep apnea has provided some of the most

important scientific discoveries about sleep in the last decade. According to Dr. M. Safwan Badr, the chief of sleep medicine at Wayne State University in Michigan, studies show that patients with severe sleep apnea have a higher mortality rate. Short of that, sleep apnea can impair cognitive function and spatial memory, the sort we use every day to remember where we left our keys or the route we take to a favorite restaurant for lunch.

Sleep apnea has been linked to depression as well as cardiac problems, including heart attacks and heart failure. And a UCLA study from 2015 revealed that obstructive sleep apnea can weaken the blood-brain barrier, a critical defense mechanism that keeps infections, bacteria, and chemicals from entering the brain. Epilepsy, meningitis, multiple sclerosis, Alzheimer's, and other conditions have all been linked to disruptions of the blood-brain barrier.

Nor is sleep apnea limited to adults. Researchers at the University of Chicago studied the connection between obstructive sleep apnea and asthma, which afflicts more than 9 percent of children in the United States and 14 percent of children globally. They found that among asthmatic children who had surgery to remove their tonsils and adenoids to treat sleep apnea, hospitalizations for asthma dropped by more than a third.

So given sleep apnea's role in such a wide array of serious medical problems, if you think you might be experiencing it, it's important that you get yourself checked out. The primary treatment for sleep apnea is CPAP—continuous positive airway pressure. Patients wear a mask hooked up to a machine that provides pressure to keep the airways open. And there are now lighter, less cumbersome masks than those originally available.

INSOMNIA

I can't sleep; no light burns;
All round, darkness, irksome sleep.
Only the monotonous
Ticking of the clock,
The old wives chatter of fate,
Trembling of the sleeping night,
Mouse-like scurrying of life . . .
Why do you disturb me?
What do you mean tedious whispers?
Is it the day I have wasted
Reproaching me or murmuring? . . .

—ALEXANDER PUSHKIN, "LINES WRITTEN AT NIGHT DURING INSOMNIA"

We've all found ourselves caught in the dreaded sleeplessness spiral: the more we try to will ourselves to sleep, the further away sleep seems to get. So we lie awake thinking about how awful the next day is going to be because . . . we're lying awake thinking about how awful the next day is going to be. A third of adults have a hard time falling asleep, and about 10 percent meet the diagnostic criteria for chronic insomnia.

Music and fashion editor Sophie Eggleton wrote on HuffPost UK that a decade of on-and-off struggle with insomnia has turned her into a "bedraggled, weather beaten, Stig of the Dump–like character—never polished, and always with more than a few hairs out of place." She went on to describe a typical day: "Half way through today a stranger on the tube kindly informed me that I was wearing my jumper inside out. A little embarrassing, particularly due to the size of the budget brand's garish label, but no big deal in the grand scheme of things. But this type of incident is a little insight into insomnia's influences on everyday life. . . . I'm currently teetering on the edge. I've been typing my debit card pincode into the microwave."

Many of us have walked in her shoes, if not her inside-out jumper. But insomnia can be serious—both a symptom of a larger medical problem and a condition in its own right. In its most common form, insomnia is called psychophysiological insomnia, which means having difficulty falling asleep because of worry, anxiety, stress, and the resulting inability to calm the mind. But, as Patrick Fuller of Harvard Medical School told me, insomnia is not easy to diagnose: "Self-diagnosed insomnia or the provision of prescriptions for sleeping pills by well-intentioned, but not fully informed, physicians remains a problem. Patients with primary insomnia, i.e., insomnia that is not associated with any other identifiable medical condition, account for only 15 percent of all insomnia patients. The diagnosis issue is complicated by the fact that insomnia is often a symptom, and not the cause, of many disorders—it is, for example, a common symptom of anxiety disorders."

Researchers are now turning to a new source of data to help identify insomniacs—Twitter. Tracking hashtags such as #cantsleep and #teamnosleep, Boston Children's Hospital and Merck are creating a map of insomnia based on patterns observed in Twitter users with sleep problems, including posting few tweets during the day but being active on Twitter at night and posting more negative tweets than average.

Several people in The Huffington Post Healthy Living Facebook community shared anecdotes about their sleep struggles—although, as Professor Fuller made clear, whether these qualify as insomnia or not would require a medical diagnosis.

> "I think about everything! Work, bills, dealing with certain family members or friends. My health, the health of my husband. My cats. The future. The weekend." —Sharlene Stenseth

> "Take things I can't change from the past, toss them with present concerns, then blend it all with future possibilities (anything from what I should make for dinner tomorrow, to where I'll be in a year, to what if a loved one gets sick, etc.) and my brain is like a horse race in quicksand." —Shany Conroy

> "Oh God, I have to get up in however-many hours. Why couldn't this happen on the nights before my day OFF? Ugh, tomorrow is going to absolutely SUCK." —Amanda Guilford

In her 2014 memoir, *Yes Please*, Amy Poehler devotes an entire chapter to her lifelong struggle with sleep: "A good night's sleep is my white whale," she writes. "Like Ahab, I am also a total drama queen about it. I love to talk about how little sleep I get, . . . as if it is a true indication of how hard I work. But I truly suffer at night." Since she was born, Poehler has chased sleep, and if the thoughts running through her head weren't enough to keep her awake, anxiety over what would happen if she *did* actually fall asleep—sleepwalking, sleep talking, snoring—did the trick. That meant the childhood ritual of slumber parties with friends—"girl summits"—was especially agonizing. "At sleepovers I would often be the last girl standing. Everyone would fall asleep while I stared at the ceiling," she writes. And sometimes it would last all night: "I watched more than one sunrise in a strange suburban driveway. Then I would sleep late and wake up to an empty house and a mother who would reluctantly mix up a new batch of pancakes." Years later on *Saturday Night Live*, she lived "a vampire life," collapsing in bed at 3 a.m. and waking up late the following day. "I am always tired," she laments. "I now read articles about how great sleep is and how important it is and I cry because I want it so bad." Let's hope that in volume two we can read about how she finally finds her sleepy white whale!

We associate insomnia with sleep eluding us at night, but it is often connected to a state of hyperarousal throughout the day. "Although hyperaroused insomniacs complain of fatigue and tiredness, . . . their problem is that they cannot relax," said Dr. Alexandros Vgontzas, a professor of psychiatry at Penn State. But there are treatments. Dr. Gregg Jacobs developed cognitive behavioral therapy (CBT) for insomnia after studying the meditative practices of Tibetan monks and seeing the control they have over their brain waves. After participating in the therapy, more than 75 percent of insomnia patients experienced sleep improvements; 90 percent stopped or reduced their use of sleeping pills. "After a few weeks of lying awake at night, frustrated and anxious about insomnia," Jacobs told me, "people start to anticipate not sleeping and become apprehensive about going to bed. They soon learn to associate the bed with sleeplessness and frustration; consequently, the bed quickly becomes a learned cue for wakefulness and insomnia." The behavioral therapy, which helps patients identify harmful habits and optimize bedtime conditions, aims to change those associations—something, Jacobs notes, sleeping pills can't do.

A trial evaluated the results of cognitive behavioral therapy versus taking temazepam, the active ingredient in Restoril, in adults fifty-five and older. The amount of time spent awake after sleep onset was reduced by 55 percent for cognitive behavioral therapy patients, as opposed to 46.5 percent for those taking the sleep drug. And those treated with behavioral therapy sustained the benefits at three-, twelve-, and twenty-four-month follow-ups, while those treated with drugs alone did not. Two other trials tested CBT versus Ambien and zopiclone, respectively, and in both cases therapy proved more effective and was the patient's preferred choice for treatment.

OTHER SLEEP DISORDERS

Other common sleep disorders include restless legs syndrome, which causes uncomfortable sensations in sufferers' legs, leading to the need to kick or stretch the legs for relief; sleep paralysis, in which sufferers report feeling paralyzed as they wake up, some feeling as though they are being pinned down by an unseen force; and exploding head syndrome—a booming, deafening sound, like a bomb exploding or a gunshot, sometimes accompanied by flashes of light, when falling asleep or waking up. Though people suffering from these symptoms should certainly seek medical advice, improving sleep habits and lowering stress are, predictably, key steps to managing sleep disorders.

6.

DREAMS

DREAMS HAVE always been an important part of my life. In my twenties, fascinated by the work of Carl Jung, I started keeping a daily dream journal. The majority of my dreams were garbled, sometimes surreal versions of my daily life, but there were also flashes of genuine insight. As I recounted in *Thrive*, one particular dream was so clear and so powerful that it has stayed with me ever since—and with the passage of time has even become clearer and more significant. In the dream, I was on a train going home to God (bear with me!). It was a long journey, and everything happening in my life was scenery along the way. Some of it was beautiful; I wanted to linger over it awhile and perhaps hold on to it or even take it with me. Other parts of the journey were spent grinding through a barren, ugly countryside. Either way, the train moved on. And pain came whenever I would cling to the scenery, beautiful or ugly, rather than accept that it was all grist for the mill, containing some hidden purpose, a hidden blessing, or a bit of wisdom. Over the years, as I've revisited variations of this dream again and again, I've come to see it as a great lesson for living life as if—as the poet Rumi put it—everything is rigged in our favor.

Through our dreams, sleep opens up a pathway to other

dimensions, other times, other parts of ourselves, and to deeper insights that lie beyond the reach of our waking consciousness. As the Tibetan Buddhist Tarthang Tulku put it, "Dreams are a reservoir of knowledge and experience, yet they are often overlooked as a vehicle for exploring reality." Max Planck, the winner of the Nobel Prize for Physics in 1918, considered matter as "derivative from consciousness" and consciousness as fundamental. And consciousness includes dreams. The timelessness of dreams, the wildly different narrative rules, the ways we move through the dream world—all of these allow us a unique access to our intuition and inner wisdom.

We live in a world in which we relentlessly track our time, revere data over wisdom, and are consumed with our work and our devices, from the moment we get up to the second we drift off to sleep. That's why the mental real estate that our dreams occupy is more valuable than ever. Technology may let us travel across time and space in an instant, but our dreams allow us to span deeper parts of ourselves.

> *The dream is a little door in the innermost and most secret recesses of the soul.*
>
> —Carl Jung, "The Meaning of Psychology for Modern Man"

Though cultures throughout history have revered dreams—and some still do—ours has tended to dismiss them. As Roger Ekirch writes, this has come at significant cost:

> Unlike the experience of non-Western cultures that have institutionalized their dreams, our assimilation of nocturnal visions has gradually waned, and with it, a better understanding of our deepest drives and emotions. If not the "royal road" to the unconscious posited by Freud, dreams nonetheless afforded innumerable generations a well-traveled if winding path to self-awareness. It is no small irony that, by turning night into day, modern technology, while capable of exploring the inner sanctums of the brain, has also helped obstruct our oldest avenue to the human psyche.

Fortunately, new scientific findings, and a growing longing to stop living in the shallows, can help us regain access to that winding path.

FREUD, JUNG, AND THE PSYCHOLOGY OF DREAMS

Our modern understanding of dreams has long been dominated by Sigmund Freud. With his work, dreams went from being a unique way of accessing divine knowledge to being a unique way of accessing self-knowledge. Dreams were still a journey, but they became less of a sacred journey and more of a personal one.

In Freud's *The Interpretation of Dreams*, published in 1900, he argued that dreams are symbolic manifestations of repressed desires, fears, and wishes that are often too painful to experience or remember directly and are thus sublimated into our subconscious through "psychic censorship." "The dream is a psychic act full of import," he wrote; "its motive power is invariably a wish craving fulfillment; the fact that it is unrecognizable as a wish, and its many peculiarities and absurdities, are due to the influence of the psychic censorship to which it has been subjected during its formation." As important as listening to our dreams was to Freud, understanding them required a certain decoding process. "The psychodynamic dream theories were about wish fulfillment and also substitutions, so that often people or objects stood for something else entirely," Yale University psychology professor John Bargh told me. "This was in part a kind of defense mechanism to protect you from disturbing content."

But whether we understand them or not, our dreams are constantly manifesting themselves in our waking lives—because the relationship between the subconscious and the conscious is ongoing and intense. "I believe," Freud wrote, "that these unconscious wishes are always active and ready to express themselves whenever they find an opportunity of allying themselves with an impulse from consciousness."

Certain kinds of unconscious wishes were more likely to be repressed than others. "The wishes for Freud were mainly sexual, and the substitutions were for blatant, explicit sexual content and also for taboo partners such as mother or father," Bargh told me. We use the term "Freudian slip" to describe when we accidentally reveal a subconscious thought or feeling which, usually relegated to the world of dreams, finds expression in our waking life.

To Freud, dreams were only the end product of an ongoing process in the subconscious: "It is like fireworks, which require hours for their preparation and then flare up in a moment." Making use of our dreams, by integrating their subconscious secrets into our consciousness and thereby being able to deal with the fears and wishes they represent, involves first making sense of them. And with Freud, dream interpretation, which had been in the hands of the priestly class in ancient times, fell to psychoanalysts. It was a new approach to a very old idea: that dreams represent a highly valuable and unique kind of knowledge, if only we can properly decipher them.

According to Freud, the meaning of a dream is often elusive and has to be teased out, through analysis, over time. What we think are the most important details of our dreams might not be. To find the way in, the analyst needs to listen for subtle clues in the recounting of a dream: "If the first report of a dream seems not very comprehensible, I request the dreamer to repeat it. This he rarely does in the same words. But the passages in which the expression is modified are thereby made known to me as the weak points of the dream's disguise. . . . These are the points from which the analysis may start."

Of course, we never remember all the parts of our dreams. But to Freud, forgetting is a kind of repression, and it's the forgotten parts that hold the keys. "The forgetting of dreams," he wrote, "remains inexplicable until we seek to explain it by the power of the psychic censorship. . . . This part of the dream that has been wrested from forgetfulness is always the most important part. It lies on the shortest path to the solution of the dream, and for that very reason it was most exposed to the resistance." Memories, especially painful ones, can be forgotten. But they remain in our subconscious, echoed and projected as dreams, and through the analysis of our dreams we can help resurrect them.

British prime minister Winston Churchill once wrote an essay entitled "The Dream." In his dream, Churchill is about to paint in his studio, and suddenly notices that his father,

Randolph, who died more than fifty years prior, is sitting in the room with him. Churchill takes the opportunity to catch his father up on all that has happened in the world since his death—the rise of socialism, the two world wars, the new rulers of various countries. As London mayor Boris Johnson wrote in *The Churchill Factor:* "Randolph never quite understands what his son has accomplished. The father gathers that the son is now a part-time painter, of indifferent ability, that he appears to live in a small cottage, and that he never rose above the rank of major in the yeomanry." When Churchill finishes updating him on current events, Randolph says, "Of course you are too old now to think about such things, but when I hear you talk I really wonder that you didn't go into politics. You might have done a lot to help. You might even have made a name for yourself." And he disappears.

Imagine Churchill's frustration! There he stands, one of the greatest political leaders of all time, with an opportunity to tell his father all he has achieved during the war and as prime minister, yet his father hears none of it. Churchill had a tumultuous relationship with his father, and the dream reflects his lifelong yearning to make his father proud—and his continuing feeling that he had failed him.

To Freud, dreams are a journey inward and back in time, sometimes through simple, forgotten memories and sometimes through dark, painful episodes in our lives. By making that journey and figuring out the meaning of our dreams, we can both heal and truly know ourselves.

Freud's slightly younger contemporary Carl Jung, the founder of analytical psychology, saw dreams less as the result of repression and more as a manifestation of the collective unconscious. As Jungian analyst Pittman McGehee told me, "Carl Jung saw the unconscious as a wellspring of creativity and a conduit for the divine. He called the dream a 'voice of God.' If one pays attention to one's dreams, one can use the dream as a vehicle for transformation."

Jung's autobiographical *Memories, Dreams, Reflections*, first published in 1963, is still one of my all-time favorite books. To understand Jung's view of dreams, we first have to understand what he meant by the collective unconscious. "As scientific understanding has grown," he wrote in *Man and His Symbols*, "so our world has become dehumanized. Man feels himself isolated in the cosmos, because he is no longer involved in nature." A gap has opened up between the conscious mind, "characterized by concentration, limitation and exclusion," and the "original mind" and its "primitive psychic energy." It's in this gap that modern anxieties, fears, mental illnesses, and psychological disturbances have grown and flourished:

> In our conscious life, we are exposed to all kinds of influences. Other people stimulate or depress us, events at the office or in our social life distract us. . . . The more that consciousness is influenced by prejudices, errors, fantasies, and infantile wishes, the more the already existing gap will widen into a neurotic dissociation and lead to a more or less artificial life far removed from healthy instincts, nature, and truth.

So for the sake of our mental, emotional, and spiritual health, he says, the two realms must "integrally connect" and "move on parallel lines." This is where dreams come in. To Jung, dreams "are the essential message carriers from the instinctive to the rational parts of the human mind" and fill in the "forgotten language of the instincts." They "restore our psychological balance" by reestablishing a "psychic equilibrium." "What we consciously fail to see," he wrote, "is frequently perceived by our unconscious, which can pass the information on through dreams." Or as he put it in *Modern Man in Search of a Soul*, "The dream gives a true picture of the subjective state, while the conscious mind denies that this state exists, or recognizes it only grudgingly."

Though he agreed with Freud that dreams can represent repressed wishes or fears, Jung believed they can also carry "ineluctable truths, philosophical pronouncements, illusions, wild fantasies, memories, plans, anticipations, irrational experiences, even telepathic visions, and heaven knows what besides." He differed with Freud regarding the symbolic nature of dreams. Since dreams are not always a manifestation of repression, their messages are not necessarily disguised and thus don't need to be decoded. "Why should they mean something different from their contents?" he wrote. "Is there anything in nature that is other than what it is? The dream is a normal and natural phenomenon, and it does not mean something it is not. The Talmud even says: 'The dream is its own interpretation.'" Indeed, he warned, "it is plain foolishness to believe in ready-made systematic guides to dream interpretation, as if one could simply buy a reference book and look up a particular symbol. No dream symbol can be separated from the individual who dreams it."

Many of his patients, Jung wrote, especially those who had been "educated—or rather miseducated—by their reading," mistakenly believed that the elements of their dreams were simply stand-ins for other things: "They wish at once to get behind the dream in the false belief that it is a mere facade concealing the true meaning. Perhaps we may call the dream a facade, but we must remember that the fronts of most houses by no means trick or deceive us, but, on the contrary, follow the plan of the building and often betray its inner arrangement."

God has given you dreams to show your inner state.

—Rumi, "Moses and Pharaoh"

Jung didn't want to replace the ancient understanding of dreams but rather to build on that understanding with modern scientific methods. "It is only through comparative studies in mythology, folklore, religion and language," he wrote, "that we can determine these symbols in a scientific way."

This integration of the ancient and the modern, of the individual and the collective natures of our dreams, and the connection between dreams and myths and other cultural narratives, continues to have a powerful relevance. "Jung's central contribution to our understanding of the unconscious," writes Christopher Booker in *The Seven Basic Plots*, "was one of the greatest intuitive discoveries of the twentieth century, ranking alongside those of Einstein and other nuclear physicists, or Watson and Crick's double helix."

Booker was a close friend of mine when I lived in London in my twenties. I had just finished my second book, *After Reason*, which was in the process of being rejected by, yes, thirty-six publishers (a different sort of nightmare). As I waited for the responses, including the response from the thirty-seventh, who finally said yes, Booker insisted that I read Jung. And that's what I did, locking myself in my little apartment and reading Jung's collected works. The immediate impact on me was that I started meticulously recording my dreams. As a result, all these years later I still have a pile of dream books from that period, which came to an abrupt end when I left my Jungian cave and reentered the world. But though I've never again been as diligent at recording my dreams, at various stages of my life I've continued to write them down and share them with family and friends, taking advantage of their collective interpretation of the collective unconscious.

Like Freud and Jung, Edgar Cayce, known as "the Sleeping Prophet," believed that we have multiple levels of consciousness: the everyday consciousness we experience in waking life; our subconscious, which Cayce saw as a source of profound insight into the self; and the superconscious, which parallels Jung's collective unconscious.

Cayce, who was born in Kentucky in 1877, acknowledged that some dreams were simply the result of the body's digesting certain foods or other physical upsets—a bit of rancid beef, in the words of Charles Dickens's Ebenezer Scrooge. But he considered most dreams meaningful on multiple levels, a kind of nightly diagnostic report, reflecting "conditions in the body that need attention; dynamics in our relationships; opportunities that need to be seized; dangers that need to be avoided; non-physical experiences in other dimensions of life that help us expand our consciousness." The two purposes of dreams, Cayce believed, are to solve problems in a dreamer's everyday life and to help dreamers be less consumed by their worldly problems so they can connect with a spiritual dimension and a higher reality. Cayce, like Jung, brought the interpretation of dreams squarely back into the hands of the dreamer.

DREAMS AND THE ARTS

Dreams have been a favorite theme of the great storytellers throughout history, in literature, art, and music. In *Hamlet*, Shakespeare plays on the long association between dreams and death, seeing dreams as a kind of staged rehearsal for death:

To die, to sleep.
To sleep, perchance to dream—ay, there's the rub,
For in that sleep of death what dreams may come
When we have shuffled off this mortal coil,
Must give us pause.

In *Julius Caesar*, Caesar's wife, Calpurnia, has a prophetic dream about his murder and begs him not to go to Rome:

Calpurnia here, my wife, stays me at home:
She dreamt to-night she saw my statue,
Which like a fountain with an hundred spouts
Did run pure blood, and many lusty Romans
Came smiling and did bathe their hands in it.

Shakespeare returned to the theme of dreams many times, including in *The Tempest*, giving life to one of the most commonly referenced lines about dreams in literature: "We are such stuff as dreams are made on, / And our little life is rounded with a sleep."

Sometimes dreams are prophetic. At other times, as

Roger Ekirch writes, they are an "escape from daily suffering." He quotes a character in one of Jean de La Fontaine's fables:

> *Fate's woven me no life of golden thread*
> *nor are there sumptuous hangings by my bed*
> *my nights are worth no less, their dreams as deep*
> *felicities still glorify my sleep.*

The power of dreams was beautifully captured by the nineteenth-century English novelist Emily Brontë: "I've dreamt in my life dreams that have stayed with me ever after, and changed my ideas," she wrote. "They've gone through and through me, like wine through water, and altered the color of my mind."

In 1888, in "A Chapter on Dreams," Robert Louis Stevenson attributed some of his work, particularly *The Strange Case of Dr. Jekyll and Mr. Hyde*, to "little people" in his mind he called "Brownies," who inspired his ideas when he was asleep:

> That part [of my work] which is done while I am sleeping is the Brownies' part beyond contention. . . . For two days I went about racking my brains for a plot of any sort; and on the second night I dreamed the scene at the window, and a scene afterward split in two, in which Hyde, pursued for some crime, took the powder and underwent the change in the presence of his pursuers. All the rest was made awake, and consciously, although I think I can trace in much of it the manner of my Brownies.

The Beatles' "Let It Be," an ode to acceptance that I fell in love with while studying at Cambridge, was inspired by a dream Paul McCartney had while the Beatles were in the middle of breaking up. As McCartney recounts, "One night during this tense time I had a dream I saw my mum, who'd been dead 10 years or so. It was so wonderful for me and she was very reassuring. In the dream she said, 'It'll be all right.' I'm not sure if she used the words 'Let it be' but that was the gist of her advice, it was, 'Don't worry too much, it will turn out OK.' So that got me writing the song 'Let It Be.' I literally started off 'Mother Mary,' which was her name, 'When I find myself in times of trouble,' which I certainly found myself in. The song was based on that dream."

Salvador Dalí described many of his surrealist paintings as "hand-painted dream photographs." His dreams were the source of many works. "I am the first to be surprised and often terrified," he said, "by the extravagant images that I see appear on my canvas. In truth I am but the automaton which registers, without judgment and with all possible exactitude, the dictates of my subconscious, my dreams." In *The Persistence of Memory*, one of Dalí's most famous works, melting clocks symbolize how arbitrary time becomes while we're dreaming.

In popular culture, dreams are often taken to be the truer expression of ourselves, a vision of the people we want to be and the lives we long to live. In the 1950 animated classic *Cinderella*, the heroine echoes the more familiar pop-culture take of dreams as inspiration, singing, "A dream is a wish your heart makes / When you're fast asleep . . ."

In movies and literature, dreams are often a gateway to other worlds. One of the most famous examples is *The Wizard of Oz*, where, after a tornado, a yellow brick road, and three heel taps, Dorothy's adventures in Oz (and Toto's, too) come to a close as she stirs in bed, waking as though from a dream.

DOROTHY: But it wasn't a dream. It was a place, and you and you and you . . . and you were there. But you couldn't have been, could you?
AUNTIE EM: We dream lots of silly things . . .
DOROTHY: No, Aunt Em. This is a real, truly live place.

Yes, we do dream lots of silly things, but we also visit some places that seem very "real, truly live." And then we wake up, like Alice at the end of her adventure in Wonderland. "Oh, I've had such a curious dream!" she tells her sister. In *Harry Potter and the Prisoner of Azkaban*, Dumbledore asks Snape not to wake Harry: "Let him sleep. For in dreams, we enter a world that is entirely our own. Let him swim in the deepest ocean or glide over the highest cloud."

In our everyday discourse, we often use the idea of dreams as expressions of a better reality or a goal we should aim for. They represent what our best selves are capable of, what we can become if we can throw off the fears, prejudices, compromises, cynicism, and resignation of our everyday (waking) lives. There's Martin Luther King Jr.'s "I Have a Dream" speech in 1963, for example, and the American ideal of achieving the "American dream" as the ultimate fulfillment of middle-class life.

Our dreams, necessarily, have elements and images particular to the dreamer. But the foundations underlying them are shared by everyone. "It is true that dreams are more obviously than stories the products of the dreamer's own personal unconscious," writes Christopher Booker. "But the real key to understanding stories lies in seeing how they are ultimately rooted in a level of the unconscious which is collective to all humanity."

"WHEN A REALLY GREAT DREAM SHOWS UP, GRAB IT!"

These interior vistas, wandering narratives, and inner sources of inspiration are accessible not just to artists but to all of us, simply by sleeping. The self-doubts that plague us during the day become quiet during sleep, and our creativity can find expression without fear, censorship, or judgment. Harvard Medical School psychiatrist Dr. J. Allan Hobson summed it up: "Dreaming may be our most creative conscious state, one in which the chaotic, spontaneous recombination of cognitive elements produces novel configurations of information: new ideas."

Indeed, dreams have been credited with inspiring several scientific breakthroughs. In the mid–nineteenth century, American inventor Elias Howe struggled to figure out how to build a sewing machine. Then, according to a published family history, he had a dream in which he had to build a sewing machine for "a savage king in a strange country," under punishment of death if he failed. When Howe's time ran out and the king's warriors came to execute him, he noticed that their spears had holes near the pointed end. When he awoke, he realized that the missing link for his invention was moving the eye of the needle to the pointed end instead of the blunt end, where it is located for hand sewing. So next time you awake from a nightmare, don't forget to go back over the details—just in case they contain the key to your game-changing invention.

The periodic table of elements, the brainchild of the Russian chemist and inventor Dmitri Mendeleev, also came to him in a dream-inspired breakthrough: "I saw in a dream a table where all elements fell into place as required. Awakening, I immediately wrote it down on a piece of paper—only in one place did a correction later seem necessary."

Dr. Otto Loewi, the German-born psychobiologist, had a dream about the way to structure an experiment proving that nerve impulses are actually chemical. He scribbled down some notes when he awoke and went back to bed. The next morning, to his horror, he could not read his own writing. He spent the whole day desperately trying to remember the dream. That night, in a twist of fate, he had the same dream again. This time he got up and went right to his lab to perform the experiment. The results won him the Nobel Prize in 1936. The lesson: if your subconscious plays your dream a second time, pay attention to it. And write carefully—good penmanship is an underrated virtue.

In 1865, a dream about a snake eating its own tail led the German chemist Friedrich August Kekulé to envision the structure of the benzene molecule—a chemical compound with many industrial uses—as a ring. It led him to the revolutionary discovery that, as Arthur Koestler wrote in *The Act of Creation*, "the molecules of certain important organic compounds are not open structures but closed chains or 'rings'—like the snake swallowing its tail." Koestler heralded Kekulé's dream as "the most important dream in history since Joseph's seven fat and seven lean cows."

In the 1890s, Sarah Breedlove, who worked as a laundress and dishwasher, mysteriously began to lose her hair. Distraught, she prayed for a cure, and an inspiration came to her in a dream: "A big, black man appeared to me and told me what to mix up in my hair. Some of the remedy was grown in Africa, but I sent for it, mixed it, put it on my scalp, and in a few weeks my hair was coming in faster than it had ever fallen out. I tried it on my friends; it helped them. I made up my mind to begin to sell it." And that's how Madam C. J. Walker's Wonderful Hair Grower was born, which ultimately led her to found the Madam C. J. Walker Manufacturing Company of beauty products for African-Americans, which made her a multimillionaire. Indeed, her 1919 obituary described her as the wealthiest African-American woman in the United States, "if not the world."

"Yours is the truest dream,
because it had immediate effect in your waking life."
What matters is how quickly
you do what your soul directs.
—Rumi, "Three Travelers Tell Their Dreams"

More recently, Google, that repository of our entire waking world, was conceived in a dream. Here is how Larry Page described its creation in his 2009 University of Michigan commencement speech:

> Well, I had one of those dreams when I was 23. When I suddenly woke up, I was thinking: what if we could download the whole web, and just keep the links and . . . I grabbed a pen and started writing! Sometimes it is im-

> portant to wake up and stop dreaming. I spent the middle of that night scribbling out the details and convincing myself it would work. Soon after, I told my adviser, Terry Winograd, it would take a couple of weeks to download the web—he nodded knowingly, fully aware it would take much longer but wise enough to not tell me. The optimism of youth is often underrated! Amazingly, I had no thought of building a search engine. The idea wasn't even on the radar. But much later we happened upon a better way of ranking webpages to make a really great search engine, and Google was born. When a really great dream shows up, grab it!

Arthur Koestler described dreams as a "period of incubation" and made the case for why they can be a more fertile place for new ideas than our rational, linear, task-driven daytime lives. The creativity of dreams comes from "the displacement of attention to something not previously noted, which was irrelevant in the old and is relevant in the new context. . . . The creative act is not an act of creation in the sense of The Old Testament. It does not create something out of nothing; it uncovers, selects, re-shuffles, combines, synthesizes already existing facts, ideas, faculties, skills." By including dreams in our definition of consciousness, Koestler helps us to see that to dismiss the content of our dreams is to diminish our vast potential.

THE SCIENCE OF DREAMS

So what exactly is happening inside our brains when we dream? In 1977, Dr. J. Allan Hobson and Dr. Robert McCarley proposed the "activation-synthesis hypothesis." According to the theory, the circuits in the brain stem activate when REM sleep begins. This in turn triggers activity in the limbic system of the brain, which is involved in a range of functions, including emotions, memories, and behaviors. During waking hours, these brain structures help us register and understand our environment. But during sleep, the brain is reacting to internal signals, and without external stimuli for context, it turns to our emotions and memories to create meaning: "Dreams are dripping with emotional salience, even when they are cognitively delirious."

In 2000, the Finnish psychologist Antti Revonsuo proposed the "threat simulation theory." According to this theory, dreams are not random but part of an evolutionary defense system that plays out frightening events in a safe way. For Revonsuo, dreams let us rehearse dangerous situations in a safe space, allowing us to develop skills to deal with threats in real life or to define and disarm them if they serve no purpose.

Dreams are also essential for learning and memory, as the findings of scientists at Beth Israel Deaconess Medical Center in Boston reveal. Participants in an experiment spent an hour learning how to navigate a complex virtual maze. Some were then allowed to take a ninety-minute nap, while the rest engaged in various activities. Five hours later, the participants were retested. Those who did not nap showed little improvement. Those who did nap and didn't report any maze-related dreams also showed little improvement. But those who napped and dreamed about the maze improved ten times more than their napping counterparts who did not dream about the maze.

Erin Wamsley, one of the study's authors, explained,

"The subjects who dreamed about the maze had done relatively poorly during training. . . . Our findings suggest that if something is difficult for you, it's more meaningful to you and the sleeping brain therefore focuses on that subject—it 'knows' you need to work on it to get better, and this seems to be where dreaming can be of most benefit." It's as though we're bringing in another brain with a different skill set to work on the problem, except the extra brain is our own.

. . . dreams in their development have breath,
And tears, and tortures, and the touch of joy;
They leave a weight upon our waking thoughts,
They take a weight from off our waking toils,
They do divide our being; they become
A portion of ourselves as of our time,
And look like heralds of eternity. . . .
The mind can make
Substance, and people planets of its own
With beings brighter than have been, and give
A breath to forms which can outlive all flesh.

—LORD BYRON, "THE DREAM"

Researchers from the University of California, Berkeley, have also found a connection between dreams and emotional intelligence. Participants were asked to distinguish among various facial expressions, ranging from friendly to threatening. Those who had had sufficient REM sleep correctly read the faces; the sleep-deprived group failed. According to Matthew Walker, the study's author, "Dream sleep appears to reset the magnetic north of our emotional compass.

One question is whether we can now enhance the quality of dream sleep, and in doing so, improve emotional intelligence." Dreams also help us process our emotions, since when we don't process our negative emotions, we are likely to experience an increase in stress and anxiety. As social psychology researcher Sander van der Linden put it in *Scientific American*: "Dreams help regulate traffic on that fragile bridge which connects our experiences with our emotions and memories."

As Rubin Naiman, a sleep and dream specialist at the University of Arizona Center for Integrative Medicine, told me, "Just as updating a computer requires temporarily shutting down its operating programs, REM sleep also takes us offline by inhibiting the use of most of our senses and voluntary muscles. Consciousness is much like water, changing its form depending on the environment it flows through. In waking life, consciousness is contained and framed by our physical being. Like a river moving across a landscape, it is shaped and directed by the banks of sensory input (seeing, hearing, touching, etc.) and motor output (movement, speech, etc.). In sleep, the river of waking opens into the sea of dreams. As a result, we find ourselves in an extraordinary world where we experience emotions, ideas, and images on their own wild terms. Dreams offer us a personal encounter of the world behind the world—the expansive and mysterious home of the unconscious . . . the source of all art and spirituality."

The Walker study echoes another by Hobson, who found that "REM sleep may constitute a protoconscious state, providing a virtual reality model of the world that is of functional use to the development and maintenance of waking consciousness." (Not a bad study to cite next time someone chides you for sleeping in.)

The nature of our dreams differs depending on what part of our sleep cycle we are in. As part of a study in the United Kingdom, researchers woke participants throughout the night and asked them to describe their dreams. The later in the night the dreams occurred, the more bizarre and distant from reality they were likely to be. And neuroscientists in Kyoto have discovered a correlation between the content of our dreams and our brain activity—a dream-reading machine of sorts. Participants slept in an MRI scanner and described their dreams after they woke up. Researchers categorized the dream reports into twenty different groups, such as "male," "female," "food," "book," "furniture," "street," "building," and "car," then matched them to the brain patterns. The correlation between the dream content and the brain patterns was so strong that they could predict with 80 percent accuracy which of the twenty categories the participants had dreamed about by looking at their brain activity.

Some dreams occur over and over again. Common themes in recurring dreams include falling, failing or missing an exam, being chased, finding yourself naked in embarrassing circumstances, or—and this is my most common recurring dream—being late. My personal variations on this last dream theme include being late for a meeting, late for a dinner, late for a plane, even late for my own wedding—all of which, except the wedding one, have come true at one point or another. Such dreams that represent unresolved conflicts or stressors in our lives are often associated with worries and fears, and when they cease, it may be a sign that the underlying conflicts or anxieties have been resolved.

Recurring dreams may have positive effects, too. A French study that looked at the dreams of medical students before an important exam found that those who dreamed about the exam scored higher than those who didn't. In fact, the frequency of the students' dreams about the exam correlated with actual exam scores even when the dreams were negative (such as arriving late to the test or forgetting answers). These dreams could be reflective of a higher academic focus, but dreams may also help the brain rehearse for the actual exam. "The immediate benefit of dreaming was the drive to address weaknesses in knowledge after awakening, which certainly provided an advantage," said the study's authors. "Additionally, the contrast between the horrible situations experienced in the dreams (appendicitis, lateness, impossibility of competing) and the more casual reality (good health, appropriate timing and tools) the next morning may desensitize the students to anxiety, which can be reassuring and beneficial." Isn't this infinitely preferable to pulling an all-nighter in order to cram and then showing up at the exam like a hungover zombie?

THE STUFF OF NIGHTMARES

Of course, not all dreams are inspirational "Eureka!" moments, fun journeys through Oz, or helpful rehearsals for actual exams. Scientists have also been working on solving the puzzle of nightmares, which are particularly prevalent among children. Around a quarter of children aged five to twelve wake up from nightmares once a week or more. I remember once when we were vacationing in Greece and a monk at a monastery we were visiting asked Isabella, then five, if she'd slept well. "No, I had a nightmirror," she replied. "A big mosquito in tennis shoes running all over me." We loved that malapropism, "nightmirror," and we have adopted it in our family.

And if you need a reason to ban television before bedtime for your child, a study from Santiago, Chile, found that children who watched television late at night reported disturbed sleep and more episodes of nightmares. Though the terms "nightmares" and "night terrors" are often used interchangeably, there actually is a difference: nightmares always awaken the dreamer, while night terrors result in only a partial awakening. Children in the middle of a night terror often have their eyes open but are unaware of their surroundings in the room. Common behavior during a night terror includes screaming and kicking, but most often children will have no memory of these episodes in the morning.

Golden slumbers fill your eyes
Smiles awake you when you rise

—The Beatles, "Golden Slumbers"

Thankfully, the frequency of nightmares lessens as we get older. "Nightmare rates climb through adolescence," science journalist Natalie Angier wrote, "peak in young adulthood, and then, like so much else in life, begin to drop. The average fifty-five-year-old has one-third the number of nightmares as the average twenty-five-year-old. At nearly every age, girls and women report having significantly more nightmares than do boys and men." In fact, the word "nightmare" dates back to 1300 and used to refer to "a female evil spirit thought to lie upon and suffocate sleepers." And gender can also influence the content of our dreams. A study by researchers at the University of Montreal found that men are more likely than women to have nightmares about natural disasters and wars, whereas women reported twice as many nightmares about interpersonal conflicts.

Why are nightmares so frightening when they often involve things that couldn't possibly happen or be real? According to Patrick McNamara, an associate professor of neurology at Boston University School of Medicine, the answer lies in the brain, specifically the amygdala, where we process negative emotions. "Over-activation of the amygdala during REM can create intense fear-responses in the individual." And while the amygdala is firing on all cylinders, our prefrontal cortex, which allows us to engage in rational thought, is, like the rest of the body, asleep.

Of course, some nightmares do become real. After Michael and I had been married for five months, I found out I was pregnant. I was thirty-six and ecstatic at the prospect of becoming a mother. Night after night, I dreamed of the baby—it was a boy, and we'd already named him Alexander—but in my dreams his eyes wouldn't open. Early one morning, barely awake myself, I asked out loud, "Why won't they open?" My dreams had told me what the doctors later confirmed: the baby's eyes were not meant to open; he died in my womb before he was born.

LUCID DREAMING

Though dreams are mysterious and outside our control, there is a phenomenon called lucid dreaming, when we are aware of dreaming while inside the dream. The concept was the basis of the hit 2010 movie *Inception*, in which people called "extractors" infiltrate and manipulate people's dreams to extract information. But long before Leonardo DiCaprio took lucid dreaming mainstream, Freud had been exploring the phenomenon in *The Interpretation of Dreams*: "Dissatisfied with the turn taken by a dream the dreamer breaks it off without waking, and begins it afresh, in order to continue it along different lines, just like a popular author who, upon request, gives a happier ending to his play."

Proponents of lucid dreaming list a slew of benefits. We can, they claim, overcome nightmares by realizing that what we are experiencing isn't real and cannot harm us. Lucid dreams can also be used as a rehearsal for real-life events. Just as athletes use visualization as part of training, lucid dreamers can use their dreams to practice skills they need in waking life—from public speaking to dreaming up a family occasion in order to rehearse a difficult conversation. Others use their ability to dream to fulfill wishes like spending time with a loved one who has died or to fulfill fantasies—sexual fantasies, flying fantasies, celebrity fantasies.

This may sound like the stuff of science fiction, but there has been ample research on lucid dreaming going back to 1975, when the British psychologist Keith Hearne instructed a lucid dreamer to perform a sequence of left-right eye movements upon achieving lucidity. Stephen LaBerge, another pioneer in the field, replicated these results five years later at Stanford and went on to found the Lucidity Institute. LaBerge believes that with practice you can take control of the dream clicker. I personally have no interest in lucid dreaming, since what I love about dreaming is surrendering to the unexpected. But many who embrace lucid dreaming say that it has the additional benefit of leaving them feeling less at the mercy of events and circumstances when they're awake.

I have frequently wondered if the majority of mankind ever pause to reflect upon the occasionally titanic significance of dreams, and of the obscure world to which they belong. . . . Sometimes I believe that this less material life is our truer life.

—H. P. Lovecraft, "Beyond the Wall of Sleep"

"The sage dreams," says the Indian spiritual teacher Ramana Maharshi, "but he knows it to be a dream, in the same way as he knows the waking state to be a dream." In that sense, those who are spiritually awake can be described as the ultimate lucid dreamers. "Established in the state of supreme reality," Maharshi continues, "the sage detachedly witnesses the three other states—waking, dreaming, and dreamless sleep—as pictures superimposed onto it. For the sage, all three states are equally unreal. Most people are unable to comprehend this, because for them the standard of reality is the waking state, whereas for the sage the standard is reality itself."

THE ENDURING PRESENCE OF DREAMS IN OUR LIVES

Despite the many scientific studies showing how important our dreams are, the prevailing view in our culture continues to be dismissive. "We view dreams the way we do stars,"

Rubin Naiman told me. "They come out at night and are certainly magnificent, but they're far too distant to be of any relevance to our real, waking lives. We devalue, avoid, and overcompensate for dream loss."

That has not always been so. Throughout history, dreams have been at the center of religions and ancient spiritual practices, treated as a special, and sacred, part of who we are. As Robert Moss writes in *The Secret History of Dreaming*, "Among ordinary folk as well as in royal palaces, across most of history, dreamwork has never been separated from other ways of reading the sign language of life. . . . In the ancient world, dreaming was 'a nightly screening of the gods,' who might show themselves in many forms."

According to many traditions, our entire existence came about in the dream of a creator. "One of the great Hindu images," as the mythology expert Joseph Campbell puts it, is of Vishnu dreaming the universe. "We are all parts of Vishnu's dream. . . . We see the world dream coming from Vishnu in the form of a lotus growing from his navel."

Like many ancient societies, the Egyptians engaged in a practice called dream incubation, in which one would sleep at a temple or other sacred place in order to receive divine guidance, wisdom, insight, or healing through one's dreams. In ancient Greece, pilgrims would trek to the temples of Asclepius, the god of healing, and after rites of purification and sacrifice they would go to sleep in the most sacred parts of the temple in the hope that healing dreams would be sent their way by the god. In the morning, priests would interpret the dreams and translate them into treatment recommendations.

The practice of dream incubation is as old as culture itself and can be seen in Paleolithic cave paintings in Europe.

"It seems," dreams researcher Kelly Bulkeley told me, "that every culture and religious tradition around the world—from Tibetan Buddhists to Plains Native Americans, from Australian Aborigines to Sufi Muslims—has developed its own methods and techniques." Dream incubation was also widely practiced in the Ming and Qing dynasties in China and in ancient Japan.

Today, for the first time, scientific findings are validating ancient wisdom about the importance of dreams. Those flimsy, often contradictory and absurd dream stories, with no beginning, no middle, and no end, may contain seeds of deep mysteries—the everyday sense of time is lost and windows to other worlds are revealed. As Carl Jung wrote: "I have found again and again in my professional work that the images and ideas that dreams contain cannot possibly be explained solely in terms of memory. They express new thoughts that have never yet reached the threshold of consciousness. . . . No one doubts the importance of conscious experience; why then should we question the importance of unconscious happenings? They also belong to human life, and they are sometimes more truly a part of it for weal or woe than any events of the day. . . . Great innovations never come from above; they come invariably from below; just as trees never grow from the sky downward, but upward from the earth, however true it is that their seeds have fallen from above."

WHEN OUR DREAMS CHANGE OUR LIVES

While writing *The Sleep Revolution*, curious about other people's experiences with dreams, I tweeted and posted on Facebook a request for people to send me accounts of times in their lives when dreams had been particularly meaningful or useful. I was surprised by the deluge I received. What follows are just a few examples.

Sandra Shpilberg is a biotechnology executive from Palo Alto, California. She credits a dream with helping save her marriage. "We had been married for 14 years with two lovely children, but there were cracks in the foundation of our relationship," she wrote. "In my waking life, I had put all my energy to try to understand the cracks, measure them, analyze them and try to fix them." But in her dream it was different: "The dream had a yellow-orange hue of a sunrise, of new energy, of new life." And that dream was worlds apart from all the analyzing she had done during her waking time. "When I woke up, I understood that I was missing the bigger perspective," she wrote. "Yes, there were cracks in the foundation of our relationship, but we had now become part of a bigger unit—a family. And that family was functional, happy, a sunrise. The dream had shifted my consciousness to stop focusing on the cracks and start seeing the beautiful sunrise in my life."

The Los Angeles–based writer Elizabeth Kirk had a recurring dream about a giant tsunami that knocked her out of a boat and into the ocean. "Once I was underwater, I reached the bottom and just took a deep breath in," she wrote. "I found I could breathe underwater perfectly, and I remember thinking to myself what a gift this was, and I swam away." To her the tsunami was about the chaos in her life. "And my 'super power' was a reminder that I had all the power I needed within myself to overcome, conquer, or ultimately allow the circumstances to transform me into something much more than I was. Not only did I survive, but I came out the other side stronger."

David H. wrote that several dreams helped him stop abusing drugs and alcohol. One was about being caught in a hurricane, the other a tornado, and the third was set at a nearby waterfall where he'd had many drug experiences with friends in the past: "There was a slippery, steep precipice where the land dropped and the force of the water pouring over the cliff had bored out a deep hole of churning water. One after another, my friends slipped over into the water and I followed. It was really scary but became terrifying when I realized there were alligators or crocodiles in the water and one got hold of my foot and pulled me under. I got free and came back to the surface at the edge where I could hold on. I felt this crystal clear awareness of a conflict between getting myself to safety, or risking myself to help my friends. All the while I could see they weren't really trying to help themselves. I felt they were going to just let themselves be savaged by the beasts and I felt guilty for not wanting to go along with them. But I wanted to save myself. I don't remember the dream ending but I believe I woke up with a new understanding." That dream started the process in which he did in fact save himself. "I still to this day believe a deeper part of myself (some may call it God) was speaking to me through my dreams," he wrote.

Dreams, as we all know, are very queer things: some parts are presented with appalling vividness, with details worked up with the elaborate finish of jewellery, while others one gallops through, as it were, without noticing them at all, as, for instance, through space and time.

—Fyodor Dostoyevsky, "The Dream of a Ridiculous Man"

Linda Jacobsen, the director of the English as a Second Language program for a Missouri school district, told me that a stubborn dream saved her life. A few months after giving birth to her third child, she came down with what she thought was the flu. "That night," she wrote, "a voice woke me, saying, 'Linda, wake up. You have to call 9-1-1. You're going to die.'" She looked at her husband, but he was sound asleep. She went back to sleep herself but was soon awakened by the same voice saying the same thing. "Again I sat up, irritated, and poked at my still-sleeping husband," she wrote. "He didn't move and kept up his snoring. I lay there, wondering what was going on." But this time she didn't go back to sleep. "I can't recall exactly what made me pick up the phone and dial, but I did. I threatened them with hell to pay if they woke my kids with sirens, too." It turns out her appendix had ruptured. Had she not called 911, she could have died. "The voice I heard was not of anyone I could identify," she wrote. "I often wonder if it was my own subconscious urging me to get help, but I prefer to think some loving angels on watch intervened in their own way to avoid losing a loving wife and mother of three young children."

Ron Hulnick, the president of the University of Santa Monica, told me of a particularly meaningful dream he had a few years ago: "I had been pondering the question, 'What would life be like if I dared to live more fully from within a spiritual perspective?' And here is the dream I had: I'm driving at normal speed along a 2-lane country road in New Mexico and all of a sudden my car veers off the road and onto the desert floor. I attempt to gain control since there are many large cactus plants where I'm driving and I need to avoid them. I'm aware that the car is picking up speed so I step on the brake. The pedal goes down to the floor—no brakes—and the car is going faster and faster. I'm steering like mad around the cactus plants and then the steering mechanism becomes dysfunctional. The car is picking up speed and I have no way of steering it. And then I notice that regardless of what I do, the car is steering itself just fine regardless of how fast it's going. I take a deep breath, relax, and enjoy the ride. The metaphorical message of the dream for me was about letting go of the illusion of control and learning to live with more trust in harmony with whatever spiritual plan was unfolding in my life."

THE POWER OF DREAMS—AND WHY YOU SHOULD RECORD THEM

Those who have integrated dreams into their lives have found that the "otherworld" of sleep has become more real—something to be welcomed rather than resisted. For me, it is way more than just feeling recharged. There is also a sense of freedom that comes from less attachment to daily battles, successes, failures, and illusions. My daughter Isabella has a recurring dream that beautifully illustrates this. She is a living stop sign, forcing people to come to a complete stop before moving on with their lives. And instead of dissolving when she wakes up, the dream takes on new relevance when she revisits it during the day, reminding her to pause, reflect, and keep all the demands of her life in perspective.

There are some simple steps we can take before we go to sleep to reinstate dreams to a central place in our lives and experience firsthand why they matter. After we put our devices aside, wind down, and let go of the day, we can learn from the practices of ancient temples and do a modern-day version of dream incubation. Synesius of Cyrene, a Greek bishop living around the year 400, called dreams oracles, always ready to serve as our "silent counselor." And dream incubation is a process of preparing our consciousness to receive guidance from our inner counselors. It can be about big life decisions, but also about anything that we want more clarity and wisdom around, however trivial it may seem.

I love how the Rubin Museum in New York, which houses Asian art, brings dream incubation into our modern lives. It hosts an annual "Dream-Over," where participants spend the night sleeping among the artworks. A Tibetan Buddhist teacher leads a discussion about the significance of dreams in Tibetan culture, and in the morning "dream gatherers" start a conversation about what everyone dreamed of.

Of course, Tibetan Buddhist teachers and thought-provoking artworks aren't required to get the dream-incubation process going. I asked Mary Hulnick, the chief creative officer of the University of Santa Monica, who teaches dream incubation as part of the Spiritual Psychology course, for specific steps to facilitate the process. She suggested asking ourselves these key questions before going to sleep:

"In what area of your life would you like to receive guidance? What question do you want answered? Word your question carefully and precisely, write it down, and focus on it as you drift off to sleep. Since the language of dreams is metaphorical and symbolic, ask that the answer to your question be given in a way that you can recognize and understand. Set an intention to remember your dreams. Then go to sleep. When you awake, and this is very important, remain totally still—do not move your body. This allows you greater access to your dream—better dream recall. Once you have your dream secure in your mind, your first movement is to get your pen and paper and begin writing any dreams or parts of dreams that you recall. Sometimes you'll have and recall a dream the very first night that you ask your dream incubation question. Sometimes, you may find that you need to ask your question for several nights. I encourage you to be patient and let go of any pressure or attachment to receiving a dream."

From breakfast on through all the day
At home among my friends I stay,
But every night I go abroad
Afar into the land of Nod.

All by myself I have to go, . . .
All alone beside the streams
And up the mountain-sides of dreams.

The strangest things are there for me. . . .

Try as I like to find the way,
I never can get back by day,
Nor can remember plain and clear
The curious music that I hear.

—Robert Louis Stevenson, "The Land of Nod"

If I wake up in the middle of the night, even if I have not asked for specific guidance in any part of my life, I write down whatever I remember from my dreams with a pen that has a flashlight attached to it. I find that when I don't turn on the lamp on my nightstand, it is easier not to lose the thread of my dreams. (And if you're not sleeping alone, you're less likely to wake your partner.) When you wake up in the morning, if you want to remember your dreams, don't grab your cell phone the moment you open your eyes and become inundated with news, texts, and emails. Before letting the outside world in, taking a momentary pause and a few deep breaths can help you recall more of your dreams, reliving the paths traveled while in your dream world. As we learn to recognize the hidden meanings beneath the surface of the everyday, it becomes easier to listen to the inner whisperings that tend to get drowned in the cacophony of our waking life.

Even if you remember just one image or one word, write that down. If you wake up and have only a vague impression of a feeling, capture that: "I woke up feeling a little sad or anxious or excited." And if you wake up and remember nothing, write that down, too: "This morning I remember nothing." I have found that the very act of writing something down has encouraged my subconscious to pay attention and remember more—or at least remember something—the following day.

No matter how much of the curtain is pulled back on dreams, no matter what new studies and discoveries bring us closer to understanding them, the mystery will remain. Their elusiveness is part of their beauty. Our dreams are, and always will be, a gateway to another world, a timeless journey to other inward dimensions.

PART TWO

THE WAY FORWARD

7.

MASTERING SLEEP

Sleep that knits up the ravell'd sleave of care
The death of each day's life, sore labour's bath,
Balm of hurt minds, great nature's second course,
Chief nourisher in life's feast.

—William Shakespeare, *Macbeth*

SO, WHERE do we go from here? We've seen sleep's profound importance in our lives. We've seen the overwhelming scientific evidence on the benefits of sleep. From highways to runways, from the halls of power to our hospitals and schools, we now know the dangers of not getting enough sleep. But how do we move from awareness to action? How do we incorporate this knowledge into our lives? It's not easy, even when we know what we should do. "I think that public awareness is there," says Dr. Willis H. Tsai of the University of Calgary. "The problem is in the execution. It's like eating at a fast food restaurant. You know it isn't really good for you, but you end up doing it anyway." When it comes to our similarly unhealthy sleep habits, how can we stop "doing it anyway"? What are the first steps we can take to make changes in our lives?

In a study on what made babies better at walking, scientists discovered that more than height, brain development, or any other variable, what made the difference was simply how much time babies spent trying to walk. As Daniel Coyle wrote in *The Talent Code*, "Baby steps are the royal road to skill," and this is as true for sleep as it is for any other habit.

And it's not just time, but also how we respond to ourselves when we try. "When a little child is learning to walk or talk," Louise Hay, the author of *You Can Heal Your Life*, wrote, "we encourage him and praise him for every tiny improvement he makes. The child beams and eagerly tries to do better. Is this the way you encourage yourself when you are learning something new? Or do you make it harder to learn because you tell yourself that you are stupid or clumsy or a 'failure'?" For those of us who have neglected sleep, reintegrating it into our lives is akin to learning a new skill. The key to our success will be practice and encouraging ourselves along the way.

Changing all our bad habits regarding sleep is not something we can achieve quickly. As with any other self-destructive pattern, making a lasting change requires taking small daily steps toward our goal. And the steps that will work for each of us are unique; we may need to try out a few different practices and rituals before landing on the right combination.

In the same way that a good day starts the night before, learning how to deal with stress throughout the day will impact how we sleep at night. As Marcus Aurelius put it, "Do not remain out of tune longer than you can help. Habitual recurrence to the harmony will increase your mastery of it." Gradually, we'll be able to make relaxation as familiar to our bodies and minds as our stresses are to us now. And this will make it much less likely we'll find ourselves awake in the middle of the night trapped in our mind's continuous loop, obsessively reliving the past or worrying about the future.

When we wake up in bed on Monday morning and think of the various hurdles we have to jump that day, immediately we feel sad, bored, and bothered. Whereas actually, we're just lying in bed.

—ALAN WATTS, *The Philosophies of Asia*

As the psychologist Neil Fiore reminds us, much of our worrying doesn't do us any good: "Calling up the stress response to deal with dangers that are not happening now is similar to pulling a fire alarm for a fire that happened twenty years ago or to fearing a fire that may happen next year. It would be unfair to the fire department and a misuse of its time and energy to ask firefighters to respond to such an alarm, just as it's unfair to demand that your body continually respond to threats of danger from events that cannot be tackled now."

Lying in bed putting out imaginary fires is one of the most draining things we can do. In this section, you'll find steps big and small you can take that will help you let go of those worries, free up that energy, and fall asleep. You'll find a path to better sleep that winds through scientific advances, policy proposals, hard-earned personal anecdotes, and both expert and crowd-sourced tips. You'll also find suggestions on how workplaces can better support employees and on policy changes that can help accelerate the sleep revolution. The best way to start is to go straight to the source, where so many of our sleep habits are formed: our families.

OUR FIRST SLEEP TEACHERS

In recent years, there's been a lot of attention paid to family nutrition, and it's become clear that it's easier to practice healthy habits if we're surrounded by others doing the same. That's why, as author Tom Rath writes, "We need to rethink sleep as a core family value."

When I was growing up, my mother would regularly stay up all night cooking, reading, and organizing because, as she explained to my sister, Agapi, and me when we would protest, it was at night, when the world had gone to bed, that she could be most creative and productive. When we lived together again years later, she would often stay up all night, and it was only after cooking my daughters' breakfast in the morning that she would finally put herself to bed. And when her granddaughters would come home from school in the late afternoon, Agapi and I would tell each other, "Darling, wake up Mom, the girls are home." Plenty of grandmothers have lives that revolve around their grandchildren, but leave it to my mother to go a step further and actually adjust her entire circadian rhythm around them!

Agapi modeled her sleep habits after my mother, though thankfully she didn't go to quite the same extremes. For most of her life, she also stayed up late, getting things done. Then she'd usually wake up tired. "But when nighttime rolled around," she says, "my mind was fully alert, ready for work." A few years ago, when I started talking about the importance of sleep and sending her articles and studies, she began to rethink things and to make some changes. But, as is the case for most of us, her progress was not linear. "It was always hit-and-miss," she says. "So many times I'd come back from a great night out with friends—and my energy would be high, and I would feel I had emails to answer and things to complete."

She realized that what she'd assumed was a time of great productivity actually wasn't: "Almost the way a parent imparts lessons to her child, I'd have to tell myself, 'Darling, it's time to put your phone down. We're going to have a cup of tea and take a bath.'" She then moved beyond putting her phone down to taking all her devices out of the bedroom. And instead of watching TV in bed, she started recording her favorite late-night shows. Eventually she developed a new routine that was all her own—as, of course, it has to be—and she learned not to judge herself when she went offtrack. As a natural late-nighter, she says it's important to have a support system around her. "We night owls need our own sleep tribe if we're going to change," she says.

For most people, the most natural sleep tribe is the family. One of the first steps in promoting good family sleep habits is changing the way we talk about sleep. In many families, sleep is meted out as a punishment to children: "If you don't eat your vegetables at dinner, you're going straight to bed." Children are taught early on that sleep is something to avoid as long as possible—a sword of Damocles hanging over their heads every night—and that with sleep comes the end of play and fun. What a terrible message to send! We need to do a much better job of framing sleep in a positive way for our children, letting them know that sleep is a vital part of being *able* to play and have fun, and teaching them healthy sleep habits, including naps and transitions to bedtime, that will last a lifetime.

HOW MUCH IS ENOUGH?

The universal, most asked question to end all questions about sleep is inevitably: How much sleep should we be getting? In 2015, experts from the American Academy of Sleep Medicine and the Sleep Research Society examined thousands of peer-reviewed articles and determined that for individuals between the ages of eighteen and sixty . . . (drumroll, please!) a *minimum* of seven hours of sleep a night is essential for optimal health. And since age is a determining factor for how much sleep we need, the National Sleep Foundation has broken it down accordingly:

Newborns (0–3 months):	14–17 hours
Infants (4–11 months):	12–15 hours
Toddlers (1–2 years):	11–14 hours
Preschoolers (3–5):	10–13 hours
School-age children (6–13):	9–11 hours
Teenagers (14–17):	8–10 hours
Young adults (18–25):	7–9 hours
Adults (26–64):	7–9 hours
Older adults (65+):	7–8 hours

(I'm compelled to point out that there is no bracket reading "Super-important, super-busy macho man: 3–5 hours." Yet we all know people, of all ages, who insist on placing themselves in this category—and most of us, including me, have been that person.)

ROCK-A-BYE, BABY . . . KIDS AND SLEEP

"Sleep," says Dr. Harvey Karp, a pediatrician who specializes in child development and the author of *The Happiest Baby on the Block*, "is the primary activity of the brain during early development. Infants with poor sleep grow into toddlers with poor sleep. Lack of sleep impairs a child's ability to learn, their emotional well-being (mood swings, anxiety, depression, hyperactivity and other behavioral problems) and even leads to many health problems like infections, high blood pressure and obesity." And in a long-term study completed in April 2015, researchers in Norway found that toddlers who consistently slept less than ten hours a night developed more emotional and behavioral problems by age five.

The most meaningful predictors of children's sleep are their parents' education (better-educated parents have better-rested children) and, according to a 2014 National Sleep Foundation "Sleep in the Modern Family" poll, whether the family has rules about caffeine intake, how much TV children are allowed to watch, and whether family members use electronic devices in their bedrooms at night. And, of course, a family's sleep life is often deeply intertwined, with each member's sleeping patterns affecting the others'.

Few questions kindle a more heated debate—or as massive a deluge of posts and comments on a parenting blog (just look at our HuffPost Parents section)—than how we should handle our babies' sleep. What worked for me was to keep Christina in my bed or in a bassinet by my bed from the moment she was born. That way, when she woke up, I could immediately feed her. But no matter what method you arrive at, I cannot overstate the importance of having a little tribe of support in the first few months after your baby is born. In addition to Michael, who was a very involved dad, I was blessed to have my mother, the ultimate Greek Yaya, living with us. She would regularly take care of Christina (and later Isabella), allowing me the chance to get some badly needed sleep. I got pregnant with Isabella while still nursing Christina (birth control alert: don't believe those who tell you this can't happen), and by the time Isabella was born, her sister was on a more regular sleep schedule and Yaya could prioritize helping me with Isabella. This was a real blessing, because baby Isabella and two-year-old Christina were on very different sleep schedules.

As controversial as it can be on parenting blogs, sleeping with one's infant was the norm throughout history and remains so to this day in many parts of the world. In developed countries, many believe that sleeping with your baby impedes the baby's ability to become independent. Others, however, see sleeping together as part of "attachment parenting," a term coined by Dr. William Sears, referring to the idea that when parents foster a strong emotional bond, children grow up to be more emotionally secure and less likely to develop behavioral problems.

The practice of sharing a bed with your children has become more visible in recent years. For example, Angelina Jolie and Brad Pitt are such strong supporters of what they call "family sleep" that they built a custom-size bed to accommodate all their children. "Everybody crawls into our bed," Jolie says. "We had sheets specially made. When we had two kids, the nine-foot bed was extraordinary. . . . Now, at six, it's tight. We end up pulling the couches to the sides. We're thinking of building a room just for family sleep."

Beyond the emotional bond, James McKenna, an expert on mother-baby sleep at the University of Notre Dame, told me that because an infant is born with only 25 percent of its adult brain volume, "its physiological systems are unable to function optimally without contact with the mother's body, which continues to regulate the baby much like it did during gestation." McKenna explained how the baby and the mother interact during sleep: "The breathing of the mother and infant are regulated by the presence of each other—the sounds of inhalation and exhalation, the rising and falling of their chests. This is one more signal to remind babies to breathe, a fail-safe system should the baby's internal breathing transitions falter. The mother's body is the only environment to which the human infant is adapted."

Sweet dreams, form a shade
O'er my lovely infant's head;
Sweet dreams of pleasant streams
By happy, silent, moony beams.

Sweet sleep, with soft down
Weave thy brows an infant crown.
Sweet sleep, Angel mild,
Hover o'er my happy child.

—William Blake, "A Cradle Song"

The American Academy of Pediatrics, while encouraging room sharing, discourages bed sharing due to the risk of suffocation if a parent accidentally rolls over onto an infant. Regardless of whether you place your baby in a crib or keep your baby in your bed, as I did, precautions should be taken. For those who choose to sleep with their babies, here are some tips from Dr. Karp: "You can reduce the risks of bed-sharing by swaddling your baby (to reduce the chance he'll roll and fall or get wedged against the headboard or wall), breastfeeding, avoiding drugs and alcohol, removing pillows and blankets from the bed, and making sure no one smokes in the house."

Of course, no matter how a baby sleeps, the parents are likely to be on a guided tour through the forbidding land of sleep deprivation. In a memorable episode of *I Love Lucy*, Lucy was so exhausted from caring for newborn Little Ricky that she fell asleep bent over with her head in the crib. But as many new parents know, this isn't a case of comic exaggeration. It's a state sometimes called "mommy brain," though it's not limited to mommies. Stuart Heritage, a reporter for *The Guardian*, wrote about his experience as a new parent: "Parenthood has worn me down, and I have become obsessed with sleep. . . . Sleep is now automatically where my mind goes when it doesn't have anything else to do. . . . Two consecutive nights spent working late have thrown my equilibrium out of whack, and I'm spiraling. By the time I've done a day's work and cooked dinner, I'm quite often seeing double." He's hardly alone. A 2014 *Today* show survey found that 54 percent of parents of newborns said lack of sleep made it hard to function during waking hours. Given the effect of sleep deprivation, Dr. Karp calls this "drunk parenting"—with major implications for parents' health. "Many studies show exhaustion is a top trigger for postpartum anxiety and depression," he told me, "affecting half a million to a million new moms every year (and many new dads, too)." It can lead to marital stress, child neglect, and accidents.

Mika Brzezinski, the cohost of MSNBC's *Morning Joe*, had her own wake-up call, which she recounts in her 2010 memoir *All Things at Once*. She writes about frantically rushing to the emergency room with her four-month-old daughter, who was conscious but not moving from the chest down. As doctors huddled around the baby, Mika heard the words "spinal cord damage" and then collapsed in tears on the floor of the hospital. She then describes what led up to the scene: sleep-deprived, she'd been carrying her daughter in her arms and tumbled down a flight of stairs. As she waited for news from the doctors, she began to reexamine her life:

> How could I have let myself get so run down, so exhausted at work that I would fumble over my own feet and fall down a steep flight of stairs with my newborn in my arms? It made no sense to me—and yet, here I was, waiting for word about what her life would look like now. Wondering if she'd ever be able to move. All for what? A blind ambition to be all things to all people? To be a super hockey mom?

Fortunately, there was no spinal cord damage, only a broken femur. But the experience had a lasting effect on Mika. "I'm starting to hear a new message," she writes. "This one doesn't come from my mother, or grandmother, or any mentors I've collected on my journey, but from within. From me. A message I am still working to put in play before my children move on into adulthood: pace yourself." That's the lesson she wants to pass on to her own daughters. "Go your own way. Narrow your focus. Breathe," she says. "Your job can be a big part of who you are, but it shouldn't be the whole package."

PLEASE, LORD, LET HER SLEEP THROUGH THE NIGHT!

Now that we know how much sleep our babies should be getting, how do we get our precious little ones to (please, Lord!) sleep through the night? Debates surrounding the various kinds of "sleep training" methods can be even more divisive than those about where the baby sleeps. A *New York Times* article caused controversy with the headline "Sleep Training at 8 Weeks: 'Do You Have the Guts?'" Though some say that self-soothing, or letting a baby "cry it out," is safe and effective, others call it heart-wrenching. What experts agree on is that, as Kim West, the author of *Good Night, Sleep Tight*, put it, "It's important that you pick a sleep coaching method that aligns with your philosophies and your child's temperament and you do it consistently."

My philosophy was to hold my babies when they cried, and as they grew older to read them bedtime stories. But as I found out, this actually isn't so simple if the parent reading the bedtime story is chronically sleep-deprived. My daughters often laugh as they remember me reading books to them to put them to sleep—through the years graduating from Dr. Seuss to Harry Potter—and falling asleep in midsentence ("One fish, two fish, red fish . . . *zzzzzzzz*"). As my younger daughter, Isabella, recounts, "My mom would begin to slur her words, and I would have to shake her and repeat over and over again, 'Wake up, Mom, wake up, Mom! Finish the story!'" (At least the stories worked on one of us.) I had also become famous for falling asleep at other inappropriate moments—in the car with a friend (I wasn't driving!), at dinner, and without fail in any darkened auditorium, concert hall, or theater. You name it, I fell asleep in it.

The Swedish author Carl-Johan Forssén Ehrlin used psychological principles to write a book that aims to put children to sleep within minutes. While reading *The Rabbit Who Wants to Fall Asleep*, parents are encouraged to read slowly and yawn frequently. The author describes the book as "the verbal equivalent of rocking a baby to sleep." One mother wrote in an Amazon review that the audiobook version worked just as well for her: "I thought I'd listen to it to see what it was like. I set up my phone beside my bed and began playing it. Next thing I knew, it was morning."

GIVING WORKING MOMS AND DADS A BREAK

Even when their baby begins sleeping through the night, different pressures can impact a family's sleep. According to one study, the children of mothers who worked between twenty and forty hours a week got insufficient sleep. The study included a large sample of single and lower-income mothers, but in today's world mothers from all income levels will be working outside the home at some point in their children's lives. In the United States, approximately 70 percent of mothers are in the workforce. Only three states, however, have laws providing for paid parental leave, while countries like Sweden and Norway offer forty and thirty-eight weeks of full paid family leave, respectively.

The Family and Medical Leave Act (FMLA), signed into law by President Clinton in 1993, grants twelve weeks of unpaid leave, but only for those in the public sector or in companies with more than fifty employees. As a result, 40 percent of the American workforce is ineligible right from the start, and that doesn't include the millions who can't bear the financial burden of unpaid time off even if they're eligible. Forced to juggle work and children, frazzled and sleep-deprived parents often feel like they have to choose between their job and their new family. Some large companies have taken the lead in changing this unhealthy dynamic. Netflix announced in 2015 that it will offer unlimited paid leave in its video-streaming division for new parents during the first year after their child's birth or adoption. New parents can choose to return full-time or part-time, or return and leave based on what works best for their family. The British telecommunications company Vodafone offers at least sixteen weeks of paid leave to new mothers and allows them to work thirty-hour weeks for the next six months while receiving full pay and benefits. These policies will likely benefit Vodafone's and Netflix's bottom lines, as they will retain more talent and spend less money on recruiting and training new personnel—to say nothing of the boost in employee well-being and the accompanying decline in health-care costs.

The importance of supporting working parents extends to other aspects of health. As Dr. Clifford Saper, a professor of neuroscience at Harvard Medical School, told me, "There is an epidemic of obesity, and good evidence that sleep loss in young people can cause glucose intolerance and overeating." Researchers from the University of Illinois highlighted this connection as they looked into the link between how much mothers worked and their children's weight, as well as at possible mediators such as diet, television watching, mealtime habits, and sleep. Surprisingly, the only factor that actually mediated that link was sleep. Three- to five-year-old children of mothers who worked full-time not only got less sleep than those whose mothers worked less than twenty hours a week, but they also had higher body mass index (BMI) readings. Only 18 percent of the participating preschoolers in the study got the recommended amount of sleep. Sleep is so crucial to so many aspects of our lives that often what looks like one kind of problem—child obesity—is actually not a diet problem but a sleep problem. When mothers leave early for work, kids get up early for day care or school. On the positive side, each additional hour of sleep a child in the study got was associated with a nearly 7 percent drop in BMI at their next weigh-in.

The lesson, of course, is not that women shouldn't be working—that ship has, rightly, sailed. Most mothers work outside the home. No, the lesson is that, as challenging as it is, it's vital that we establish policies—like paid family leave and access to affordable quality child care—that will allow everyone to prioritize sleep.

THE MORNING BELL

For many young people, schools have become burnout zones where along with history, math, and science, we teach our kids the worst habits of our destructive work culture. But happily, many schools around the world are responding to the latest science on sleep, taking creative steps to restructure the school day in ways that can make a big difference in academic performance and overall well-being.

Right now the average start time for public high schools is around 8 a.m. But in 2014, the American Academy of Pediatrics recommended that middle and high schools not start before 8:30 a.m. Currently, only 14 percent of schools follow those guidelines. When and how we start the day really matters, setting the stage for everything that follows. And when you add pre-class activities—like sports practice and student-council meetings—you can see why so many high-schoolers resemble extras from *The Walking Dead*.

When schools do make changes, the results are clear. A 2011 study from the Technion-Israel Institute of Technology found that students who started school at 8:30 a.m. slept nearly an hour more and performed better on tests measuring attention levels than peers who began school at 7:30 a.m. In the United Kingdom, one high school in North Tyneside, England, moved the school's start time from 8:50 a.m. to 10 a.m. and found that student test scores improved significantly. And during the 2016–17 school year, nearly thirty-two thousand students from one hundred secondary schools in the United Kingdom will take part in "Teensleep," an Oxford experiment to study school times.

The stakes are not merely academic. In 2015, Japan's education ministry conducted its first survey on the sleeping habits of students and found that 46 percent of the children who went to sleep between 9 and 10 p.m. said that they "like or somewhat like who they are," while the number dropped to 30 percent among those who went to sleep between 1 and 2 a.m.

Brown University professor Mary Carskadon and her team ran a study on school start times in 1998. They looked at teens in the ninth grade with a start time of 8:25 a.m. and followed their progress to tenth grade with a start time of 7:20 a.m., logging the students' sleep schedules and daytime alertness. When they were evaluated at 8:30 a.m., half of them showed what Carskadon describes as "pathological levels of sleepiness," falling asleep in just three and a half minutes and going directly into REM sleep, a pattern normally associated with narcolepsy patients. "This study," Carskadon told me, "indicated that half of the students experiencing this early start time in 10th grade were having to wake up and be in school at a time when their brains—driven by the circadian timing system and by having too little sleep—were prepared for REM sleep, not for the classroom."

Thankfully, some policymakers are taking this to heart. In August 2015, New Jersey passed a law that requires the state's Department of Education to conduct a study of the health benefits of later school start times and of the consequences of sleep deprivation on academic performance.

In Singapore, a school district is experimenting with a new kind of bus service that, instead of shuttling a load of up to forty children, will pick up no more than four and drive them directly to school, allowing them to sleep later. One student, Sydney Tang, now leaves her house at 6:40 a.m. instead of 5:55 a.m. "She was always so tired and groggy," her father said, "but she is much more well-rested now."

Small changes in schools can have big results. Deerfield Academy, a boarding school in Massachusetts, enacted several reforms to improve students' sleep, including starting school thirty-five minutes later and reducing sports commitments and homework assignments by 10 percent. The results were remarkable. As reported by the Associated Press, Deerfield saw "20 percent fewer student visits to the health center (in a bad flu year); 17 percent more students taking time for a hot breakfast; and a record increase in GPA."

Aside from start times, one way for students to improve their sleep habits is to study somewhere other than their beds. Eighty-two percent of British teens surveyed said that their bed was where they studied the most. Unfortunately, that makes it much harder to fall asleep when they turn out the lights. "We know that a good bed is a comfortable and comforting place to be, but we would rather students sleep in it than study on it," says Lisa Artis of the UK Sleep Council. "It's really important to associate the bed with sleeping."

As parents around the world—including me—have long realized, adolescence is always going to involve battles over independence. But at least some of what we think of as typical teen bad judgment may actually be about sleep. "This is not just about teens not sleeping enough and then feeling a bit grumpy the next day," Dr. Maida Chen of the Seattle Children's Hospital said. "Sleep really affects their ability to function and make good decisions."

SLEEP 101: THE SLEEP REVOLUTION GOES TO COLLEGE

Since so much of the current revolution in the science of sleep is coming from our colleges and universities, it's only fitting that our institutions of higher learning are beginning to put these in-house-generated insights into practice. This is a big departure from the past, because for far too long our colleges and universities have been laboratories not only for learning but for burnout.

This association of college life with sleep deprivation is deeply ingrained in our culture. The defining ingredients of college life—the pressure to perform and get good grades, the newfound freedom, the yearning to fit in socially, and the endless digital distractions—aren't exactly a recipe for great sleep. Especially when you throw in other damaging habits that have become an accepted part of college life, like bingeing on energy drinks and alcohol.

With the rise of a new campus sleep consciousness, that's all beginning to change—well, maybe not the alcohol part. A growing number of colleges are beginning to build a culture that both supports healthy sleep habits and educates students on what exactly healthy sleep habits are. UCLA, for example, provides sleep education through "Sleep Week." Kendra Knudsen, who works with the UCLA Mind Well initiative, described the problem she sees on campus: "There's a weird pride in certain students when they pull all-nighters." During Sleep Week, the university holds lectures on the effects of sleep deprivation, provides yoga and meditation sessions, and offers free fifteen-minute sleep assessments.

The dreaded early-morning class is something many students will instinctively avoid. And that's getting easier, because, like many high schools, colleges are also rolling back start times. Duke University eliminated 8 a.m. classes in 2004, making the earliest start time 8:30 a.m. Penn State followed suit in 2005, reducing the number of 8 a.m. course offerings. "We found if you try to teach at 8 a.m.," said Richard Cyr, a professor of biology, "people aren't as motivated as they are at 9 a.m. It's easier to engage students when they're more awake."

At Stanford, students in the 200-level psychology course study the neuroscience of sleep and sleep's physical and mental effects. And in 2011, the university began looking beyond the classroom, launching its "Refresh" initiative, designed to teach students cognitive behavioral therapy techniques and mindfulness exercises. By the end of the program, students who reported poor sleep going in experienced improvements in sleep quality and a reduction in depressive symptoms.

At Dartmouth, computer-science professor Andrew Campbell collected data from students using a mobile app called StudentLife and discovered that the average bedtime for students was 2:30 a.m. It's no wonder that a Dartmouth health survey showed that more than half of the students had experienced sleep difficulties within the past year. Freshman Kristin Winkle said, "I think sleep is seen as the enemy of fun, or of productivity." Freshman Rob Del Mauro cited FOMO as the reason sleep was sacrificed, calling sleep a "taboo practice" at Dartmouth. And sophomore Ke Zhao tells her roommate that "the trade-off for A's are Z's."

Clearly, Dartmouth—like most colleges—had a problem on its hands, with a student culture that not only accepted but celebrated sleep deprivation. Recognizing this, the college implemented its own version of Stanford's Refresh program in 2014. Now the health service actively screens students for sleep problems, provides tips and tools, and refers students with more serious problems to the medical center. Refresh is also being replicated at the University of Iowa and the University of Chicago, and sleep-education programs are spreading to colleges across the country, from a private liberal arts school like Hastings College in Nebraska to a large state school like the University of Georgia.

If you can't get students to go to bed earlier—and as the mother of two recent college graduates, I know what a tall order that can be—there's always napping. Of course, napping during class is a time-honored tradition, but many colleges are trying to make it easier for students to nap in a more productive way.

At the University of Michigan, a senior noticed other students falling asleep in the library and collaborated with the administration to set up a nap room outfitted with cots and pillows. The library has also begun trying out MetroNaps EnergyPods, ergonomically designed reclining chairs with a privacy shield and built-in speakers. Placing the cots and nap pods in a twenty-four-hour library may have the unintended consequence of discouraging students from going back to the dorm for some longer shut-eye, but the hope is it will remind them of the link between sleep and learning.

Nap rooms have become so popular that at Berkeley, Melissa Hsu campaigned and won her seat in the student senate on a sleep platform. One of her posters showed a triangle of "Good grades," "Social life," and "Enough sleep" with "Choose two" crossed out and "Have all three!" written on top. And her campaign slogan was "Keep calm & NAP on!"

And schools are raising awareness about sleep in creative ways. At the University of Arizona, students working at the campus health service produced sleep-advocacy videos highlighting the importance of sleep—including a rap video of tips for getting better sleep. Illinois State University launched a "zombie campaign," with theater students dressed up as zombies handing out sleep kits. And James Madison University has the "Nap Nook," a room filled with plush beanbag chairs that can be reserved for forty minutes at a time, the brainchild of Caroline Cooke, a psychology major and sleep researcher. "Heavy workloads," she said, "make you choose between A's and sleep, and I wanted to change the perception that napping was a lazy behavior." It's been a huge success: more than 2,500 naps were logged in the Nook in a nine-month period.

The college sleep movement is a global one—from the University of East Anglia, which in 2015 became the first UK school to install a nap room equipped with beanbags and sofa beds, to the Institute of Advanced Media Arts and Sciences in Ogaki, Japan, which offers a sleeping room and showers.

Of course, when you're tired enough, you don't need an actual, school-sanctioned nap room or state-of-the-art sleep pod—you just need somewhere quiet to stretch out. And on most campuses, there are spots all over the place—you just have to know where they are. So students have leveraged technology to map out the best spots for a quick snooze based on noise levels and crowds. These "nap maps," now found on many campuses, are essentially Google maps with pins on crowdsourced sleep-friendly locations. At the University of Texas, students can consult their handy Healthyhorns (a play on the school's Longhorn mascot) Nap Map, which shows the favored napping spots around campus as voted on by students. The online version shows them all on a Google map, each one marked "Zzz." When you click, you see photos and a description.

One common thread in these stories is the initiative of college students. The growing number of students who have not only identified the problem of sleep deprivation but are actively taking part in its solution is a key driver of the sleep revolution. This spirit is perfectly exemplified by Christina Kyriakos. In 2011, while a senior at Holy Cross in Massachusetts, she was inspired by a psychology course she took, Sleep and Behavior, to help local children sleep better. Kyriakos used tools and training from Sweet Dreamzzz, a nonprofit dedicated to improving the well-being and academic performance of economically disadvantaged children through better sleep. The program's motto is "Get A's and B's by getting more Zzzs!" and it has provided sleep education to more than 45,000 children around the United States. "We delivered the REM (Rest, Educate, and Motivate) sleep education program," Kyriakos explained, "to over 250 children at a local elementary school, where over 80 percent of the students were eligible for free or reduced school lunch. We also fundraised to provide each child with a sleep kit that contained all the essentials for a good night's sleep—a sleeping bag, nightshirt, socks, toothbrush, toothpaste, book, crayons, and a stuffed animal."

TEACH YOUR CHILDREN WELL

Parents spend an enormous amount of time preparing kids to succeed in the world—helping them with homework, schlepping them to endless sports and extracurricular activities, hectoring them to study, policing their social-media habits, teaching them responsible sexual behavior. But we don't teach them much, if anything, about sleep, a key building block of all those other things. And, of course, the best way to teach them is less by telling than by showing—by modeling the very behavior we want to encourage. Preparing them to counter the effects of stress and anxiety begins with showing them how we're doing it.

We must also remove unnecessary roadblocks to better sleep, which means not only working to change the structure of the school day but also helping our children use the rest of their time better. Are our kids overscheduled? Do they have enough time for unstructured play and downtime? Are they spending too much time on their laptops, their smartphones, or watching TV, especially in the hour or so before bedtime? Asking them to get more sleep without helping them to make changes in their day won't work; only by changing some of the factors in the equation will they arrive at a different result.

8.

SLEEPING TOGETHER

FOR MANY PEOPLE, decisions about sleep—when to go to sleep, where to go to sleep, how to sleep—involve another person. And for a couple, these decisions can make for a delicate dance. It's an angle that gets ignored in much of the literature about how to get better sleep.

So why do most of us sleep in the same bed as our partners anyway? According to Roger Ekirch, the custom was born less out of intimacy than necessity: "Among the lower classes in pre-industrial Europe, it was customary for an entire family to sleep in the same bed—typically the costliest item of furniture. . . . Genteel couples, for greater comfort, occasionally slept apart, especially when a spouse was ill."

And without being able to flick on a light switch, nighttime was also a time of fear. "Never did families feel more vulnerable than when they retired at night," says Ekirch. "Bedmates afforded a strong sense of security, given the prevalence of perils, real and imagined—from thieves and arsonists to ghosts, witches, and the prince of darkness himself."

The crowded bedroom had some other advantages as well. "Often a bedmate became your best friend," he explains. "Not just married couples, but sons sleeping with servants, sisters with one another, and aristocratic wives with mistresses. Darkness, within the intimate confines of a bed, leveled social distinctions despite differences in gender and status. Most individuals did not readily fall asleep but conversed freely. In the absence of light, bedmates coveted that hour when, frequently, formality and etiquette perished by the bedside." Further evidence of sleep as the great equalizer.

> *No man prefers to sleep two in a bed. . . . I don't know how it is, but people like to be private when they are sleeping. And when it comes to sleeping with an unknown stranger, in a strange inn, in a strange town, and that stranger a harpooner, then your objections indefinitely multiply. Nor was there any earthly reason why I as a sailor should sleep two in a bed, more than anybody else; for sailors no more sleep two in a bed at sea, than bachelor Kings do ashore. To be sure they all sleep together in one apartment, but you have your own hammock, and cover yourself with your own blanket, and sleep in your own skin.*
>
> —Herman Melville, *Moby-Dick*

But as the bed got less crowded, devolving to one couple per bed, we came to realize that there are different ghosts and witches haunting us. Like a horror movie in which the police dramatically announce that the menacing phone call is coming from inside the house, we now realize that the primary nighttime danger to our sleep is all too often coming from inside the bedroom, in the form of a partner with very different sleep habits.

It makes sense that many people sleep better alone—if only because there's less chance of being woken up in the night by snoring, a stray leg, a partner with a cold or getting up to go to the bathroom. And there are differences between how men and women sleep alone versus together. A study from the University of Vienna found that women woke up more frequently throughout the night when they slept in the same bed as their partner, while men's sleep did not change. When asked about the quality of their sleep, the men said they had slept better with their partner, while women said they had slept better only on nights they had sex.

But the connection between sleep and relationships is, like everything about relationships, complicated. Even though our sleep might benefit from separate beds, there are many reasons why couples are reluctant to go their separate nighttime ways. "The main issue is if you're not sleeping in the same bed, the perception is you're not having sex and people are afraid to admit to sleeping apart," said couples therapist Lee Crespi.

And the decision of where to sleep can affect more than just the sexual side of relationships. Studies show that relationship satisfaction is intricately interwoven with our sleep. A 2014 study from the University of Hertfordshire in the United Kingdom looked at the positions in which couples began their sleep. What they found was that 94 percent of the couples who slept with their bodies touching were "happy with their relationship." Of the couples who didn't touch when they went to sleep, 68 percent were happy. Indeed, the farther apart a couple slept, the more unhappy they were in their relationship. Of course, it's hard to distinguish between correlation and causation. In other words, we don't know what came first, the unhappy chicken or the sleep-deprived egg. Couples who are unhappy are much more likely to start the night farther apart. And if your sleep is easily disrupted by someone else's presence, being tired all the time because you're losing sleep from sleeping too close to your partner isn't going to do your relationship (or any other part of your life) any good.

What about couples for whom the starting sleep position isn't even an issue because they go to bed at different times? As *The Wall Street Journal*'s Elizabeth Bernstein reports, these couples "have more conflict, spend less time in shared activities and serious conversation, and have sex less frequently than couples with similar sleeping schedules."

The connection between sleep and relationship satisfaction is different for men and women. A study from the University of Pittsburgh found that women slept better when they reported being happy in their relationship, while for men it was a night of good sleep that translated into more relationship happiness. "Women are more sensitive to the highs and lows of relationships, so women show a link between relationship functioning and sleep," said Wendy Troxel, a psychologist at the RAND Corporation and a coauthor of the study. "For men, sleep has an effect on their functioning, so that affects their relationships." Another study of Troxel's found that when women slept at the same times as their partners, they were more likely to report being happy in their relationship the next day.

Of course, wanting to avoid going to bed at the same time as your partner might just as likely be a symptom of a dysfunctional relationship as a cause. But for couples who want to sync up their schedules but can't, one option is to sleep separately. The key, says Troxel, is communication. "Some couples end up sleeping apart out of desperation, because one partner is not sleeping at all," she says. "But there is no conversation involved. When that happens, the other partner may feel abandoned." At which point it might be time to bypass the sleep consultant and go straight to a couples therapist. This can be especially fraught because the time after climbing into bed, when couples are decompressing and telling each other about their day, is an important source of intimacy. Troxel's advice? "Don't sacrifice the quality couple time before bed."

LET'S TALK ABOUT SEX

Then there is sex: one of the obvious reasons that couples sleep in the same bed is the fear of becoming a couple that doesn't have sex. On the other hand, if you're not getting enough sleep, that can start a chain reaction that results in less sex. "If one partner is not sleeping well because of the other, it can lead to resentment, bitterness, arguments, and other troubles in the relationship," says sex expert Nikki Ransom-Alfred. "If you can compromise to resolve your issues and remain in the same bed, great! However, if you do need your own space just to sleep, be sure to do what's needed to maintain the love, romance, and intimacy in the relationship before retreating off to your own bed."

Regardless of where you sleep, getting more sleep can lead to getting more sex, at least for women, according to a 2015 study. Researchers measured the duration of women's sleep and compared it to their level of sexual desire the next day. They found that every additional hour of sleep brought with it a 14 percent rise in the likelihood of having some kind of sexual activity with her partner. So more sleep is better—especially if you want more sex.

In terms of men, a 2010 study from Drexel University and

the University of Pennsylvania found that nearly 70 percent of men who had serious breathing problems during sleep reported having decreased sexual desire, and nearly half had lower rates of arousal. Though we can't say that improving our sleep will magically translate into a better sex life, it's clear that when we're sleep-deprived and exhausted, sex isn't the first thing on our minds.

SAWING WOOD: WHAT TO DO WHEN YOUR PARTNER SNORES

One of the biggest barriers to getting a good night's sleep with another person in the bed is that rhythmic, bed-shaking hum known as snoring. Experts estimate that one-third of adults snore. And we are more likely to snore as we get older. According to a 2015 survey by the American Academy of Dental Sleep Medicine, a quarter of respondents said that a partner's snoring has made them angry or annoyed; 20 percent have actually been forced to get out of bed by the racket. Among women, 40 percent said snoring is a turnoff in a possible mate, and 10 percent of both genders said snoring had damaged a relationship.

Hope suddenly cries out angrily in the darkness, claiming that my "snoring" is making it impossible for her to fall asleep, and insisting that I either turn on my side or else leave . . . and to "for God's sake" grant her some "peace." The sudden vehemence of her crying out floods my nervous system with adrenaline, cortisol or other stress related hor-

mones . . . which, subsequently, make it nearly impossible for me to fall asleep, sometimes for hours or even more.

—David Foster Wallace, *Oblivion*

The costs of sleeping next to someone who snores are high, but silencing a snorer is no easy task. Snoring happens when your airways narrow, resulting in a vibration of your throat's soft tissue as you breathe. "When you are snoring, you're spending too much energy to breathe," says Dr. M. Safwan Badr. "Snoring is like fever for a general internist—it tells you something is going on, but it doesn't tell you what." According to the American Sleep Apnea Association, half of America's 90 million snorers are actually suffering from obstructive sleep apnea.

For the 45 million whose snoring is not linked to sleep apnea, there are tips worth trying, including changing sleep positions. Badr finds that fancy pillows and the nasal strips from your local drugstore rarely work. Instead he suggests skipping your evening nightcap (alcohol weakens the throat muscles, making it harder to keep your airways open at night), sleeping with a humidifier (particularly helpful if your snoring is connected to congestion or allergies), and losing weight (those extra pounds add tissue to your neck, which can restrict airways). Some of these are harder to implement than others, but each method illustrates the same point: snoring is connected to aspects of our lives that we have at least some control over.

If trying to get the snorer to stop doesn't work, you can try changing how you react to snoring. How? Through hypnosis! "Most people like sleeping next to the sound of waves," says Joy Martina, a coauthor of *Sleep Your Fat Away.* "The snoring also comes in waves. So through hypnosis, you can give people the suggestion that every time they hear their spouse snore, it lulls them into deeper sleep." Think of it as having a free white-noise machine (albeit one without an off switch, or even a volume knob).

And of course there are always earplugs and noise-canceling headphones. If even those fail, you may have to resort to the only guaranteed way to stop being woken up by your partner's snoring: sleep in a different room. In 2014, *Huffington Post* reporter Yagana Shah asked readers on Facebook how they deal with a snoring partner. We were surprised by how many couples were opting to sleep apart: "It's the new way of creating a long-lasting and happy marriage," wrote Pinsey Christensen. "Being woken up constantly all night long listening to hubby snore like a moose caused me to have anxiety issues and severe headaches during the day from never getting a full night's sleep. This is society's 'last taboo.' People are afraid to admit it, because others think that the couple is having marital problems." As Jamie Greco put it, "Lying awake because it's a sign of trouble to sleep soundly in separate rooms is tantamount to avoiding stepping on cracks to save your mother's back. . . . If you have to be a few feet away from each other while you are sleeping in order to remember to have sex, you've got bigger problems than snoring."

The prejudice associated with couples sleeping separately, whether regularly or occasionally, needs to be updated beyond the 1950s sitcom version of a chaste "Good night, dear" peck on the cheek and retiring to twin beds. Perhaps it's time to reclaim the term "sleeping around" to refer not to sex but to finding a place to get the sleep we need.

9.

WHAT TO DO, WHAT NOT TO DO

TIPS, TOOLS, AND TECHNIQUES

FROM THE beginning of time, people have struggled with sleep. As a result, we've accumulated a staggering body of wisdom about it—techniques and tips passed down from generation to generation. And we could fill a decent-size library (or a really spacious thumb drive) with all the sleep advice that's been amassed in just the last decade in the wake of all the new scientific research.

There is no silver sleeping bullet that's going to do the trick for everybody. People's reasons for not getting enough sleep are deeply personal, specific to their lives and circumstances. And those reasons shift over time. Still, for those looking to improve their sleep life, it makes sense to begin with some of the scientifically proven general principles for good sleep habits.

LET THERE BE (LESS) LIGHT!

On the first day, God proclaimed, "Let there be light," and separated the light from the darkness (which no doubt helped in getting some well-deserved rest six days later). To get a good night's sleep, we should all follow the Almighty's lead by minimizing the former and maximizing the latter. As I discussed in the Science chapter, light suppresses the production of melatonin, which signals us to sleep. So we should take steps—even before we climb into bed—to turn down the lights and make our bedroom the kind of calming, quiet, dark space that will coax us toward sleep. The National Sleep Foundation advises using low-wattage incandescent bulbs in your bedroom. Dr. Mathias Basner of the University of Pennsylvania echoed this advice. "Turn off the lights in the bathroom and instead use the light from the hallway while grooming before bed," he told me. "Bathroom mirror lights can be excessively bright and thus suppress melatonin excretion. Also, turn the lights down during the late evening, and try not to expose yourself to bright light from the TV, e-readers, etc., late at night."

Sensing a shift in the market, some lightbulb companies, such as the Lighting Science Group Corporation in Florida, are now creating bulbs designed to be in sync with our circadian rhythms instead of disrupting them. One type of bulb is to be used in the daytime, the other at night.

THE BLUE LIGHT THAT IS KILLING YOUR SLEEP

We also know that blue light, the sort given off by our ubiquitous electronic devices, is especially good at suppressing melatonin—which makes it especially bad for our sleep. Staring at a blue-light-radiating device before you go to bed can serve as "an alert stimulus that will frustrate your body's ability to go to sleep later," said George Brainard, a circadian-rhythm researcher and neurologist at Thomas Jefferson University in Philadelphia. "When you turn it off, it doesn't mean that instantly the alerting effects go away. There's an underlying biology that's stimulated."

When we ignore this fact, says Dr. Dan Siegel, a clinical professor of psychiatry at UCLA, the result can be a vicious cycle: "People are exposing their eyes to this stream of photons from these objects that basically tell your brain, 'Stay awake. It's not time to go to sleep yet.' So it's 10 p.m., it's 11 p.m., it's midnight—you're checking for emails, you're looking for texts—those light beams tell your brain, 'Don't secrete melatonin, it's not time to sleep.' And you're up at 12:30, 1, you're checking some more because you're up, so why shouldn't you check? Now, you go to bed at 1, you wake up at 6 because it's time to go to work, that's five hours of sleep." Sound familiar?

The problem is that our relationship with our devices is still in that honeymoon phase where we just can't get enough of each other—we're not yet at the stage where we're comfortable being apart for a few hours or taking separate vacations. In fact, a 2015 survey showed that 71 percent of Americans sleep with or next to their smartphones. We should think of light, especially blue light, as an anti-sleeping drug or a stimulant—something few of us would willingly give ourselves each night before bed, especially when so many of us are using sleeping pills or other sleeping aids in a desperate effort to get some sleep. There are some new technologies, such as f.lux software, that help mitigate blue-light exposure, as I'll discuss in the Technology chapter. But gently escorting our smartphones out of our bedrooms at least thirty minutes before we fall asleep is still the best option.

It's not just the screens that are potential problems but what's on them. Heather Cleland Woods, a sleep researcher at the University of Glasgow, coauthored a study on how social-media use affects teens. "If we're all on social media and we have this 24-7 culture," she asked, "are we raising a generation of kids that are not going to be able to get a quality night's sleep?" She and her team set out to answer that by looking at the social-media practices of adolescents, their "emotional investment" in social media, and their mental health, including histories of depression or anxiety, in which sleep plays a role.

Participants who said they had the highest emotional investment in their social-media lives also reported having low sleep quality—as well as increased anxiety and depression and decreased self-esteem. Woods is not recommending that parents force their teens to go cold turkey, but rather to help them think through their use of social media.

IT'S GETTING HOT IN HERE

Then there's the matter of temperature. According to a study by researchers from the Clinique du Sommeil in Lille, France, the ideal sleeping temperature is 60 to 66 degrees Fahrenheit. The National Sleep Foundation recommends 65 degrees and says that sleep is actually disrupted when the temperature rises above 75 degrees or falls below 54 degrees. As the French study confirms, our bodies have a temperature cycle much like our circadian sleep cycle: our body temperature drops throughout the night, bottoming out a few hours before waking and going up as we approach morning.

As Natalie Dautovich, an environmental scholar at the National Sleep Foundation, said, a small drop in body temperature can prompt sleep signals to our brains: "We know that a cool bedroom environment is key to getting a good night's sleep. We also know there are a lot of positive associations between fresh air and relaxation, and when we feel relaxed and comfortable in our environment, we're more likely to feel sleepy."

LET'S GET PHYSICAL: EXERCISE AND SLEEP

We also sleep better when we make time for regular physical activity in our lives. A 2014 study from the University of Georgia found a strong connection between sleep problems and cardiorespiratory fitness. "Staying active won't cure sleep complaints," said lead author Rodney Dishman, "but it will reduce the odds of them." I find that on the days when I've biked or hiked or walked or done yoga, it's much easier to unwind and fall asleep.

In fact, there's plenty of science confirming the direct relationship between exercise and sleep. A study from Bellarmine University and Oregon State University found that "regular physical activity may serve as a non-pharmaceutical alternative to improve sleep," at least for those who meet the basic recommended guidelines of 150 minutes per week of moderate exercise. And researchers at the University of Pennsylvania showed that those who walked for exercise got better sleep and that, as lead author Michael Grandner put it, "these effects are even stronger for more purposeful activities, such as running and yoga, and even gardening and golf." In other words, move your body! Even when you have a jam-packed day, try taking a longer route to your subway stop, or take the stairs instead of the elevator, or park at the outer edge of the parking lot. Or if you can, set up a walking meeting at work. When we were launching *The Huffington Post*, some of our best ideas came up while hiking in the hills of L.A.

For so many of us, sleep and exercise feel like mutually exclusive choices. If we want to catch up on our sleep, setting that early alarm for the gym seems to conspire against it. If we try to make time for an evening workout, we worry about sacrificing an extra hour of sleep to fit it in. It's a thought process familiar to a lot of us; we have become masters at this kind of self-negotiation, this either/or thinking. The key is making exercise a habit. Rather than trying to add an occasional long workout to our day (which demands a big time commitment), try exercising just twenty or thirty minutes at least five days a week. "The real danger," says the Mayo Clinic's Dr. Edward Laskowski, "is when you only make adequate time for one of them."

But don't get discouraged if the gains aren't apparent right away. A 2013 study from Northwestern University found that exercise added around forty-five minutes of extra sleep, but it took around four months for the full benefits to kick in. This street runs both ways: researchers also found that after a bad night of sleep, participants had bad workouts, while they had better workouts after a good night's sleep.

What about the timing of exercise? Is exercising close to bedtime a bad idea? As it turns out, exercise is so beneficial to sleep and overall health that we should attempt to fit it in whenever our lives allow. "The timing of exercise ought to be driven by when the pool's lap lane is open, or when your tennis partner is available or when you have time to get away from work," says the University of Kentucky's Dr. Barbara Phillips.

EAT RIGHT, SLEEP TIGHT (EAT WRONG, UP ALL NIGHT LONG)

So can we eat our way to better sleep? Not really, but we can eat our way to bad sleep. With food and drink, it's more a matter of what to avoid than what to take in. The obvious and all-too-common obstacle to a healthy sleep diet is going between caffeine and sugar all day so we end up tired but wired at night.

"Don't talk to me until I've had my coffee" is practically our national refrain, muttered daily by heavy-lidded men and women as they get out of bed and begin to brave the day. Caffeine—the key ingredient in a morning cup of joe—is a stimulant that wakes us up or revives us during the day. But a caffeine jolt late in the afternoon or in the evening can seriously disrupt our sleep.

Most people know not to have coffee after dinner, but in fact caffeine's power has a longer effect on our bodies than we think. A 2013 study from Wayne State University and Henry Ford Hospital in Detroit, Michigan, concluded that when taken even six hours before bed, caffeine can decrease sleep by as much as one hour. "The risks of caffeine use in terms of sleep disturbance are underestimated by both the general population and physicians," the researchers concluded. In other words, our caffeine cutoff time should begin well before evening.

What about those drinks that might actually help us sleep, like the fabled glass of warm milk? Studies have not shown a connection between drinking milk and sleep, but if drinking warm milk before bed is a ritual that relaxes you—perhaps because of childhood associations—then by all means, do so. And for those who are dairy-intolerant, try switching to almond or coconut milk, or a soothing cup of chamomile tea. Anything that puts you in a calm frame of mind can help you fall asleep (provided it does not contain sugar).

Also, milk does give us calcium, and calcium, along with magnesium and B vitamins, is involved in sleep regulation (while calcium deficiencies are sometimes associated with sleep problems). So although foods that contain calcium won't put us to sleep, there are key nutrients they include that provide the necessary building blocks for sleep. The same is true of foods that contain magnesium (such as nuts, seeds, leafy greens, and bananas), B6 (such as fish, beans, and poultry), and tryptophan (an amino acid found in foods like chickpeas, seaweed, egg whites, pumpkin seeds, halibut, and most famously, turkey). Another food that may help us sleep is cherries, which are rich in melatonin. A 2014 study from Louisiana State University found that participants who drank a glass of tart cherry juice twice a day for two weeks slept an average of eighty-five minutes more each night than those who drank the placebo.

Is it true that we shouldn't eat big meals right before bed? Yes—that bit of conventional wisdom is true, especially if you suffer from acid reflux, which afflicts an estimated 40 percent of Americans. This can be a particular problem given our modern-day work schedule, says Dr. Jamie Koufman, who specializes in acid reflux: "Over the past two decades, I've noticed that the time of the evening meal has been trending later and later among my patients. The after-work meal—already later because of longer work hours—is often further delayed by activities such as shopping and exercise." She considers eating earlier to be the "single most important intervention" in avoiding acid reflux. She found that this lessened symptoms of sleep apnea in many of her patients as well.

Since it can take us two or three hours to digest a meal, even those who don't suffer from acid reflux should pay attention to the time they eat dinner. Christopher Colwell, a professor of psychiatry at UCLA, says that eating late or at odd times can disrupt our circadian rhythms and therefore our sleep-wake cycle: "We have this illusion that with the flip of a switch, we can work at any time and part of that is eating at any time. But our biological systems . . . work based on having a daily rhythm."

I know the times when I've turned to food to help me power through to complete a project at night—when my body was actually craving sleep—I would often wake up feeling dehydrated and heavy. Of course, no two people are alike, so it's exciting to become scientists specializing in ourselves, observing, analyzing, and experimenting with what's best for our own sleep.

Another thing best to avoid before bedtime is spicy foods, which can cause heartburn and bloating. Australian researchers found that participants who ate food containing Tabasco sauce and mustard before bed took longer to fall asleep and slept less. They also found that the participants' body temperatures increased after eating spicy food, another factor that leads to poor sleep. Eating too many fatty foods can be another culprit in disrupting our sleep. Researchers found that rats put on a high-fat diet suffered from more fragmented sleep. They ended up sleeping more, but the extra sleep occurred mainly during the daytime. The researchers also linked high-fat diets to excessive daytime sleepiness, something often found in overweight and obese people.

Understanding the link between food and sleep means swallowing some (decaf, non-spicy, low-fat) hard truths. "The number one weakness reported by my patients in over twenty years of practice," HuffPost wellness editor and founder of the Santa Monica Wellness Center Patricia Fitzgerald told me, "is late night ice cream. No close seconds." She recommends avoiding not just ice cream but sugar in general before bedtime.

And while there may not be much scientific research on it, I can provide some anecdotal evidence on the need to avoid the combo of salty foods and scary movies before you go to sleep. I remember the night my daughters, then eight and six years old, sat down with a big bag of salty popcorn and watched *Ghostbusters*—a comedy to adults but another thing entirely, as I found out, to my girls. It was not a fun night; it was past midnight by the time we finally got them to sleep. So as far as I was concerned as a parent, salty foods and scary movies were immediately moved to the Not Before Bedtime list!

WOULD YOU LIKE TO COME UP FOR A NIGHTCAP?

The next stop on our tour of sleep-related misconceptions is the nightcap. Many people believe that a quick drink before bed helps them get to sleep—and the ritual has been endorsed by authorities from Winston Churchill to James Bond. What they don't realize is what happens in their body afterward. According to a 2015 study from the University of Melbourne, alcohol does indeed initially act as a sedative. But later in the night, it changes allegiances and acts as a sleep disrupter. "The take-home message here is that alcohol is not actually a particularly good sleep aid, even though it may seem like it helps you get to sleep quicker," said study author Christian Nicholas. "In fact, the quality of the sleep you get is significantly altered and disrupted." A study from the London Sleep Centre confirmed this, finding that "at all dosages, alcohol causes a more consolidated first half sleep and an increase in sleep disruption in the second half of sleep."

We all respond differently to alcohol, but for me, waking up with a dry mouth in the middle of the night made it very clear that a nightcap too close to bedtime was just too hard for my body to process. Again, the key is to experiment with what works for you.

NATURE'S ARSENAL: ACUPUNCTURE, HERBAL REMEDIES, AND OTHER SLEEP AIDS

Acupuncture has a long history as a sleep aid, and now modern science confirms what practitioners and patients have known for centuries. According to a review from Emory University that analyzed thirty studies of insomnia treatment, 93 percent of them found that acupuncture had positive effects on sleep. In addition, several studies have found that auricular acupuncture (needles placed in the ear) works particularly well. Another study, this one from Peking University, found that acupuncture was just as effective a treatment for insomnia as medication. Digging deeper into how acupuncture reduces insomnia, researchers from the Center for Addiction and Mental Health in Toronto found that acupuncture increased nighttime secretion of melatonin and lowered anxiety levels.

Acupuncturist Janet Zand told me that "in Traditional Chinese Medicine we know sleep as yin—nourishment—essential for restoration." Overstimulation, on the other hand, which she singles out as a driver of our sleep-deprivation crisis, "is considered excessive yang—heat/inflammation." In her practice, Patricia Fitzgerald has found that "a treatment plan including acupuncture, a Chinese herbal formula, or supplements like holy basil and magnesium, tailored for the patient's specific sleep problems, brings dramatic results without the side effects." For an at-home option, she recommends acupressure—holding pressure points on the heel, ankle, and wrist while breathing deeply to help you prepare for sleep.

One of the most popular herbs for sleep is lavender, which has been used throughout history for healing and relaxation. The Greek physician Dioscorides wrote about lavender's many medicinal benefits as early as the first century. The herb was a staple of Greek and Roman baths, and in ancient Egypt it was used frequently for incense. And again, there is scientific evidence to support what the ancients knew. A Thai study found that smelling lavender helps us relax by slowing down our heart rate, decreasing our blood pressure, and lowering skin temperature. Other studies have found sleep quality improved in a room scented with lavender or when lavender oil was sprinkled on pajamas or pillows. And in Germany, lavender tea has been approved by their equivalent of the FDA as a treatment for insomnia.

Those who want to explore herbal sleep aids—and especially those who want to wean themselves off sleeping pills—have many options to consider. Valerian root, for example, is a natural sedative whose use dates back to ancient Greece, where Hippocrates prescribed it in the fourth century BC. In recent years, its effectiveness has been supported by research. In addition to valerian root, Dr. Frank Lipman also recommends other nutrients that can improve sleep, including gamma-aminobutyric acid, or GABA (a naturally occurring chemical that dampens brain activity), and L-theanine (an amino acid found in green-tea leaves that induces brain waves connected to relaxation).

Interior designer Michael Smith, who spends a large part of his life on planes, told me he sprays orange essential oil on the T-shirt he sleeps in at night. He finds the scent calms his mind and has a humidifying effect. The lesson here is that it is important to experiment. And the mere fact that you're taking any deliberate action to improve your sleep means that you likely will.

RETREAT INTO YOURSELF: MINDFULNESS, MEDITATION, AND SLEEP

Sleep is the best meditation.

—The Dalai Lama

The most common nonmedical causes of insomnia are stress and anxiety, or a state of hyperarousal. Here's how those afflicted by chronic insomnia are described in a joint study by Penn State, the University of Athens, and the Autonomous University of Madrid:

> They generally tend to handle stress and conflicts through internalization of emotions, which leads to emotional arousal. At bedtime, they are characteristically tense, anxious, ruminative about issues associated with health, work, personal affairs, death, etc. Since the emotional arousal causes physiological arousal, they face difficulties in sleep initiation or returning to sleep after awakenings during the night. As a result, they develop a "fear of sleeplessness," which intensifies their emotional arousal perpetuating their insomnia.

In other words, people who can't sleep are stressed out, and their stress makes it harder to sleep, which gives them another thing to be stressed out about. For those caught in this spiral of sleeplessness and next-day grogginess—and at some point in our lives that describes most of us—anything that can help us de-stress can help break the cycle.

As Jon Kabat-Zinn, the founder of Mindfulness-Based Stress Reduction, put it, "If you are having a lot of trouble sleeping, your body may be trying to tell you something about the way you are conducting your life. As with all other mind-body symptoms, this message is worth listening to." Far too often the message is that we go through our days on autopilot, reacting to everything that comes our way and forgetting to pause and recharge once in a while—the cumulative stress making it harder to wind down at night.

One thing keeping us up at night is worrying about our never-completed to-do lists. We lie in bed thinking of all that was not done today and all that needs to be done tomorrow, and it seems impossible to shut our minds off. "I would stress three words: calm the mind," USC professor of gerontology Jennifer Ailshire told me. "If we can't slow our thoughts and disengage our minds from the daily stress and strain we experience, we have little chance of getting restful sleep. Strategies for doing this will vary from person to person, but yoga and meditation are good options." So is qigong, an ancient Chinese practice of physical postures and breathing that can help us prepare for sleep.

I have a quote by Ralph Waldo Emerson by my bed that helps me silence my mind: "Finish every day, and be done with it. . . . You have done what you could—some blunders and absurdities no doubt crept in, forget them as fast as you can, tomorrow is a new day. You shall begin it well and serenely, and with too high a spirit to be encumbered with your old nonsense."

One way to finish every day and be done with it is what Joey Hubbard, who directs our Thrive workshops, calls the "mind dump." Before bed, write down all the things you can think of that you need to do. This can empty your mind and reassure you that you don't need to remember your tasks through the night—your to-do list will be waiting for you in the morning.

When we walk through the door of our bedroom, it should be a symbolic moment that marks leaving the day, with all of its problems and unfinished business, behind us. When we wake up in the morning, there will be plenty of time for us to pick up our projects and deal with our challenges, refreshed and recharged. I treat my transition to sleep as a sacrosanct ritual. Before bed, I take a hot bath with epsom salts and a candle flickering nearby—a bath that I prolong if I'm feeling anxious or worried about something. I don't sleep in my workout clothes as I used to (think of the mixed message that sends to our brains) but have pajamas, nightdresses, even T-shirts dedicated to sleep. Sometimes I have a cup of chamomile or lavender tea if I want something warm and comforting before going to bed. Think of each stage as designed to help you shed more of your stubborn daytime worries.

And when I'm really having trouble sleeping, or wake up with thoughts crowding my mind, I've found meditation to be a great remedy. Instead of stressing out about how I'm staying awake and fearing I'll be tired the next day, I prop a few extra pillows under me and reframe what's happening as a great opportunity to practice my meditation. If it's in the middle of the night, I remind myself that that's precisely when many avid meditation practitioners, like the Dalai Lama, wake up to get in two or three hours of meditation; this both takes the stress out of my wakefulness and adds an extra layer of gratitude to my practice. Just by reframing it from a problem to a blessing that allows me to go deeper without a deadline or any distractions, I find that I both have some of my deepest meditation experiences and, inevitably, drift off to sleep at some point.

As Marcus Aurelius wrote in *Meditations*, it's a journey that's always available to us: "People look for retreats for themselves, in the country, by the coast, or in the hills, when it is possible for you to retreat into yourself any time you want. There is nowhere that a person can find a more peaceful and trouble-free retreat than in his own mind . . . so constantly give yourself this retreat and renew yourself." Since we find it harder and harder to retreat into ourselves in the middle of our busy days, the retreat in the middle of the night—whether through sleep or meditation—can be reframed as a precious luxury. This certainly didn't come easily to me. But I was able to train myself to see the time spent meditating in the middle of the night as productive and enriching instead of lying awake in bed resenting the fact that I was wasting time lying awake in bed.

Another practice that my older daughter, Christina, has been using, and that I've borrowed, is making a gratitude list part of our bedtime routine. I find that it focuses my mind on the blessings in my life—large and small—rather than on the running list of unresolved problems. For all of us, every day has its blessings and its setbacks, but it's the setbacks and stresses that seem to take center stage in our minds once our head hits the pillow. They are the preening, attention-seeking, spotlight-hogging divas of our bedtime hours, ignoring the stage manager begging them to exit. And if we don't stop them, they'll drag the whole production down with them. A gratitude list—whether written in a notebook, spoken aloud, or just recited silently—is a great way to knock them down a peg, shift the spotlight, and make sure our blessings get the closing scene of the night.

Jim Gordon, the founder of Edgewater Funds, a multibillion-dollar private equity fund, has his own gratitude-based sleep ritual that's better than any sleeping pill (and with none of the destructive side effects). He told me that when he wakes up in the middle of the night and can't get back to sleep, he starts counting his blessings (literally) in the form of his children and grandchildren jumping over a picket fence. When he described this to one of his daughters, who is a psychologist, she told him it sounded like classic cognitive behavioral therapy, but he had come to it by himself.

The science is loud and clear: meditation and sleep make splendid bedfellows. A 2009 Stanford study found that a six-week mindfulness meditation course helped people who have trouble sleeping fall asleep twice as quickly, in fifteen instead of thirty-three minutes (in Appendix B, you will find a list of my recommended guided meditations).

Richard Davidson, a neuroscientist at the University of Wisconsin who has worked closely with the Dalai Lama on the connection between meditation and science, explained to me that emotions like kindness and gratitude help us sleep because they have a calming effect on the mind and reduce disturbing emotions. And he puts them to use in his own life. "I usually do a short meditation before I go to sleep where I reflect on the day and express my gratitude for the opportunities I've been given to help others and make a difference," he told me. "When I wake up, I also reflect on how I can best serve others in the various meetings and events I have scheduled that day." If dwelling on our problems is a hindrance to sleep, what better way to ease our transition to sleep than reflecting on all that we are grateful for?

As Matthieu Ricard, the French Buddhist monk and molecular geneticist who's been deemed the happiest man in the world based on neuroscientific experiments that showed exceptional gamma-wave levels in his brain, put it, "Those who do contemplative retreats in hermitages are far from doing nothing, since they are constantly engaged in training their minds, but there is no 'noise,' no 'waste' to eliminate, no stress to cure, no chaos to reorganize. This means that there is less to repair during sleep and the sleep quality of meditators is deeper."

Here is how Clark Strand, a former Buddhist monk and

the author of *Meditation Without Gurus*, describes his experience with meditation. It's very much the way I experience sleep when I let go of my thoughts and my worries: "Like dropping through a hole in everything that the world said was important. . . . Like discovering that nothing else mattered and all I needed was now. . . . Temporarily removed from the game. . . . Like floating weightless on the Dead Sea and looking up at an empty sky."

In 1976, on an episode of the number-one–rated TV show in America, *The Mary Tyler Moore Show*, Mary's boss, Lou Grant, afraid that Mary is becoming addicted to sleeping pills, dumps them all down the drain. When Mary cries, "Now I'll never get to sleep!" he leads her to the sofa and tells her "just breathe deeply, as if you were asleep, and before you know it, you will be asleep." She tries it, and it works. In fact it works so well that Lou, with his arm around her, is trapped on the sofa beside the snoring Mary, fearing that if he moves he'll undo all his good work. Mr. Grant knew what he was doing.

Breathing is a favorite "sleep hack" of mine. Counting out a few slow breaths is one of the techniques I use when I'm having trouble falling asleep. One such version, the 4-7-8 method popularized by Dr. Andrew Weil, is rooted in the ancient Indian practice of pranayama. I love its simplicity: you inhale quietly through the nose for four counts, hold for seven counts, and exhale with a whooshing sound through the mouth for eight counts. Weil says that with practice and regularity it can put you to sleep in one minute—and anything that can help you get to sleep that quickly is worth a try. Even if it doesn't immediately put you to sleep, it can help calm and relax you—which is both a necessary precursor to sleep and a technique you can use to reduce stress during the day. If you tend to respond better to visual cues, you can try what psychiatrist Brent Menninger recommends: "Visualize images that evoke serenity, like a picture of the Mona Lisa. . . . The half-smile relaxation response is available to you as you breathe. Inhale as you visualize serenity. As you exhale, express a half-smile. Inhale the serenity. Exhale with a half-smile. . . . The half-smile starts with relaxed lips which turn slightly upward and a loose jaw and the eyes are soft and relaxed. Then the half-smile spreads to the whole face as your scalp and neck relax and your shoulders drop." It's crucial, of course, to exercise your judgment and imitate only relaxing paintings. (And definitely avoid Edvard Munch's *The Scream*, which would not only keep *you* up but also wake the neighbors.)

One of the most ingenious new sleep tips I've discovered comes from a study by researchers at the University of Glasgow. Participants suffering from insomnia were divided into two groups. One was told to go about their normal routine to try to fall asleep, while the other was instructed to deliberately try to stay awake (though without getting up and turning on the computer or TV). The group told to stay awake, using what's called "paradoxical intention," had "a significant reduction in sleep effort, and sleep performance anxiety," the study's authors wrote. "Patients realize when they try to remain awake, they feel sleepier, which is what normal sleepers do—people who sleep well don't try to sleep," said study author Colin Espie. "Paradoxical Intention Therapy re-creates the blasé attitude towards sleep that normal sleepers have in those in whom anxiety about sleep is causing insomnia." It reminds me of the scene in

Mary Poppins when the children want to stay up and play and Mary sings to them, "Stay awake, don't rest your head. . . . / You're not sleepy as you seem. / Stay awake, don't nod and dream"—promptly putting them to sleep.

MY SLEEP GOODY BAG

I'm not a sleep scientist (though I've certainly talked to as many of them as I could find), but we're all conducting our personal longitudinal study on our own sleep patterns. The trick is to not get so caught up in the day-to-day ebb and flow of our lives that we forget to look back, find patterns, isolate variables, make sense of our lifetime's worth of knowledge, and then make adjustments. So here is my personal bag of tricks. For me, changing my relationship with sleep meant first coming to terms with the idea of shutting down the day. I had to appreciate the concept of stillness. "When we feel like there isn't enough time in the day for us to get everything done, when we wish for more time," wrote sociologist Christine Carter, "we don't actually need more time. We need more stillness."

For most of my life, I'd never thought of stillness as anything but absence—the absence of noise, the absence of other people, the absence of activity. But here is another way to experience stillness—as a force, as something present, as something so powerful that it can actually burn through all the worries and fears that consume us and leave behind only essence, ease, and grace.

I discovered that when I was not wasting energy, and burning up my nighttime hours on mind chatter, it was much easier for me to fall into a deep sleep and thus have the energy and enthusiasm to deal with the inevitable challenges in the morning.

Stillness—our ability to pause and connect with our deeper selves—is a skill that can be learned and cultivated. And this is all the more important when the world is coming at us at an increasingly frantic pace. So for me, becoming comfortable with stillness—without a constant stream of external stimulation—was a prerequisite to becoming comfortable with sleep.

My appreciation of stillness, and the better sleep that comes with it, did not happen overnight. Once I was clear about the overall change I wanted to make in my life, getting there was a matter of taking small steps in the right direction, every day and every night (okay, almost every night). And no matter how old you are or how many hundreds of nights you've spent tossing and turning, it's never too late to head in a new direction and get back to your natural state of sleep and relaxation. Each night is a fresh chance to begin.

So I tried different meditations, breathing exercises, and visualizations, noting the results and making adjustments. I tried to go from being an amateur, one who simply crashed every night and hoped for the best, to being a sleep pro. According to Steven Pressfield, the author of *Turning Pro*, when we turn pro, things become much simpler. "It changes what time we get up and it changes what time we go to bed," he writes. "It changes what we do and what we don't do. It changes the activities we engage in and with what attitude we engage in them. It changes what we read and what we eat. It changes the shape of our bodies. When we were amateurs, our life was about drama, about denial, and about distraction. Our days were simultaneously full to the bursting point and achingly, heartbreakingly empty."

For me, going from sleep amateur to sleep pro meant trying a lot of things and seeing what worked. Here is a list of things I've tried. If any of these resonate with you, give them a try, too, keep what works, and discard the rest. It doesn't matter how hokey or unsophisticated a particular technique might feel; all that matters is, did it help you get a good night's sleep?

One image I like to use is that of a calm lake. Any thought, worry, or concern that comes up I think of as a stone dropping into the lake. There may be a ripple or two, but quickly the lake returns to its smoothness and calm. As more thoughts or worries or fears come up, I let them drop like stones and let the lake return to its natural tranquillity.

Another technique that works for me is conscious breathing—using my breath to slow myself down and relax any tense areas in my body. As our breath flows in and out, our tensions gradually give way, as if our breath is massaging us from the inside out, releasing the stresses of the day we're still needlessly holding on to. As we get ready for sleep, we can practice seeing ourselves not as a closed, contracted fist but as supple and relaxed as a sleeping baby.

One way we can use our breath to relax and put ourselves on the path to sleep is to breathe while focusing on love, grace, peace, or joy. Relax your eyes, relax your jaw, drop your shoulders, and feel yourself floating on a bed of air. Imagine yourself drifting on a raft down the Mississippi or floating on your back in a calm sea, trusting the gentle rocking of the waves to carry you somewhere safe.

It may seem morbid to some, but one thing that never fails

to work for me when worry is keeping me from sleeping is to remember that at some point I'm going to die. I tried this for the first time after I read the commencement speech that Steve Jobs gave at Stanford in 2005. "Almost everything—all external expectations, all pride, all fear of embarrassment or failure—these things just fall away in the face of death, leaving only what is truly important," he said. "Remembering that you are going to die is the best way to avoid the trap of thinking you have something to lose. You are already naked. There is no reason not to follow your heart." And there is certainly no reason not to fall peacefully asleep—if all these earthly worries eventually "just fall away," there's no reason you can't let them fall away each night.

Of course, the ideas of sleep and death have long been intertwined. We saw in the History chapter the very American belief that we can somehow conquer sleep, and as Lewis Lapham wrote, there is also a very American belief that we can somehow conquer death: "Military and economic command on the world stage fostered the belief that America was therefore exempt from the laws of nature, held harmless against the evils, death chief among them, inflicted on the lesser peoples of the earth. The wonders of medical science raked from the ashes of the war gave notice of the likelihood that soon, maybe next month but probably no later than next year, death would be reclassified as a preventable disease."

This idea of death as something deeply frightening, to be avoided at all costs, also affects people's ability to surrender conscious control over their lives every night and go to sleep. Ira Glass, the host of *This American Life*, described this fear of sleep—formally called hypnophobia, somniphobia, or clinophobia: "I would lie awake at night, scared to fall asleep, because sleep seemed no different than death. . . . You were gone, not moving, not talking, not thinking, not aware—not aware. What could be more frightening?" As Philip Larkin wrote in his poem "Aubade," when he wakes up in the middle of the night all he sees is: "Unresting death, a whole day nearer now, / Making all thought impossible but how / And where and when I shall myself die."

The opposite view—one I fully embrace—was summed up by Montaigne: "To practice death is to practice freedom. A man who has learned how to die has unlearned how to be a slave." Being a slave to our job and our status in the world makes it much harder to put our day behind us and surrender to sleep.

If death is too heavy a sleep aid, a much less fraught tool is to find a sleep talisman, an object that sends a clear signal to both your body and your mind that it is time to slooooow down. Some of these I have used, others friends have told me about: an old-fashioned music box (a friend of mine has a miniature version she travels with; it plays "Silent Night": "Sleep in heavenly peace . . ."); a weighted eye pillow lightly scented with lavender; a special little pillow with an image or a saying that resonates with you; a cozy robe or fluffy slippers.

Or maybe your sleep talisman is an image that brings you peace and serenity, one that you can keep on your nightstand. It could be photos of your children, your pets, or a soothing landscape—anything that helps you exhale the tensions and incompletions of the day. I have two Gordon Parks photographs in my bedroom that help bring me a sense of calm. One is of a little boy lying in the grass with his eyes closed and a june bug resting on his forehead, the other is of a deep forest with a mother and child walking in the distance. Another photograph in my bedroom, this one by Jeffrey Conley, is of a single figure standing in front of the endless ocean. It helps me put the problems of the day I'm leaving behind into perspective.

Finally, I want to reemphasize the two very tangible suggestions that have had the biggest impact on my sleep: First, banish all tech devices from your bedroom at least thirty minutes before you turn off the lights—smartphones are like anti-sleep talismans. And second, if you've been in bed struggling to sleep for twenty minutes, try switching to meditating or reading a book (not on a tablet, which gives off blue light and also often has your emails on it, but a physical book or an e-reader) that has nothing to do with work (a novel, a biography, a book of poetry or spirituality).

THE BEDTIME DRESS CODE: WHAT TO WEAR, WHAT NOT TO WEAR

So what should you wear to bed? The short answer is, anything you feel comfortable and relaxed in—except what you wear to work out. Clare Sauro, a fashion historian and the curator of the Fox Historic Costume Collection at Drexel University in Philadelphia, explained to me that throughout most of Western history people simply wore their daytime undergarments to bed. But the centuries spanning the Renaissance to the Baroque period were a turning point, as the wealthier class started to distinguish between day clothes and sleepwear. With the advent of the Industrial Revolution, sleepwear became more affordable as linen was superseded by cotton. And in the twentieth century, pajamas as we know them really gained traction. Since the 1920s, as Sauro put it, "Pajamas for men have remained fairly consistent, while those for women have followed the shifts in fashion." It seems that women can't escape the pressures of fashion even when we sleep.

I have my own pajama story. In 2010, Cindi Leive, the editor-in-chief of *Glamour* magazine, joined me in a New Year's resolution to get more sleep. Cindi admitted that with her work at the magazine, her two young children, and her TV habit, she was averaging just more than five hours a night. We committed to getting a full night's sleep for a month—which for Cindi meant seven and a half hours and for me eight.

As we found out, resolving to get a good night's sleep is easier said than done. We had to tune out a host of temptations—from Jon Stewart to our email in-boxes. As the month wore on, my favorite sleep aid became the yummy pink pajamas Cindi sent me as a gift. Just putting them on made me feel ready for bed—so much more so than the cotton T-shirts I usually wore. Something switched in my brain when I put the pajamas on; they were unmistakably "going-to-bed clothes," not to be confused with "going-to-the-gym clothes." Slipping on the pj's was a signal to my body: time to shut down.

According to a 2012 poll, 74 percent of Americans prefer to sleep in pajamas and nightgowns, 8 percent sleep naked, and the rest sleep in "something else" (hopefully not their work clothes). In another poll, 57 percent of those who sleep naked said they were happy in their relationships. There is even some science behind that finding. "When you and your partner both sleep naked, the skin-to-skin contact will release the feel-good hormone [oxytocin]," said Fran Walfish, a psychotherapist and the author of *The Self-Aware Parent*. "Even further, you may have more sex and we all know orgasms are Mother Nature's best answer to insomnia . . . better than bottled milk and Ambien!" And with no side effects (or, in this case, I guess falling asleep is the side effect).

10.

CATNAPS, JET LAG, AND TIME ZONES

ONE QUESTION I get all the time is, what do you do when, for whatever reason—a sick toddler, a bad cold, jet lag, a project deadline, or a late night out—you just can't get the recommended seven to eight hours of sleep? Fortunately, there's a great remedy to that problem: the nap. Naps are a cheap and readily available way to enjoy what the National Sleep Foundation calls "a pleasant luxury, a mini-vacation."

In fact, as it turns out, naps are great for us even when we are getting good sleep at night. According to David Randall, the author of *Dreamland*, even a short nap "primes our brains to function at a higher level, letting us come up with better ideas, find solutions to puzzles more quickly, identify patterns faster and recall information more accurately."

While chronic poor sleep can have long-lasting effects on our health, naps can help mitigate some of those effects, at least in the short term. According to a study by the Sorbonne University in Paris, short naps were found to lower stress and boost the immune system. "Our data suggests a 30-minute nap can reverse the hormonal impact of a night of poor sleep," said one study coauthor, Brice Faraut. "This is the first study that found napping could restore biomarkers of neuroendocrine and immune health to normal levels." Short of time travel, a next-day nap may be the closest we can get to a second chance at a good night's sleep.

But the benefits of naps don't stop there. In a study by Allegheny College in Pennsylvania, participants who napped for forty-five minutes during the day were found to have lower blood pressure after completing a stressful task than those who didn't nap. A study from Greece confirmed these findings: participants who took a noontime nap had a 5 percent decrease in blood pressure, enough to make an impact in reducing heart attacks. According to a NASA report, "Studies have demonstrated . . . strategic naps can be used effectively to promote performance and alertness in operational settings."

Let me tell you about the nap. It's absolutely fantastic. When I was a kid, my father was always trying to tell me how to be a man, and he said to me, I was maybe 9 . . . "Philip, whenever you take a nap, take your clothes off, put a blanket on you, and you're going to sleep better." Well, as with everything, he was right. . . . Then the best part of it is that when you wake up, for the first 15 seconds, you have no idea where you are. You're just alive. That's all you know. And it's bliss, it's absolute bliss.

—Philip Roth, on NPR's "Weekend Edition"

Naps can also help you increase your learning power. A study from Saarland University in Germany had participants learn single words and word pairs. After that, half of the group watched a DVD and the other half napped. Members of the group that napped retained significantly more word pairs than their DVD-watching counterparts, resulting, as the study put it, in "a five-fold improvement in information retrieval from memory."

A study from Georgetown University Medical Center showed that during a nap the right side of the brain, the side associated with creativity, was highly active, while the left stayed mostly quiet. In fact, Yo-Yo Ma told me he always tries to take a nap before playing a concert. "It's one way to press the reset button, to restart the day," he said. "I find that being in an in-between state of consciousness and unconsciousness is best for performing, when the pathways between the analytical self and the intuitive self are most open."

And the benefits of napping multiply as we age. A study of older adults by researchers from Japan found that, along with moderate exercise, a thirty-minute nap increased the quality of nighttime sleep, and decreased daytime grogginess.

So when is the best time to nap? Experts say that the best "circadian timing" for a nap is the early afternoon. But you don't have to worry about nailing the timing to get the benefits, so nap as soon as you can after you feel your energy flagging, and don't overthink it. In the course of our overstuffed days, there aren't many opportunities to nap. Take them when you can get them. In other words: *Carpe dormio!*

Our workdays, especially in the afternoon, have a way of taking on a survivalist tinge—how, we ask ourselves, are we going to make it through the rest of the day, trekking with flagging energy through enemy territory mined with meetings, emails, and expanding to-do lists? So we squirrel away provisions—usually unhealthy ones—and, like addicts, we think about where that next shot of caffeine or that next sugar bomb is going to come from. But there are other options. Rather than reach for our fifth cup of coffee or third doughnut to deal with the usual post-lunch lull, consider a twenty- or thirty-minute nap. In fact, if you're deciding between the two—caffeine or nap—the science is clear that, in a productivity version of rock-paper-scissors, naps trump caffeine. Sara Mednick, professor of psychology at the University of California, Riverside, compared the relative beneficial effects on memory and problem solving of 200 milligrams of caffeine (about what we get from a cup of coffee) to a long nap. The two were equal on perceptual learning, but naps outscored caffeine in word recall *and* motor learning (which caffeine actually impaired).

When I feel in need of a nap, I use the couch in my office—so that I don't occupy our highly publicized nap rooms at *The Huffington Post*, which are always in high demand. I used to close the curtains of the glass wall in my office that looks out over the newsroom, but one day it dawned on me that leaving the curtains open sends a clear message to the newsroom that not only is there no stigma—at least at HuffPost—attached to napping, it's also the best thing we can do to recharge ourselves. So now the curtains stay open.

The practice of napping still suffers from our collective delusion that equates sleep with weakness and laziness, but the performance-enhancing benefits of naps have been no secret to many leaders throughout history. Margaret Thatcher used to tell her staff not to bother her during her 2:30-to-3:30 p.m. nap. John F. Kennedy took a long nap after lunch, with no interruptions or telephone calls from the staff allowed (though, given what we know now about

JFK, it's unclear how broad his definition of "taking a nap" was). And while traveling, Kennedy would nap on a big bed installed in Air Force One. Charlie Rose, who swears by up to three naps a day to be at his best on the air, even napped in the car (complete with eye mask) on his way to interview Vladimir Putin in Moscow in 2015. He called it "my Putin prep." Night owl Bill Clinton made up for his famous late-night gab sessions with some restorative naps, while Winston Churchill is credited with coining the term "power nap." Here he is, with typical oratorical flourish, on the joys of napping: "You must sleep sometime between lunch and dinner, and no halfway measures. Take off your clothes and get into bed. That's what I always do. Don't think you will be doing less work because you sleep during the day. That's a foolish notion held by people who have no imaginations. You will be able to accomplish more. You get two days in one—well, at least one and a half."

Pope Francis isn't just a global spiritual leader, he's also a globe-trotting napping ambassador. "I take off my shoes," the pope said, "and I lie on my bed for a rest." During his visit to the United States in 2015, downtime was crucial to allow the seventy-eight-year-old pontiff to keep a whirlwind schedule of speeches, meetings, Masses, and other public appearances. As Vatican officials told HuffPost's Jaweed Kaleem, each day intentionally included unscheduled time so that the pope could take a midday nap—usually about forty minutes.

And another spiritual leader, the Dalai Lama, understands the power of both napping and sleep in general. "For me, sleep is very important," he said when I interviewed him in London in 2012. "The other day in Delhi," he added, "I had a new driver, and I asked him, 'How many hours do you sleep?' 'Four hours,' he replied. 'Four hours is not adequate,' I told him. As for me, I sleep—sound sleep—usually eight hours, sometimes, like last night, nine. Very sound sleep." Here's hoping the driver took his enlightened passenger's advice.

TRAVEL, TIME ZONES, AND JET LAG MINUS THE JET

Even for those who normally sleep well, nothing can disrupt sleep like travel. Our circadian rhythms didn't evolve with jet planes and air travel in mind, so if you've flown long distances, you've almost certainly experienced jet lag at some point.

According to the Smithsonian's *Air & Space Magazine*, the term "jet lag" was first used in 1966. "If you're going to be a member of the Jet Set and fly off to Katmandu for coffee with King Mahendra," wrote the travel writer Horace Sutton, "you can count on contracting Jet Lag, a debility not unakin to a hangover. Jet Lag derives from the simple fact that jets travel so fast they leave your body rhythms behind."

In other words, when we change time zones, we also change sleep zones. But it takes a while for our body clocks to sync up with the clocks where our bodies currently are. Though we mostly associate jet lag with being groggy, in some extreme cases I've experienced something closer to a sleep-deprivation coma. And according to researchers from Rush University Medical Center in Chicago, jet lag can lead to depression, gastrointestinal problems, impaired judgment, and long-term problems such as cognitive impairment and menstrual-cycle disturbances. Flight attendants, whose working lives are defined by constant travel across time zones, even show a higher risk of cancer.

Weary with toil, I haste me to my bed,
The dear repose for limbs with travel tired;
But then begins a journey in my head,
To work my mind, when body's work's expir'd.

—William Shakespeare, "Sonnet 27"

Till Roenneberg, an expert on sleep cycles, is so convinced of their importance that he makes sure in his own life he never needs an alarm clock in the morning. As he has shown, jet lag goes beyond air travel, which is why he coined the term "social jet lag." He explains, "A biological clock is ticking in every person, producing an individual daily timing. This defines a person's unique 'chronotype,' which can vary greatly between individuals. For some people, internal midday may coincide with external midday. Others can reach their internal midday several hours before or after external midday. Social jet lag measures this difference between our external social timing and that of our internal clock."

This internal clock is located in a part of the brain that controls circadian rhythms of all kinds throughout the body—including sleep, temperature, and the digestive system, among others. It does this by processing light from the retina and by the expression of so-called clock genes. A study by researchers from the Beth Israel Deaconess Medical Center in Boston found a helpful tool to beat jet lag: food—or, more accurately, the absence of it. "When food is plentiful," they wrote, "circadian rhythms of animals are powerfully entrained by the light-dark cycle. However, if animals have access to food only during their normal sleep cycle, they will shift most of their circadian rhythms to match the food availability." Studying mice, they discovered a "master clock" in a region of the brain (the dorsomedial nucleus) that can reset the circadian rhythm when faced with a shortage of food. The thinking is that when food is not an issue, lightness and darkness synchronize our sleep cycle. But when food is scarce, another system kicks in to synchronize our sleep cycle with our ability to find food.

So they suggest we can adjust our eating schedules to trigger our circadian rhythms to adapt more quickly. "A period of fasting with no food at all for about 16 hours is enough to engage this new clock," says the study's senior author, Dr. Clifford Saper. For example, for a fourteen-hour flight the researchers suggest that you stop eating two hours before flying and continue your anti-jet-lag fast during the entire flight, aiming for a total of sixteen hours. For those who can't go that long without food—especially those prone to fainting—there are other steps to take to ease the transition between time zones while still avoiding that $14.99 dry turkey on dry rye: bring your own nourishing snacks. My own travel kit includes salt-free almonds and walnuts, cut vegetables, and on long flights my favorite: goat cheese and honey-baked turkey in a small container with an ice pack. If you don't have anything to eat, it is going to be much harder to resist the airline's offerings of salty pretzels, chips, and "freshly baked" cookies. And of course the most important thing for me is to continue to drink a lot of water throughout the flight. In fact, depending on the length of the flight, I buy a bottle or two once I get through security, so I'm not dependent on the kindness of the flight attendants.

Or, if you prefer, there's an actual diet for jet lag called the Argonne Anti-Jet-Lag Diet, named for the Argonne National Laboratory near Chicago, where it was formulated by the biologist Charles Ehret. With this method, four days before your trip you alternate two cycles of feasting and fasting, switching every two days, making sure to link up the last fasting day with the day you travel. The diet was tested in 2002 by U.S. National Guard troops going to and from South Korea. The anti-jet-lag group was 16.2 times less likely to experience jet lag on their way home from South Korea than the control group was.

Dr. Charles Czeisler, former chairman of the board of the National Sleep Foundation, raises a red flag about another common travel misstep: starting off already tired. "Most people are usually running around a day or two before their trip," he said, "so they tend to be preloaded with sleep deprivation even before they set foot on the plane, which will further complicate the condition." And try to avoid the aptly named red-eye flights altogether. Instead, Czeisler advises, fly in the afternoon if you're headed west and in the morning if you're going east. "The airlines have finally woken up to this issue," he says, "so there are now plenty of earlier flights to Europe." If you have to take a night flight, he suggests at least trying to get in a nap the day before. "Taking a nap before you're exhausted can actually reduce the adverse effect of being awake at the wrong time of day. This is what we refer to as prophylactic napping."

Not surprisingly, technologies are being created to help us beat jet lag. Researchers at the University of Michigan are developing an app called Entrain, which uses sophisticated math and data analysis to tell users how and when to utilize light to more quickly shift their sleep cycle in a new location. And then there is Re-Timer, an eyeglasses-like piece of headwear that can be used not just by travelers but also by shift workers who need to make regular adjustments to their circadian rhythm, especially in the winter. Worn over the eyes, it exposes the wearer to a simulation of outdoor light, which, when used in the morning, can help reset our body clock so that we can fall asleep at the right bedtime.

Another way to try to beat jet lag is to not adjust to local time at all. "For a quick trip, it probably does not make sense to try to adjust to the new time zone," says Dr. Chris Winter, medical director of Charlottesville Neurology and Sleep Medicine. "Instead, you want to try to do things to make it feel like the trip never happened." Depending on which way you're going, this just means sticking to your home time zone and staying up later or going to bed a few hours before the locals, with corresponding wake-up times. "If you're on vacation, you should ask yourself this question, which many people never bother to do: Is there any reason I should adjust to this new time zone?" asks Czeisler. "People feel compelled to change their routine once they change their wristwatch, but it's not always necessary—and not always a good idea."

My advice, based on what has worked for me through my many travels across multiple time zones, comes down to arranging my schedule so that I have plenty of time for sleep—even if it means building in an extra day for travel. I've talked to many executives who fly around the world and go into meetings exhausted, unable to stay awake; they often end up offending people who may have worked for weeks getting presentations ready for that meeting.

And what about on the plane itself? Though the airlines don't always make it easy, there are some things you can do to at least make sleep more likely. I'm actually a little bit obsessed—okay, totally obsessed—with trying to do everything I can to make my flights more sleep-friendly. That's because I travel so much, and I've learned over time that a little preparation goes a long way. I have my sleeping gear permanently packed in my carry-on: an eye mask, noise-canceling headphones, earplugs, herbal teas (including lavender and licorice), and my favorite neck pillow. I always like to dress comfortably, even if it is a short flight, and I wear only flat shoes when I travel. Why would women wear high heels on a flight? I have seen more than a few sprinting in stilettos through airport terminals, a sight as exotic as seeing an ostrich dash across the savanna.

The difficult truth of air travel is that a great deal of the experience is out of our control. Variables from turbulence and crying babies to chatterbox seatmates and jolting announcements can thwart even the best-laid sleep plans. As Betty Thesky, the author of *Betty in the Sky with a Suitcase*, wisely warned, it helps to set the bar low. "Passengers will often have unrealistic expectations on an all-night flight," she says. "They think, 'I'll sleep on the plane and be ready to hit the ground running' when they land at their destination many time zones away." But given that you don't know how rested you will be when you land, it's best to allow time for some real sleep before you schedule meetings or hit the tourist spots.

11.

SLEEP AND THE WORKPLACE

THE SLEEP revolution is finally hitting the workplace. It's not in full swing yet, but you can see the evidence all around. Of course, it was also in the workplace where sleep first got knocked off its pedestal in the Industrial Revolution. But now the business world is waking up to the high cost of sleep deprivation on productivity, health care, and ultimately the bottom line. We're living in a different time from when *Seinfeld*'s George Costanza had to build a custom "bed-desk" at his office to keep his napping habit a secret. Still, we often define ourselves by our work. And so we reverse-engineer the structure of our non-work lives to conform to our work lives. Because of that, it becomes much easier to change our sleeping habits when we have supportive workplace policies and a business culture that embraces sleep. I expect the nap room to soon become as universal as the conference room.

I'll never forget one morning, before I saw the light, when, completely sleep-deprived and exhausted, I was staggering through a day of back-to-back-to-back meetings. As I walked into a conference room, my eye was drawn to a table running the length of the back wall. I still remember looking at it longingly and wondering whether if I went and lay under it and fell asleep, anyone would notice. At some point in the meeting, I hallucinated that I actually did go over there and lie down—sort of like Schrödinger's Sleep-Deprived Cat. Only at the end of the meeting did I snap to and realize, with great disappointment, that I was still sitting at the conference table.

Some version of this feeling is universal. And pressure to change is coming both from employees, who are realizing that they are actually more productive when they don't drag and drug themselves through the day like workplace zombies, and from employers, who are realizing that healthy employees make for a much healthier bottom line. This link between work burnout and bad sleep was illustrated by a Swedish study that found "higher work demands predicted disturbed sleep, [and] disturbed sleep predicted subsequent higher work demands, perceived stress, less social support, and lower degree of control."

Some of the positive changes in the business world are motivated by the increasing competition for recruitment and retention, and some by business leaders who simply want their companies to succeed while creating a culture that allows their employees to thrive. Whatever the motivation, sleep makes us better at our jobs while simultaneously reminding us that we are more than our jobs.

SLOUCHING TOWARD FLEXIBILITY

Given how much time we spend working—even when we are not physically at work—it's no surprise that work and sleep are so intricately connected. Anything that affects one affects the other. Indeed, work is the number-one reason people cut back on sleep. Sleep is affected not only by how much we work but by when we work. For each hour later that we start work, we gain an average of twenty minutes of sleep.

The truth is, many companies have more flexibility than they realize. A 2015 study found that simply training managers and employees to introduce more flexibility and personal control into work schedules can increase sleep for employees. And workshops about sleep habits and screenings for sleep disorders can lead, as Dr. Carol Ash has said, to "millions of dollars in savings for companies." A 2015 Stanford University study of Chinese workers found that those who worked from home saw their productivity go up by 13 percent. The main reason was less distraction. "Our advice," study authors Nicholas Bloom and John Roberts wrote in the *Harvard Business Review*, "is that firms—at the very least—ought to be open to employees working from home occasionally, to allow them to focus on individual projects and tasks."

Working at home was once primarily associated with freelancers and small side businesses. But more and more big companies are realizing its value. According to the U.S. Census Bureau, more than 13 million people worked at least one day per week at home in 2010—an increase of 45 percent since 1997. In the United Kingdom in 2014, 13.9 percent of all workers worked from home—the highest rate for that country since such data has been collected.

For those still heading into work every day, there are many ways that the office can influence your sleep. A 2014 study by Northwestern University and the University of Illinois at Urbana-Champaign found that employees whose offices had windows got forty-six minutes more sleep every night than coworkers without access to natural light. "There is increasing evidence that exposure to light, during the day—

particularly in the morning—is beneficial to your health via its effects on mood, alertness and metabolism," said study author Dr. Phyllis Zee.

At HuffPost, there was skepticism when we first installed nap rooms in New York in 2011. HuffPosters were reluctant to be seen walking into a nap room in the middle of a bustling newsroom in "the city that never sleeps." But now they are perpetually full, and we're spreading nap rooms around the world, starting with our London office. And more and more companies are installing nap rooms, including Ben & Jerry's, Zappos, and Nike.

Even the tech world, which has been a nerve center for burnout and overwork, is now changing its way. Google's vice president of people development, Karen May, helped build the company's famous employee-friendly work culture. But for all the changes she had implemented and all the scientific studies she'd read about sleep's importance, she kept putting sleep on the back burner in her own life. "Not getting enough sleep," she said, "allowed me to get more work done, say yes more often, and meant that I didn't have to make some of the tough choices between different, important parts of my life." But a couple of years ago, after she and I started talking about sleep over dinner one night, Karen realized that it just wasn't worth it. "When I'm tired," she told me, "I'm grumpy, resentful, and reactive—and that's not how I want to live."

And so here are some of the tips she's developed for getting more and better sleep:

- Focus on quantity. You've got to get the basics first. If you're not in bed longer, you can't get more sleep. For me that meant getting to bed 10 minutes earlier, then another 10, and so on.

- Focus on quality. I found two things made a difference: paying more attention to what I eat and drink in the afternoon and evening (no more afternoon lattes!) and doing something other than work, like sudoku or a crossword puzzle, right before falling asleep.
- Be accountable. It helps to have help. In my case, I had Arianna as my sleep coach. I can picture her talking about the tough choices she's made to get enough sleep and I'm motivated to do the same. And on the delicious mornings when I wake up more rested (okay, not every day) I imagine her smiling and saying, "Oh, good, darling, you've slept!"
- Play the long game. Change is never a straight line, and trying to get more sleep has been no exception. Stuff comes up at work that I want to tackle. I'm with my family and friends, and I don't want to leave the party. Some nights I just don't sleep well—but I remind myself that this is a long game, and little incremental changes add up.

Brian Halligan, the CEO and founder of HubSpot, a maker of marketing and sales software, installed a nap room at the company's office and credits some of his best ideas to napping: "In a given month, I do a lot of very mediocre stuff, but once in a while I come up with a really good idea. Maybe I'll come up with two in a month. Those two inevitably happen when I'm either falling into a nap, or coming out of a nap, or waking up slowly on a Saturday morning. I'm trying to engineer more of those in my life."

It's a philosophy shared by Ryan Holmes, the founder and CEO of Hootsuite, a leading social-media management dashboard (which I use to schedule tweets and Facebook posts when I'm traveling so I can stay connected back home without having to stay up late). Holmes has also installed a nap room, with cots perfect for a midday rest, and he says he sees progress in terms of sleep even among his fellow techies: "Many of the same tech start-ups so notorious for workaholic culture are taking the lead in ensuring employees get adequate shut-eye." This is quite a departure in the tech world, where part of the mythology of start-up narratives is about the endless sleepless nights considered a necessary part of the road-show story.

Shampa Bagchi, the founder and CTO of two enterprise software start-ups in the Bay Area, writes about how easy it is to sacrifice sleep unless you actively prioritize it: "Between managing product releases, juggling multiple client projects, working with teams across two continents and being mom to a schoolgoing girl, life gets busy. And as it always happens in such cases, sleep takes the hit. As the businesses grew, so did my work load, and my sleep hours kept going down. I did not complain, thinking it was necessary, even normal. . . . It doesn't count as real work as long as you enjoy doing it, right? Burnout and exhaustion were for others, for those who do not like what they do. I love my work so I cannot be exhausted, right?"

She had read about the dangers of burnout and had watched a video interview in which I recounted the story of my collapse from exhaustion. But she didn't make the connection to her own life until one night, when everything changed. "I woke up in the middle of the night on the cold bathroom floor wondering how I got there," she writes. "The loud noise I heard was my head crashing on the floor and I could feel the painful bump forming. I did not know how long I lay there unconscious and was clueless on what could have happened to me. But later, as I lay on my bed mentally creating a checklist of all the illnesses I thought I had, that TED Talk of Arianna suddenly popped up in my mind and in that eureka moment I realized that I had the 'Arianna Huffington experience.' I visited the doctor to rule out any health issues, but in my heart I knew that my lifestyle needed a drastic change." Since then she's started getting more sleep and has come to the same realization I did: "I discovered that you don't have to make earth-shattering changes to see the benefits; even small steps matter a lot."

Alicia Hansen, an integrative nutrition health coach living in Australia, had an equally painful wake-up call. "In March 2014," she writes, "I woke up on the cold tiles of my kitchen floor, alone, at midnight. An intense pain throbbed through my cheekbone and head. I could not move, or see." She had fainted from exhaustion and required reconstructive surgery on her cheek and eye. "There are now metal plates holding my cheekbone and eye in place," she writes. "After the surgery I was bedridden for a month and couldn't hold or hug my children. I felt completely helpless." So she, too, made changes in her life: "I reclaimed my rest. Eight hours of sleep every night has become non-negotiable. It makes me more productive, less stressed, able to maintain a healthy metabolism, healthy immune system and gives me more energy and bounce in my step. . . . I feel connected to myself and those around me, and for the first time feel like I am living life on purpose."

And casualties proliferate in the art world, too. Hans Ulrich Obrist, codirector of exhibitions and programs at the Serpentine Galleries in London, was so fascinated by the productivity of Honoré de Balzac, who consumed up to fifty-two cups of coffee a day, that he tried to emulate that extreme way of living and working—until he suffered a total collapse. "I used to consider sleep a waste of time," he told me, "because I have this insatiable curiosity to learn, and I always feel that I don't have enough time to read and to know and to write. But I no longer consider it a waste of time, because now that I sleep, I dream. I understand now that sleep is a necessity, and it's also a necessity to discover your internal clock and then to make the best out of it, rather than try to go against it."

There is hardly a day that goes by when I don't get an email about, or read about, or meet someone who has collapsed from exhaustion and, like me, can't stop talking about the transformative power of sleep. At a lunch in Los Angeles for Jennifer Aniston, her manager, Aleen Keshishian, took me aside. "You see that mark on my nose?" she asked. "What happened to you happened to me. I collapsed from exhaustion and found myself in a pool of blood." So it seems I've managed to become the National Collapsing and Breaking Your Cheekbone Spokesperson—but, as the saying goes, if I can save one cheekbone . . .

When forced to choose, I will not trade even a night's sleep for the chance of extra profits.

—Warren Buffett, 2008 Letter to Shareholders of Berkshire Hathaway

---

Business leaders are now beginning to talk publicly about the role of sleep in making good decisions and growing a business. Sure, there is still plenty of early-morning wake-up-time braggadocio in the business world ("Can you meet for breakfast at 6 a.m.?" "Hey, sounds great, although it's kind of late for me. . . . Tell you what, I'll hit the gym and make a few calls to Europe before I meet you"). But there are more and more business leaders willing to come out about prioritizing sleep, including Microsoft CEO Satya Nadella, who said that he is at his best after eight hours of sleep.

And the changes are happening across the workplace, from CEOs to interns. Goldman Sachs has banned summer interns from staying overnight in the office, limiting working hours from 7 a.m. to midnight (in the finance world, that's progress). The bank has even brought in sleep experts. (And yes, the experts are there to help the bankers sleep more, not less.) There is still a long way to go, but it's clear that even institutions notorious for sleep deprivation are finally recognizing the need for change.

As the head of human resources at LinkedIn, Pat Wadors knows a great deal about productivity. And for her, productivity follows directly from a good night's sleep. "Waking up after eight hours sets me up perfectly for the day ahead," she wrote on HuffPost. "I can bring my best self to the entire day." Since she works in HR, she's also keenly aware of how widespread is the myth that equates sleep deprivation with work dedication. "Trust me, it's not a badge of honor to brag that you can get by on four hours or five each night," she writes. "I've heard that statement too many times. And when I hear that, what I'm really hearing is it's okay for you to harm your health and not perform your best at work or at home."

For Wadors, as for so many of us, sleep hasn't always been a priority, but unlike many of us, she was very aware of the consequences: "Without a good night's rest, I was more emotional, less resilient, less focused, and more impatient.

As a leader—that's not a good thing." So a few years ago, she decided to make sleep a priority. She says she's still figuring it out, but it's working: "I got my eight hours in last night and I feel great! I have energy, I laughed more today, and I was really 'present' to those around me. Most importantly I enjoyed my day. It showed in my smiles and my walk. It is a gift to both me and those around me."

Long before our sleep renaissance began, Amazon CEO Jeff Bezos—ahead of the curve in so many ways—was talking about getting eight hours of sleep. "I'm more alert and I think more clearly," he told *The Wall Street Journal*. "I just feel so much better all day long if I've had eight hours." In the same article, venture capitalist Marc Andreessen talked about the lessons he learned after his sleep-deprived days launching Netscape: "I would spend the whole day wishing I could go home and go back to bed." Now he knows how to get the best out of himself: "I can get by on seven and a half without too much trouble. Seven and I start to degrade. Six is suboptimal. Five is a big problem. Four means I'm a zombie."

Campbell's Soup CEO Denise Morrison is a longtime sleep advocate. "It is essential for me to get eight hours' sleep each night for peak performance—to restore my energy, rest my active brain, and wake up rejuvenated," she told me. Google Chairman Eric Schmidt gets eight and a half hours of sleep a night. As a licensed pilot, he's particularly aware of the dangers of fatigue. And at the health-care company Aetna, CEO Mark Bertolini has become famous for the well-being policies he's instituted. So far, more than thirteen thousand employees have participated in the programs, which include yoga, meditation, and mindfulness training. Employees who have taken part have reduced their stress levels by 28 percent and seen their sleep quality go up by 20 percent.

TECH PROBLEMS, TECH SOLUTIONS

In the age of smartphones, working late of course doesn't necessarily mean staying late at the office. Now we bring our work wherever we go in our pocket or our purse. The fact that the communication device we use for our personal lives is also a portal to our professional lives means it's harder than ever to stop working. Yes, you can always turn it off, but few of us do. Fortunately, policies are being adopted that can help us out.

In Germany, in the hope of inspiring companies across the country, former labor minister Ursula von der Leyen—now the defense minister—established a "crystal-clear" protocol for her staff over the use of work-related phones after hours. "It's in the interests of employers that workers can reliably switch off from their jobs; otherwise, in the long run, they burn out," she said. "Technology should not be allowed to control us and dominate our lives. We should control technology." Following von der Leyen's example, her successor as labor minister, Andrea Nahles, commissioned a study to examine the consequences, from the economic to the psychological, of work-related stress. In the meantime, Nahles has declared her support for legislation banning employers from contacting their employees after work. The German car maker Volkswagen took the step of turning off company email servers thirty minutes after the workday is finished, and other German companies such as BMW and Deutsche Telekom have similar policies.

In a deal between employers' federations and unions, France has established rules to allow employees in digital and consulting companies to turn off their phones after work. Ideally, all these changes won't have to be enforced by law but will come about as corporate cultures continue to evolve.

This new growing global consensus around our need to take time away from our always-on lives has some overlap with the labor-reform movements of the nineteenth and early twentieth centuries. Only now much of the battle isn't just against employers but against our own addiction to our devices and to constant connectivity.

This new labor movement for our digital times still awaits its slogan—its own version of "Eight hours for work, eight hours for rest, eight hours for what we will." If and when it arrives, in all likelihood it will be tweeted, Instagrammed, and Snapchatted. "Workers of the world, unplug! Workers of the world, recharge!"

We can all take steps in our own lives to accelerate this shift, but to really scale it requires change at the top. Boards of directors need to acknowledge that a CEO who's bragging about getting only four hours of sleep a night is essentially saying that he or she is making decisions while drunk. They need to see that that's not something to be applauded or rewarded. In fact, it's a massive red flag.

When venture capitalists and angel investors hear prospective pitches, along with plans for how viable and sustainable a business product is, they should also be aggressively vetting the start-up team's plans for how to keep their lives sustainable. Maybe we need a *Shark Tank* for that. I'm in!

12.

FROM HOLLYWOOD AND WASHINGTON TO HOSPITALS AND HOTELS

DISCOVERING THE POWER OF SLEEP

YET ANOTHER sign that sleep is becoming fashionable is how it's being embraced by those who *decide* what's fashionable: the fashion industry. And it makes sense that an industry dedicated to helping you look good would find its way to one of the most effective tools we have to make us both feel better and look better.

For actors, models, and entertainers, taking care of themselves is part of their work regimen. And sleep is at the heart of it. No matter how you feel about celebrities or a culture that obsesses over their every personal and professional move, their appreciation for sleep and its benefits is one thing their fans could emulate. Of course, their success gives them resources that most can't afford, but the fact remains: we can all take some steps to prioritize sleep in our lives.

Bobbi Brown, the founder of Bobbi Brown Cosmetics, is very aware of the value of sleep. While she wakes up early, at 6 a.m., she also goes to bed early. "Sleep and rest and happiness and healthy living make you your prettiest," she writes.

Supermodel Karlie Kloss agrees. "Sleep," she says, is "the best and most generous thing you can do for yourself. Sleep is such a big part of one's beauty." Asked how she maintains her health and looks, Cindy Crawford has said, "If I look back over 25 years, for sure it starts with sleep. . . . Sleep is when your body restores itself."

Christina Aguilera says that "people spend money on beauty potions, but a good night's rest makes all the difference," while reality star–turned–fashion designer Lauren Conrad says that "there's a reason they call it 'beauty sleep.' Getting 7 to 9 hours of sleep a night can actually improve your appearance." Gwyneth Paltrow calls sleep a "major thing" in her life. "I don't always get it," she says, "and when I don't, I look like I've been hit by a truck."

And if tonight my soul may find her peace
in sleep, and sink in good oblivion,
and in the morning wake like a new-opened flower
then I have been dipped again in God, and new-created.

—D. H. Lawrence, "Shadows"

"Sleep is my weapon. . . . I try to get eight hours a night," said Jennifer Lopez. "I think sometimes we get caught up in what we need to do next and forget about what are the very essential and important things in life. I treasure my time to sleep. It's just as important as eating or exercise." Beyoncé's "definition of beauty" is "having peace, happiness and healthiness. And you can't have any of that without sleep." Jane Fonda credits her age-defying looks to sleep. "It's not a secret formula," she says. "I make sure I get eight or nine hours' sleep a night."

In *The Body Book*, Cameron Diaz writes that her travel-heavy schedule taught her how essential nighttime rituals are: "I don't keep any electronics in my bedroom. I wear a sleep mask. And I need a dark, quiet space. Because sleep is when my body powers down so that it can restore, repair, and replenish. When I get enough sleep, my memory is sharper. I can focus. And my body is more capable."

In *Yes Please*, Amy Poehler puts it all into perspective. "Sleep can completely change your entire outlook on life," she writes. "One good night's sleep can help you realize that you shouldn't break up with someone, or you are being too hard on your friend, or you actually will win the race or the game or get the job. Sleep helps you win at life."

THE POLITICS OF SLEEP: WE HOLD OUR SLEEP TO BE SELF-EVIDENT

In 1940, President Franklin D. Roosevelt did something that would be inconceivable in today's political climate. To think through the monumental question of whether America should enter the war, he announced that he would be taking a ten-day vacation, sailing around the Caribbean on a navy ship. A letter from his wife, Eleanor, read, "I think of you sleeping and eating and I hope getting rest from the world."

As Roosevelt's aide Harry Hopkins later said, "I began to get the idea that he was refueling, the way he so often does when he seems to be resting and carefree." The result of Roosevelt's refueling was the $50 billion Lend-Lease program, in which the United States would lend arms and supplies to Great Britain and be paid back after the war in kind. As Roosevelt's speechwriter Robert Sherwood put it, "One can only say that FDR, a creative artist in politics, had put in his time on this cruise evolving the pattern of a masterpiece."

In 2012, when Hillary Clinton stepped down as secretary of state—having flown more than 900,000 miles to 112 different countries and, possibly even more taxing, having sat in 1,700 meetings with world leaders—she discussed her immediate plans with *The New York Times*' Gail Collins. "I just want to sleep and exercise and travel for fun," she said. "And relax. It sounds so ordinary, but I haven't done it for 20 years. I would like to see whether I can get untired." What a great word—"untired."

Further proof that sleep can make a difference in politics comes from another highly placed source, her husband Bill Clinton, himself famous for running on very little sleep during his presidency. Looking back, though, in a *Daily Show* appearance in 2007, he saw the power of sleep. "I do believe sleep deprivation has a lot to do with some of the edginess of Washington today," he said. "You have no idea how many Republican and Democratic members of the House and Senate are chronically sleep-deprived."

Politics, of course, is the ultimate sleep-deprivation machine. Much of what our political leaders face is out of their control. But that is all the more reason to optimize the factors that *are* in their control. The most basic one is to improve their decision making by getting enough sleep. Will it instantly solve the world's problems? Of course not. But will our leaders be better prepared to face those problems with more creativity and wisdom? Without a doubt.

PAGING DR. SANDMAN: HOW OUR HOSPITALS MAKE US SICK

Given that lack of sleep can make us sick and that not getting enough sleep when we are sick makes it harder to get better, it's surprising that hospitals have taken so long to come around. Our medical system is brimming with the latest technology and the most advanced medical equipment. But for too long, one of our most powerful healing tools has been completely overlooked.

If you've ever spent a few nights in the hospital, you know how hard it is to get a good night's sleep in one—with the cacophony of alarms, beeps, and buzzes, complete with glaring lights and shift changes, requiring a groggy, sleep-deprived patient to answer important questions in the middle of the night. All this on top of the pain and discomfort caused by the actual illness or injury that landed you in the hospital in the first place.

The World Health Organization, recognizing this as a health issue, recommends that the average hospital room's noise level not exceed 30 decibels. Yet studies have shown that many if not most hospitals regularly create a din far exceeding that. In 2014, researchers from Oxford found that the noise levels in the intensive care units surveyed went higher than 85 decibels. That's about the noise level of a passing motorcycle or a nearby jackhammer. And noise at that level would occur up to sixteen times per hour during the night. In a University of Chicago study, overnight hospital noise peaked at levels equal to that of a chainsaw. Welcome to the hospital, where we've created a healing environment that's a cross between an active construction site and a horror movie.

The consequences of this go well beyond an increase in the normal irritation and grogginess from getting a bad night's sleep. Poor sleep undermines recovery. A 2013 study by researchers at Johns Hopkins University found that poor sleep can cause patients in the intensive care unit to experience delirium. And University of Chicago researchers found that for each hour of sleep lost due to high noise levels, patients experienced an increase in their blood pressure of up to six points.

Thankfully, more hospitals are finding creative ways to put sleep into their top-line medical arsenal. St. Luke's Hospital in New York City, for example, launched a noise-reduction program in response to low patient-satisfaction scores on sleep. A key aspect was educating staff on how noise and disrupted sleep can lead to high stress levels, confusion, and cardiac problems. Noise levels were checked six times a day, and sound monitors modeled after traffic lights were installed to increase awareness of noise. Staff distributed earplugs to patients, installed door stoppers, turned down television and telephone volumes, and implemented "quiet times" for certain units. After the program, patient satisfaction went from the 2nd percentile (it's hard to get much lower) to the 95th percentile.

At Johns Hopkins Hospital, doctors and staff made a concerted effort to reduce nighttime noise in the ICU with a checklist for staff, which included things such as dimming hallway and room lights, more thoughtful scheduling of nighttime medical visits to the rooms, and turning off televisions. In 2009, Stanford Hospital launched the "SHHH" system, which stands for Silent Hospitals Help Healing, with each floor assigned a "noise champion" to reduce noise in the area, while the "Too Loud" initiative at Newark Beth Israel Medical Center in New Jersey offers a Noise Hotline that patients can call when noise levels are excessive.

At the Department of Veterans Affairs in New Jersey, a partnership with Planetree—a nonprofit dedicated to helping health-care providers deliver patient-centered care—starts with interviewing incoming patients about their sleep habits and giving them a "sleep menu," which lists a selection of sleep tools (eye masks, earplugs, white-noise machines, aromatherapy, and heated blankets) to choose from. These small, cost-effective changes can significantly improve patient sleep and health. As Orfeu Buxton, a professor of biobehavioral health at Penn State, put it, "Sleep is such a powerful source of resilience. . . . We need to begin grouping sleep with all the other things we do to make patients better."

The improvements in the hospital system have extended to doctors themselves. In May 2015 a patient at a hospital in Mexico took a picture of a doctor sleeping at her desk during the overnight shift and posted it on a blog. The picture went viral, and doctors around the world jumped on the bandwagon, snapping photos of one another sleeping while at work with the hashtag #YoTambienMeDormi ("I've also fallen asleep"), promoting awareness of the profession's challenging schedules.

AWAKE AT THE WHEEL

Given that, as we learned in the Crisis chapter, 60 percent of adults in the United States admit to driving while drowsy, the American Academy of Sleep Medicine launched "Awake at the Wheel," a campaign to promote education among drivers about the importance of sleep. And in the United Kingdom, drivers pass by signs on the highways reading "Tiredness Can Kill, Take a Break." Researchers at Clemson University in South Carolina are exploring using GPS technology to detect car deviations associated with drowsy driving. And similar technology is already making its way onto our roads. The Ford Fusion sounds an alarm if it detects the car going out of its lane, and Mercedes' "Attention Assist" tracks the driver's technique at the start of the trip and compares it to driving behavior later. If there is substantial deviation, it will indicate that the driver needs a rest. As Dr. Nathaniel Watson, the president of the American Academy of Sleep Medicine, said, "Drowsy driving is deadly, but it's also completely avoidable."

BEYOND "DO NOT DISTURB": HOTELS AND THE SLEEP REVOLUTION

If you really want to see what a society values, look to the marketplace. So for the clearest evidence of the sleep revolution, there may be no better example than the intensifying competition among hotels to see which hotel brand can deliver the best sleep experience. It wasn't always this way.

With the rise of hotels catering to business travelers in the last several decades, the strategic play was to try to outdo the competition with luxury amenities—the fitness center, the business center, the Wi-Fi, the robes, the concierges. Or it was all about fostering a booming social scene with a hopping bar and a high-end, famous-chef restaurant.

All that's great, but there's a reason we measure hotel stays by the night—what most guests actually want is a good night's sleep. We can find a gym or a great meal someplace else; what we can't get outside the hotel when traveling is sleep. According to John Timmerman, the chief scientist for customer experience and innovation at Gallup, a comfortable bed is one of the most sought-after features in hotels at every level. "Given that almost one out of three guests is willing to pay a premium for an enhanced bed experience," he says, "hotel brands should first evaluate if they are consistently delivering a comfortable bed experience before upgrading far less critical product attributes like a new guestroom clock-radio or bathroom amenity."

Hotels are finally getting the message, with the industry focusing its attention on the new holy grail: sleep. Options for sleep-obsessed travelers now go well beyond the classic request to be on a high floor and away from the elevators.

One of the most innovative establishments on the sleep front is the Benjamin Hotel in New York City. The Benjamin has a sleep concierge and has brought in Cornell University sleep researcher Rebecca Robbins to give the hotel's staff seminars on how to provide guests with the best sleep possible. "We're in the business of sleep," Robbins says. And for an additional fee, she offers personal sleep consultations.

The array of sleep-inducing amenities includes the choice of several pillows, ranging from one that plays lullaby music and one for pregnant guests to one for the back sleeper and one for the side sleeper; the complementary Winks' Kidzzz Club children can join, which gives them a pillow and a bathrobe, bedtime books, and a sleep certificate at checkout; and the work-down call, which is my favorite feature. This is sort of the opposite of a wake-*up* call—the front desk rings you to tell you that if you're going to make your bedtime on time, you need to start wrapping things up. And then they even offer tips for how to wind down.

After all, there are few appointments throughout the day that are as important as bedtime. (And if the word "bedtime" sounds childish or embarrassing, feel free not to use it, but remember, there's nothing childish or embarrassing about being well rested.) Yet our appointment with sleep is one we don't seem to mind missing, day after day, night after night. When we think of sleep as an actual appointment—a meeting of sorts, with ourselves—we're much more likely to grant it the time it deserves. Given that we now set alarms on our smartphones and smartwatches for things of much less importance, the work-down call is a great idea to adopt.

> *I opened the bed fastidiously, lay into the middle of it, closed it up again carefully and let out a sigh of happiness and rest. I felt as if all my weariness and perplexities of the day had descended on me pleasurably like a great heavy quilt which would keep me warm and sleepy. My knees opened up like rosebuds in rich sunlight, pushing my shins two inches further to the bottom of the bed. Every joint became loose and foolish and devoid of true utility.*
>
> —FLANN O'BRIEN, *The Third Policeman*

Other hotels, including the Four Seasons, the InterContinental, and the Marriott, have embraced sleep as well, and I've provided a longer list in Appendix C. Of course, we still have a long way to go—most of the special features and offerings are available only at higher-end hotels and spas, while the need for sleep is universal. So I look forward to the day when features that promote a good night's sleep for travelers at all levels are as standard as television and air-conditioning.

13.

THE SPORTS WORLD'S ULTIMATE PERFORMANCE ENHANCER

AS THE definition of fitness has expanded beyond how much you can lift, how fast you can run, or how far you can go, the modern gym has come to be about more than just exercise. Trainers today know that recovery is a critical element of successful training, allowing you to come back stronger. And recovery is about more than cooling down after stepping off the treadmill—it is, in a very big way, about sleep.

Equinox is working with researchers at UCLA to explore how sleep and fitness are connected. "The Equinox core philosophy," Liz Miersch, editor-in-chief of *Q by Equinox*, told me, "is that training alone is not enough. The best results are driven through a combination of proper movement, nutrition and regeneration—the key component of which is adequate sleep."

And when I visited SoulCycle, a fitness center famous for its intense spin classes, I was amazed by how committed the instructors were to sleep as part of a complete healthy routine. "The body is super busy repairing muscle and tissues and replacing dead cells while we're sleeping, and for athletes that time is crucial," said instructor Kym Perfetto. "The harder I train, the more sleep I need." Sue Molnar, another cycling instructor, constantly talks to her riders about the importance of quality sleep. "It is everything," she said. "We live in New York City. We work hard, play hard, eat and drink hard, exercise hard. We *need* to have the rejuvenation of a good night's sleep."

Joey Gonzalez, the CEO of Barry's Bootcamp, agrees. "Eating well and working well are incomplete without sleeping well," he says. And this more complete definition of fitness is spreading quickly.

REST, RESTORATION, RESULTS

Since sleep is often bundled with practices such as meditation and mindfulness, to many people it still has the feeling of something vaguely new-agey and "alternative." This perception exists despite the fact that (as with the latest findings on meditation and mindfulness) the data behind it is being supplied by the very non-new-agey, evidence-based, peer-reviewed world of science. Perhaps those who equate sleep with laziness or lack of dedication can be convinced of the benefits of sleep by looking at what's going on in a world that is the ultimate in pragmatism, where performance and winning are everything: sports. To professional athletes, sleep is not about spirituality, work-life balance, or even health and well-being; it's all about performance. It's about what works, about using every available tool to increase the chances of winning.

And by looking at these results, we can see exactly what works and what doesn't. So when it comes to new performance tools involving sleep, the sports world is like a massive lab experiment, one with a huge and ever-expanding data set from which to draw conclusions.

Those at the leading edge of the sports world have concluded that sleep is the ultimate performance-enhancing drug—one that comes with only positive side effects. And much of this is, of course, about recovery. "Just as athletes need more calories than most people when they're in training, they need more sleep, too," said sports medicine specialist Dr. David Geier. "You're pushing your body in practice, so you need more time to recover." The power of sleep in the animal kingdom is exemplified by the cheetah. It's the fastest land animal on earth—able to accelerate from zero to sixty miles per hour in just three seconds—and yet it also spends up to eighteen hours a day sleeping.

The sports and fitness worlds were slow to recognize the benefits of sleep. For those whose performance is all about movement, activity, and alertness, the idea that there could be an advantage to be gained in increasing the time spent being inactive was not obvious. That's why, until pretty recently, sleep was considered lost time—time that couldn't be spent training and practicing.

For college and professional football coaches—alpha males in a macho sport—sleep deprivation has long been a way of life. In his book, *Do You Love Football?!: Winning with Heart, Passion, and Not Much Sleep*, Jon Gruden, the youngest head coach in the NFL to win a Super Bowl at the time, attributes his achievements to sleeping only four hours per night. He boasts that he is "actually one of the older coaches in football history" if you "factor in the alert, non-sleep hours." Coach George Allen of the Washington Redskins was among the first NFL coaches to sleep night after night in his office. He put in a sixteen-hour coaching workday and once said, "Leisure time is the five or six hours when you sleep at night."

What these coaches didn't realize was that they were selling themselves short: they were most likely winning *in spite of*, rather than because of, not sleeping. Fortunately, more and more coaches, athletes, and trainers today recognize that sleep is an essential part of the winning combination. You can be as tough as nails and practice twelve hours a day, but if you disregard sleep, you'll dilute the effectiveness of all that practice. And what they're finding on the field and on the court is being backed up by what's going on in the labs.

THE COMPETITIVE EDGE

Cheri Mah, of the Stanford Sleep Disorders Clinic and Research Laboratory, is one of the foremost researchers exploring the connection between sports and sleep. In 2002, Mah was leading a study about the effects of sleep on cognitive performance. Some of the participants, who were put on a sleep schedule designed to compensate for sleep debt, also happened to be on the Stanford swimming team. And their results went past cognitive performance. "Several collegiate swimmers walked into the lab with wide grins," Mah told me, "having set multiple personal records."

As a result, Mah's focus began to shift. The negative consequences of sleep deprivation, she told me, had been well researched. But she became intrigued by the opposite question—"investigating the potential benefits of getting extra sleep, and whether improving sleep patterns can positively impact functioning and enhance performance."

She began running studies and found that "multiple weeks of sleep extension significantly reduces athletes' accumulated sleep debt and results in faster reaction time, decreased fatigue levels as well as improved athletic performance measures."

One of her most widely cited studies was published in 2011. Mah had eleven members of the Stanford basketball team wear sleep sensors for two weeks. She recorded their normal sleep patterns—they averaged just more than six and a half hours each night—along with statistics on sprints, free throws, and three-point shots. Then, for five to seven weeks, she had them aim for a minimum of ten hours in bed each night, spending as much of the time as possible asleep ("sleep extension," as it's called). The players' sleep average went up to eight and a half hours, and the increases in performance were dramatic. Sprint times were .7 seconds faster, free-throw shooting went up by 9 percent, and three-point shooting increased by 9.2 percent. That's an amazing difference for such elite athletes—and all achieved just by sleeping more. Ask any athletes you know if they're interested in shaving nearly a second off their sprint time or increasing their performance in any category by nearly 10 percent, and you'll have their attention. The study also had participants report their mood, which improved significantly as well.

Mah conducted another study to test the effects of sleep extension on Stanford football players. She found that average times for a twenty-yard shuttle sprint went from 4.71 seconds to 4.61 seconds, and average 40-yard-dash times went from 4.99 to 4.89 seconds. The players' level of daytime grogginess went down, and their vigor went up. "Some sports teams are beginning to realize there are untapped benefits in improving their athletes' sleep," Mah told me.

"Applying findings from sleep research can provide a competitive edge."

Chris Winter says he became interested in the topic as a way of getting ordinary people to take sleep more seriously. "I thought if I can get a pro athlete to really value sleep, his or her fans might do the same," he told me. It certainly worked on the athletes. "Players learn that the hours spent in the bedroom lay the foundation for their physical improvement and nutritional goals," he said.

He's been so successful at showing the connections between performance and sleep that he's now a sought-after consultant for many college and professional teams. In fact, that's one of the reasons he doesn't publish some of his research. "Teams view what I do as a way to gain an advantage and do not want to give that advantage away," he explained.

DON'T TAKE IT FROM ME: TOP ATHLETES ON WHY THEY PRIORITIZE SLEEP

One of the teams leading the way in capitalizing on that advantage is the Seattle Seahawks, who won the Super Bowl in 2013 and came within two yards of repeating their victory in 2014. Head coach Pete Carroll is known as much for his innovation off the field as on it. "When it comes to the precision and science of sleep for optimal performance," Carroll told me, "we've been fortunate to work with experts to help guide us on both the physical and mental strategies to enhance our recovery process."

Two of the experts leading his science team are Sam Ramsden, the team's director of player health and performance, and Michael Gervais, the director of high-performance psychology at the DISC Sports & Spine Center. Together, they educate both players and coaches on the importance of sleep. "Fatigue and performance are intimately linked," they told me, "and sleep is one of the important variables to get right to help athletes sustain high effort and enthusiasm for the long haul."

This isn't news to the New England Patriots' quarterback Tom Brady, who managed to beat the Seahawks in the last Super Bowl—and win the MVP title. Brady goes to bed at 8:30 p.m. and is still managing to play at the highest level even as he approaches forty. "The decisions that I make always center around performance enhancement," he says. "I want to be the best I can be every day."

The Chicago Bears are employing a similar strategy. Their sport-science coordinator, Jennifer Gibson, teaches players how to develop good sleep habits and proper napping techniques as a way to maximize performance, and provides them with memory-foam mattresses during training camp. Pro Bowl guard Kyle Long has become an enthusiastic sleep advocate. "Getting that eight, nine hours is just as important as weightlifting and studying your playbook," he says. "I can know all the plays like the back of my hand. I can lift all the weights in the world. But if I get five, six hours of sleep, I'm going to have that doubt in my head and that sluggish nature, and you can't have that when you're trying to block these elite guys. I'd absolutely say sleep is a weapon."

As former NBA All-Star Grant Hill put it, "People talk about diet and exercise," but "sleep is just as important." Four-time NBA MVP LeBron James swears by twelve hours a day when practicing. And two-time NBA MVP Steve Nash believes that "napping every game day, whether you feel like it or not, not only has a positive effect on your performance that night but also a cumulative effect on your body throughout the season." Professional triathlete Jarrod Shoemaker describes sleep as "half my training," while Usain Bolt, the world's fastest man, explains, "Sleep is extremely important to me—I need to rest and recover in order for the training I do to be absorbed by my body." Volleyball player Kerri Walsh Jennings, a three-time Olympic gold-medal winner, admits that sleep "could be the hardest thing to accomplish on my to-do list, but it always makes a difference." And tennis great Roger Federer trumps them all. "If I don't sleep eleven to twelve hours a day, it's not right," he says. "If I don't have that amount of sleep, I hurt myself." Before Wimbledon in 2015, he even rented two houses: one for his family to sleep in and one for him (and his training team), so the family activities wouldn't wake him.

This recognition of sleep's impact on performance is now a worldwide phenomenon. In the United Kingdom, the Southampton soccer club has its own sleep app, which players use each morning to log the previous night's sleep. If a player's sleep-quality level drops, team officials will intervene. The Manchester City soccer club has a new £200 million training center that includes eighty bedrooms. The team sleeps in the training center the night before home matches—a recognition by the coaching staff that sleep isn't just for training but an integral part of game-day preparation.

Nick Littlehales, a sleep coach for Manchester United as well as other top soccer clubs, rugby teams, and the UK cycling team, will often go to a venue ahead of the players to make changes to their hotel rooms. "I have been preparing with various teams for the 2016 Rio games," he told me, "and a key part of that is ensuring the hotels being used in the run-up to the games are ticking all of our recovery boxes."

At the college level, making the sleep/performance link is even more important, since the athletes are younger and even more likely to be in the "I'll sleep when I'm dead" phase of life. A 2015 *Wall Street Journal* headline read, "College Football Wakes Up to a New Statistic: Sleep." Pat Fitzgerald, the head football coach for Northwestern University, noticed in 2012 that many of his players seemed especially tired during afternoon games. It turns out the reason was that the games occurred right when his players were used to taking afternoon naps. So he started a policy of mandatory game-day naps. That year the team won ten games, for only the third time in the history of Northwestern football. "At first, we didn't really know much about sleep and we were just curious," then–defensive end Tyler Scott said. "But we really embraced it, and after a while, we got really competitive about sleep efficiency. We started checking our data every day."

Other teams are taking note. At their 2015 training camp, University of Tennessee football coach Butch Jones introduced his team to a new part of their practice routine—sleep trackers and sleep coaches. The team worked with Rise Science, which helps athletes improve performance through sleep. They paired each athlete with a sleep coach and monitored everything—from the amount of time players sleep to how long it takes them to fall asleep to the quality of their sleep—with the results sent directly to a smartphone app. The players also wear orange-tinted glasses an hour before they go to bed to help eliminate the blue light from screens that can disrupt sleep. "It was very powerful to see the cultural shift at the University," said cofounder Leon Sasson. "It went from who can sleep less and still do well at practice to it being cool if you show up to practices with nine-plus hours of sleep under your belts."

At the University of Pittsburgh, coach Pat Narduzzi makes sure his players get enough sleep by coming into their dorms and tucking them in at night himself! "We've got lights out at 10:30 and bed check at 10:45 every night, so we're trying to get them down early. . . . We can't close their eyes at night for them, but you can see it on the field that I think our kids are getting better rest."

PEAK PERFORMANCE, IN EVERY TIME ZONE

The link between sleep and performance isn't just about getting enough sleep in the days or weeks before a game. It is also about the connection between game time and players' body clocks. Fans tend to think of home-field advantage as mostly about the cheering crowds and familiar surroundings. But a bigger advantage might be that the away team's body clocks are often out of whack. No matter how well a team manages its sleep at home, travel can undercut that performance advantage.

This is one of the focal points of Chris Winter's work. The conventional thinking in sleep medicine is that it takes about twenty-four hours to normalize your body clock for each time zone you cross. To test that, Winter and his colleagues retroactively analyzed every Major League Baseball game over a ten-season period (more than twenty-four thousand games), assigning each team a measure of how jet-lagged they should be, and then used that data to predict, as the study put it, the "magnitude and direction of circadian advantage." In short, as Winter told me, "Basically, we proved what hardcore gamblers have probably known for years . . . travel impairs performance!"

A study from Vanderbilt University backs this up. Researchers studied thirty Major League Baseball teams over the course of the season. From April to September, "plate discipline"—a batter's ability to judge which pitches are worth swinging at—declined. For the baseball illiterate, like myself, let me offer a translation: the more tired the players were, the more likely they were to swing at bad pitches. "This decline is tied to fatigue that develops over the course of the season due to a combination of frequency of travel and paucity of days off," concluded lead author Dr. Scott Kutscher. So it's a kind of cumulative jet lag. But as Kutscher says, "A team that recognizes this trend and takes steps to slow or reverse it by enacting fatigue-mitigating strategies . . . can gain a large competitive advantage."

Winter has been working with the San Francisco Giants and their head athletic trainer, Dave Groeschner, since 2009. Together, they work to adjust the team's travel schedule to minimize sleep disruption. Sometimes this means having the team spend another night in the hotel after the game, instead of jetting back home right away and arriving in the early hours of the morning. "What we're trying to do is create a situation where their brain is being tricked into thinking that whatever time the game is happening, it's 4 o'clock in the afternoon," Winter said. "That's when those athletes are at their best." Peak physical performance and the lowest risk of injury usually occur between 3 p.m. and 6 p.m., according to Michael Smolensky, a leading chronobiologist. (By the way, that's my favorite title among the sleep researchers I've met. But there's still some fertile ground to be plowed. How about dozologist? Somnusist? A superhero named Siestor who puts people into REM sleep? Maybe for an action-movie franchise?) Since Winter started consulting for the Giants, they've won three World Series—2010, 2012, and 2014.

The Seattle Mariners baseball team has brought high-tech solutions to the travel problem. The team has a clear geographical disadvantage. In 2013, the Mariners flew more than 52,000 miles for their away games, while the centrally based Chicago White Sox flew less than half that—only 23,000 miles. In 2014, the Mariners began wearing sleep-monitoring devices, Readibands, produced by a local company called Fatigue Science. The Readibands monitor the players' sleep rhythms, and the data are then combined with their sports statistics, all of which is then factored into team decisions on scheduling.

A 2015 study by researchers from the University of Birmingham in the United Kingdom explored the connection between the natural rhythms of athletes' body clocks, their relative performance, and the time of day of a competition. Participants were grouped according to their body clocks, into larks (morning people), owls (late-night people), and those in the middle. When tested at the worst times for them (i.e., for an owl, during the morning), there was a 26 percent decrease in performance. "If you're an early type in a competition in the evening," said lead author Roland Brandstaetter, "then you're impaired, so you could adjust sleeping times to the competition." Using these findings, Brandstaetter now does what he calls "circadian coaching" for athletes.

For athletes, sleep isn't just about performance but also about staying in the sport over the long haul. Major League Baseball players who were fatigued were almost twice as likely to leave the sport early than their more rested teammates. "For players who want to have long, lucrative careers,"

Winter told me, "ignoring healthy sleep is not the way to go about it!"

LEARNING FROM THE PROS: CREATING A WINNING SLEEP ROUTINE

For elite athletes, the consequences of sleep deprivation become very obvious very quickly—they're literally tallied up on a scoreboard. Imagine for a moment if we all had this as an incentive. Or, worse, if sports announcers were broadcasting play-by-play color commentary on our every move:

"Well, Bob, Arianna is here at work, but she seems to be moving very slowly. She's operating on only five hours of sleep."

"And she's opened her first email. The workday has officially begun."

"But look, Bob, she's already distracted—before even reading one email she's switched over to a funny cat video."

"And what's this? She's already reaching for her second coffee."

"Bob, it's astonishing. It'll be a miracle if she can get through the morning, much less the day. But let me tell you, this crowd is ready to see what she's got."

"She's flagging, Don. She's really got to be kicking herself right now for not getting enough sleep last night."

"Clearly, she didn't bring her A-game, Bob. You have to wonder if ownership will be looking to make a change here."

"Unbelievable!"

Thankfully, we don't all live in the sports-world fishbowl and can course-correct without pundits weighing in. But athletes also face the same challenges we all face. During the 2014–15 NBA season, Jason Smith played with the New York Knicks, having just been acquired from the New Orleans Pelicans. He was eager to prove himself, but as the season began, his wife, Kristy, gave birth to their first child, Ella Rose. He described their new daughter as a blessing, but he soon found out that newborns don't exactly respect the demands of a grueling NBA schedule. "The first couple of weeks it was a lot of sleep deprivation, for sure," Smith said. He was getting five or six hours a night, often in two-hour chunks or less. At practice the next morning, he'd stagger in, "eyes glazed, just tired as can be."

Not surprisingly, his job performance suffered. He had shot 46.5 percent and averaged 9.7 points a game for New Orleans the previous season. But in the sleep-deprived first half of the season with the Knicks, he shot just 42 percent and scored an average of 7 points per game (while also playing fewer minutes). "Sleep deprivation . . . is one of the hardest things to go through when you're trying to perform at your highest level," he said.

By mid-January, Ella Rose had mercifully begun sleeping longer at night. And as her sleep time increased, so did her dad's shooting average, which rose to 11 points per game, while his assists per game jumped from 1.1 to 3.8. There are no doubt many lessons still to come from Ella Rose, but she's certainly taught her dad the value of sleep.

POSTING YOUR OWN BEST SLEEP STATS

The Golden State Warriors' Andre Iguodala also makes sleep a priority. But it wasn't always that way. Iguodala's old sleep routine didn't leave much room for actual sleep: he'd stay up late watching TV and then wake early to hit the gym. On game days he'd try to make up for it with three- or four-hour naps, but the sleep debt could not be repaid.

The pattern went on for years until, just before he turned thirty, Iguodala told Keke Lyles, Golden State's director of performance, that he needed to see a sleep therapist. And so his sleep journey began: he moved his devices out of the bedroom, set his thermostat to a cool, sleep-friendly temperature, and started wearing a Jawbone UP to track his sleep. During the season, he begins winding down at 11:15 p.m. He stretches, does deep breathing, reads for a few minutes, and is asleep by midnight. And he wakes up recharged. As he put it, "Sleep good, feel good, play good."

When Iguodala adjusted to a consistent eight hours of sleep a night, his points per minute went up 29 percent, his free-throw percentage increased by 8.9 percent, his three-point-shot percentage more than doubled, his turnovers decreased 37 percent per game, and his fouls dropped by an astounding 45 percent. He was named the 2015 Finals MVP, and he Instagrammed a picture of himself holding the MVP award—credit where credit is due—while sleeping!

For my Thrive e-course on Oprah.com, I invited basketball great Kobe Bryant of the Los Angeles Lakers to be my unlikely guest teacher on sleep. "I've grown," Bryant said. "I used to get by on three or four hours a night. I have a hard time shutting off my brain. But I've evolved. I'm up to six to eight hours now." His bedtime routine these days is a hot shower, and after that he turns the phone off. "You know the other major thing about sleep?" he says. "It gives me more energy to spend time with my family and have fun with my kids. As I got more rest, I could work and come home—and become the human jungle gym again."

Sleep is clearly the next innovation frontier in sports. And that's a good thing, because sports exert a powerful hold on American culture. Athletes speak to something aspirational in us. So the behaviors they exemplify—how they take care of their bodies, how they recharge, and how they go about performing at their best—matter. If future versions of ad campaigns telling us to "Be like Mike" were to send a message on the vital importance of getting enough sleep, it could help teach the next generation that health and fitness are impossible without that firm foundation. Imagine if NBA stars didn't just have a signature pair of sneakers but a signature pillow or alarm clock or eye mask!

Perhaps a star athlete will soon become the public face of this new revolution. Until then, sleep is the not-so-secret all-natural recipe for those seeking a performance edge. And it makes just as big a difference for us as for the pros.

14.

PUTTING TECHNOLOGY IN ITS PLACE (NOT ON YOUR NIGHTSTAND)

THE UBIQUITY of technology and its addictive nature have made it much harder for us to disconnect and go to sleep, but the news about technology and sleep is far from all bad. As technology has spread into nearly every corner of our lives, it's also begun to turn inward, expanding its reach beyond helping us connect with the world to helping us connect with ourselves. That's the new frontier of tech—not outward but inward.

At tech conferences throughout the world, the big chatter now is all about wearable technology and the "Internet of Things." The global wearables market is predicted to grow 35 percent a year between 2015 and 2019, with 148 million devices expected to be shipped in 2019. One in five Americans already owns some kind of wearable device. A big percentage of these are fitness trackers, which have been growing in popularity by the day, especially with the introduction of smartwatches. As technology has expanded what we can learn about our fitness, so, too, has our notion of fitness. And for the first time, sleep is a part of that.

We're never going to banish technology from our lives. Nor would we want to. But what we can do is get the best out of technology—and there is now plenty of it out there that promises to improve our sleep. The range of options is wide—from apps designed to help us sleep, to a universe of sleep-centric hardware like noise-blocking headphones, smart earplugs and lightbulbs that mimic the natural light of sunset and sunrise. Crowdfunding sites such as Kickstarter and Indiegogo have been a major boon to sleep entrepreneurs, with new products routinely shattering fund-raising goals. Meanwhile, entire industries—such as the mattress and bedding industries—are being disrupted, with nimble start-ups hammering the old guard.

My personal sleep revolution, which started nine years ago, did not involve any sleep-tracking devices, so I'm living proof you can make changes and get the sleep you need without them. But here are some to try out. In fact, another start-up, Lumoid, can send you five to try for a nominal fee.

Technology has given us an unprecedented ability to learn more about ourselves, and there is a widespread hunger to track how we sleep. According to a 2015 study by Sleep Number, 43 percent of respondents said they had tracked their workouts and 41 percent had tracked their diet. Only 16 percent had tracked their sleep, but look for that number to rise, since 58 percent wished they knew more about how to track and get better sleep.

James Proud is the founder and CEO of Hello, a data-science and engineering company that recently rolled out a product called Sense. It's a nonwearable sleep tracker that sits by your bedside, promising to track not only your sleep but how light, sound, temperature, air quality, and humidity affect the quality of your sleep. "This gives us a more complete understanding of how to improve things," Proud told me. The data come from a bedside orb that monitors the room conditions, a small "sleep pill" that attaches to your pillow, and an app for your phone. It also includes an alarm designed to gently wake you up during the lightest phase of your sleep cycle. Another product that's gotten a big response is Chrona, created by Ultradia. It's a memory-foam insert that you slip inside your pillowcase, where it tracks your sleep based on the movements of your head and torso. Ultradia cofounder Ben Bronsther says his goal is to build Chrona into a home polysomnography, or PSG, device, which can act as a full-fledged home sleep lab for users, with no uncomfortable wires and no overnight stays in a lab required.

Some of the bigger names in the electronics and wearables industry are also adding sleep to their product lineups. The Samsung Gear S, an Android smartwatch, includes sleep tracking in its fitness app. Jawbone's UP3 band tracks steps, meals, heart rate, and REM sleep, light sleep, and deep sleep. And as Jawbone's CEO, Hosain Rahman, told me, "The app's Smart Coach feeds you the insights, data, and guidance you need to actually change your behavior and get a better night's sleep."

Fitbit, the largest maker of fitness-tracking wristbands, measures the time you spend in bed into three categories: asleep, restless, and awake. The device also allows you to set sleep goals and track your sleep history, and its Charge HR band measures your resting heart rate while you sleep. "There's a saying," James Park, the cofounder and CEO of Fitbit, told me, "that you can't improve what you can't measure. In addition to activity, we believe that applies to sleep, too."

In 2014, Withings, a French maker of smart products and devices, released its Aura sleep system. It includes an eleven-inch bedside device that monitors light, sound, and temperature levels—and emits sound and light to help users go to sleep and wake up. The second part of the system is a sensor pad that is placed under the mattress, which tracks heart rate, breathing patterns, and movements. It's all part of a shift toward incorporating technology into our beds and bedding, so while we're sleeping, our beds will be working.

Artificial light, a problem exacerbated by technology, is now also being mitigated by technology. We know how light can suppress the body's production of melatonin, which helps regulate our circadian rhythms. But now we're finding out just how little light it takes to do that. According to Harvard sleep researcher Steven Lockley, a light of just 8 lux—which is less than most ordinary room lamps and only twice that of a night-light—is enough to affect us. And it's not just the level but the kind of light that matters. Research has shown that blue light—the kind we are bathing in as we look at our electronic screens and which is also emitted by fluorescent and LED bulbs—has an especially disruptive effect on our melatonin levels and our body's circadian rhythm.

The ideal solution, once again, is to put our screens away. But if we don't, there are some technological hacks available. The software application f.lux, for example, can automatically adjust the light composition of our devices throughout the day. "During the day, computer screens look good—they're designed to look like the sun," f.lux's cocreators, Michael and Lorna Herf, write. "But, at 9pm, 10pm, or 3am, you probably shouldn't be looking at the sun." So during the day you'll get that sunlight-like brightness. As day turns to evening, your screen's light will turn warmer, with less blue light. In August 2015, f.lux introduced a new feature, the backward alarm clock. As Michael Herf told me, "It sends a little notification every half hour from nine hours before your wake time, just so you're more aware of the time." Sort of like an electronic sleep minder, cajoling you to go to bed. Maybe next they can add an electronic shock. Some of us (including me) sometimes need an enforcement mechanism.

There's also tech help on the way for parents—since, as all parents know, if the baby isn't sleeping, neither are you. Of course, parents have been using technology to lull babies to sleep for decades: loud fans, washing machines, dishwashers, even hair dryers and the nuclear option, strapping the baby into the car and going for an aimless drive. But there are now a lot of new options, from data-tracking monitors to customizable white-noise machines.

If you want to play a guided meditation or soft music to help lull you to sleep, load them up on an iPod (there are really inexpensive versions on the market), so you avoid the temptations of having all your data and social media distractions at your fingertips if you wake up in the middle of the night. And for those of you who are going to ignore my advice (I'm a realist) and keep your smartphone by your bed—even though, remember, it's Kryptonite!—I've included a list of a few apps in Appendix B that can improve your sleep. Use responsibly and remember that there is no magic app for cramming eight hours of sleep into four.

Technology that can help us live healthier lives is good, but there are no shortcuts to sleep. The best technology in the world isn't going to help us avoid the myriad negative effects of sleep deprivation if we don't prioritize sleep in our lives.

MY SLEEP WISH LIST

It's not enough to simply know that sleep has the potential to transform our lives. All that knowledge has to be put into action. The early stages of the sleep revolution we're in have brought us a large array of things to help us do just that. But there's always room for more. So here are a few items on my wish list. Some are serious, some are whimsical, some are personal, some involve public policy, some are utopian, and some are completely within our reach.

The saying "I'll sleep when I'm dead" is unceremoniously tossed into the dustbin of history.

The day arrives when nap mats are as plentiful as the yoga mats we see poking out of people's bags as they go to and from work.

People are listing their healthy sleep habits as an item on their résumés and LinkedIn pages.

A congressional sleep committee is formed to set the agenda for sleep as the public-health issue that the CDC says it is.

Our elected leaders lead on sleep by example, starting with political candidates—at all levels—making sleep health a part of their platform.

Political candidates begin using their opponents' macho lack-of-sleep braggadocio in political ads.

A public-awareness campaign for drowsy driving comparable to the one against drunk driving is launched.

Education about the dangers of drowsy driving is added to the warnings against drunk driving in driver's education classes.

A test for drowsiness is developed—similar to the Breathalyzer—so that drowsy driving can be measured and regulated.

A wearable fitness tracker comes on the market that alerts us when we're too tired to drive and then automatically summons an Uber for us.

Health insurers offer discounts in premiums for healthy sleep habits.

Congress passes stricter laws to better enforce regulations so that long-haul truckers can get adequate sleep.

Sleeping pill TV commercials become a thing of the past. No more beautiful, happy people leading perfect lives while a narrator reads a terrifying list of side effects.

Widespread school reform is enacted, moving school start times later so that children and adolescents can get enough sleep.

A device is created that allows us to record, and play back, our dreams.

And finally, an app is launched that turns our smartphone into a dumbphone from the time we start preparing for sleep to the time we wake up—with no power to override it!

EPILOGUE

SO HERE we are in the early years of the twenty-first century, with ever-greater awareness about both the crisis of sleep deprivation and the central importance of sleep in our lives. We have more and more doctors, coaches, wellness experts, and performance gurus offering us solutions—many of them sound and scientifically proven. We also have a growing number of leaders in every field realizing that well-rested employees are better employees. In sports, in schools, in medicine, and in the workplace, sleep is finally beginning to claw its way back to the place of respect and reverence it deserves.

But if we're going to truly restore sleep to its proper role in our lives, we have to look beyond all the tools and techniques, the lavender pouches, the blackout shades, the space-age mattresses, the rules about caffeine and screens. At the end of the day (literally), being able to do something as natural as going to sleep shouldn't require chronically medicating ourselves or putting ourselves on a nightly war footing against all the screens, foods, and activities that stand between us and a good night's sleep. Rather, it starts with something as simple as it is profound: asking ourselves what kind of life we want to lead, what we value, what gives our lives meaning.

Of course, no two people's answers to these questions

will be exactly alike. But there is one thing we all have in common: how easy it is to put off that conversation with ourselves by getting caught up in our daily routines and pursuits, in accepting society's idea of success and chasing things we may later realize we don't even value. When we shrink our whole reality down to our pending projects, when our life becomes our endless to-do list, it's difficult to put them aside each night and let ourselves fall asleep and connect with something deeper.

In the centuries-old tradition of the Japanese tea ceremony, it was customary for samurai, before entering the tearoom, to remove their swords and leave them outside. It was a symbolic way of leaving the conflicts, tensions, and struggles of their daily lives outside the sacred space. In fact, the path (or *roji*) that led to the tearoom, often through a garden, was designed to begin the gradual process of leaving the outside world behind and entering a quieter, more contemplative state.

To be able to leave the outside world behind each night when we go to sleep (our swords these days are mostly electronic and handheld), we need to first recognize that we are more than our struggles and more than our victories and failures. We are not defined by our jobs and our titles, and we are vastly more than our résumés. By helping us keep the world in perspective, sleep gives us a chance to refocus on the essence of who we are. And in that place of connection, it is easier for the fears and concerns of the world to drop away.

For many of us, thinking this way is a big change. It certainly has been for me. After all, we live in a world that celebrates getting things done above all else. So who are we when we are not getting things done? If we stop emailing or texting or planning or doing, will we cease to exist? (It's not hard to imagine a modern-day Descartes declaring, "I tweet, therefore I am.")

To be sure, we can strive to get more sleep without asking these existential questions. But making the most of the third of our lives that we should be spending asleep and reaping all the benefits sleep offers in terms of our health, our clarity of thinking, our decision making, and our engagement in our lives requires reflecting on what matters most to us and then reprioritizing our days—and our nights—accordingly.

I love that we're living in a time when people seem open once again to the power of sleep on our waking lives. We're emerging from the Dark Ages of Sleep into a Sleep Renaissance. This renaissance is defined by an unparalleled sense of possibility, rooted in science but also in the knowledge that sleep is much more than just a critical building block of our daily lives—a tool to help us be better at work, give a better presentation, come up with more ideas in a meeting, score more goals, or put more points on the board. It will undoubtedly help us do all these things, and if that's your entry point to take sleep more seriously, embrace it. There's no wrong reason for rediscovering sleep and its benefits—it's not like high school math, where a teacher is going to check your work to see how you arrived at the right answer. But getting more sleep, for whatever reasons, will also likely help us realize that there is more to life than work and productivity. So yes, come for the job-enhancing benefits, stay for the life-enhancing opportunities. Because sleep is the easiest daily way to shift our focus from our worldly problems to a higher reality. It involves a sometimes meandering journey to a destination other than a corner office or a championship trophy.

But somewhere in the narrative of our long, tumultuous

relationship with sleep, we've lost track of the mystery. And I speak from experience. I'm often asked a question that goes something like this: "Arianna, it's great that you get all this sleep now, but would you have had the same career if you had done this earlier in your life?" And my answer isn't just a categorical yes—I also believe that not only would I have achieved whatever I've achieved, but I would have done it with more joy, more aliveness, and less of a cost to my health and my relationships.

Technology promises us greater control, choice, and convenience in every aspect of our lives—how we shop, whom we date, our friendships, our heart rates, our schedules. But it also sells us the illusion that minutely mapping out and controlling our lives, even if it were possible, is a worthwhile goal—which it's not. Sleep offers just the opposite. While it makes us better at things our culture celebrates—performing and doing—it also teaches us how to trust and let go.

As our days become more and more consumed by doing, by distractions and urgency, sleep, waiting for us every night, offers a surrender. Perhaps that's one reason so many of us have such difficulty falling asleep—because we can't lay down our swords. We're told again and again that we must work harder, must never let our guard down, and we must always fight on. And so we fight sleep, too. Or we stress out about our inability to control it and summon it whenever we want, at the snap of our fingers—the way that we believe we can everything else in our age of On Demand ("your Uber Sleep will arrive in five minutes").

Even as science continues to unearth the seemingly endless secrets of sleep, its mystery defiantly remains. And what a blessing that is. For what sleep and dreams offer us is increasingly hard to come by in our waking lives—

timelessness, renewal, the opportunity to make connections that have eluded our conscious brains, freedom from our everyday cares and concerns.

When we reclaim sleep, we reclaim what sleep has offered us throughout human history—a gateway to the sacred and to life's mystery.

APPENDICES

APPENDIX A

SLEEP-QUALITY QUESTIONNAIRE

This sleep-quality questionnaire—the Sleep Condition Indicator—was developed by Colin Espie, professor of sleep medicine at the University of Oxford and a cofounder of the sleep-education app Sleepio. Consider it a helpful, science-backed tool to start a conversation with yourself, your family, and your friends, and a useful reference as you take steps to renew or sustain your relationship with sleep.

To start, circle the most accurate response for each question. At the end, add up your points to get your sleep assessment, along with tips for improvement.

Thinking about a typical night in the last month . . .

1. **How long does it take you to fall asleep?**

   0–15 min. 4 POINTS

   16–30 min. 3 POINTS

   31–45 min. 2 POINTS

   46–60 min. 1 POINT

   >60 min. 0 POINTS

2. **If you then wake up one or more times during the night, how long are you awake in total?** *(Add up all the time you are awake.)*

   0–15 min. 4 POINTS

   16–30 min. 3 POINTS

   31–45 min. 2 POINTS

   46–60 min. 1 POINT

   >60 min. 0 POINTS

3. If your final wake-up time occurs before you intend to wake up, how much earlier is this?

I don't wake up too early/Up to 15 min. early	4 POINTS
16–30 min. early	3 POINTS
31–45 min. early	2 POINTS
46–60 min. early	1 POINT
>60 min. early	0 POINTS

4. How many nights a week do you have a problem with your sleep?

0–1	4 POINTS
2	3 POINTS
3	2 POINTS
4	1 POINT
5–7	0 POINTS

5. How would you rate your sleep quality?

Very good	4 POINTS
Good	3 POINTS
Average	2 POINTS
Poor	1 POINT
Very poor	0 POINTS

Thinking about the past month, to what extent has poor sleep . . .

6. affected your mood, energy, or relationships?

Not at all	4 POINTS
A little	3 POINTS
Somewhat	2 POINTS
Much	1 POINT
Very much	0 POINTS

7. affected your concentration, productivity, or ability to stay awake?

Not at all	4 POINTS
A little	3 POINTS

Somewhat	2 POINTS
Much	1 POINT
Very much	0 POINTS

8. troubled you in general?

Not at all	4 POINTS
A little	3 POINTS
Somewhat	2 POINTS
Much	1 POINT
Very much	0 POINTS

Finally . . .

9. How long have you had a problem with your sleep?

I don't have a problem/<1 month	4 POINTS
1–2 months	3 POINTS
3–6 months	2 POINTS
7–12 months	1 POINT
>1 year	0 POINTS

Now add up your total score and enter it here: ________

Use the following as a guide:

0–9 Your sleep problems seem to be severe. You should definitely try to get some help.

10–18 You have some sleep problems. It's important to examine your sleep habits and see how you can make changes.

19–27 Your sleep is in good shape, but there are still many steps you can take to make it even better.

28–36 Your sleep is in great shape. Keep doing what you're doing and spread the word!

For more information, go to the Sleepio app or www.sleepio.com.

APPENDIX B

GUIDED MEDITATIONS TO HELP YOU FALL (AND STAY) ASLEEP

To help you disengage from the stresses of the day and prepare your mind and body for sleep, here's a list of recommended guided meditations—as well as some soothing music and other relaxing audio guides.

First, here's a meditation created for *The Sleep Revolution.* You can also hear my sister, Agapi Stassinopoulos, reading it online at bit.ly/meditationforsleep (she sounds exactly like me!).

> Settle into a comfortable position. Take in a deep breath and then, very gently and naturally, exhale and let go. Now take in another breath, and this time as you exhale, breathe away the day and any worries. Gently relax your jaw and take in another breath, this time exhaling away any concerns, upsets, and irritations. Just breathe them away.
>
> Now relax more deeply and begin to breathe normally, observing the rising and falling of your breath. If a thought intrudes, just come back to your breath. Don't follow the thought, don't get caught up in the thought. Just return to your breathing—not forcing the breathing, just allowing it. It's as if you are being breathed. With each breath you take, you find yourself getting more and more relaxed, any tension dissolving away.
>
> Be aware of the sensations in your back, your arms, your shoulders, your legs—all of them relaxing more deeply into the surface of your bed. No matter how relaxed you think you are, there is always a deeper place of relaxation.
>
> As you continue to let go, you will find yourself relaxing more deeply with each inhale and exhale. In this state of relaxation, you are aware that the room you are in is filled with light. It's as if a pure white mist pervades

it. This light surrounds you and fills you, for your highest good. Feel the protection and the warmth of this mist around you and observe it as it changes color.

Right now you see this white mist turn to a beautiful red, which brings you balance.

Now this red gently turns to a vibrant orange that fills you with an inner strength.

Take in another deep breath as it now turns a bright yellow. Surrounded by this yellow mist, you let go, relax, and attune to your deeper self.

The mist now turns to a soft, natural, healing green. If any part of your body or your consciousness needs healing, let that part absorb this soft green healing color.

You find yourself relaxing even more deeply, smiling a very soft smile, for you know that all is well.

The green mist now turns to blue, signaling a spiritual attunement with your deeper self, the part of you that remains loving, peaceful, and joyful no matter what's going on. As this blue pervades the room and your consciousness, it strengthens the sense that all is well and everything is in its right and proper place.

Remain aware of the rising and falling of your breath as the mist gently turns to a rich purple that pervades the room, transmuting any negative thoughts and feelings. Be willing to release any disturbances into this purple and see them replaced by unconditional love.

Now the mist becomes a pure white light, comforting and relaxing you. You breathe in and out through your heart. You breathe in love, and you breathe out love. Continue to breathe this love in and out through your heart and feel this energy of peace and calm arc from your heart center into the center of your head. As you breathe in love and breathe out love, another arc begins to form from your heart into your belly, below your navel.

Your heart, your mind, and your whole body are now in harmony. All you need to do is follow the rising and falling of your breath, in and out, silently repeating the word "love" or "peace" or "joy"—whatever word works for you.

It's as if you've become a finely tuned instrument, and the sound you're playing is one of pure harmony. As you continue to breathe in and out of your heart, you are aware of a deep centeredness, a peace and serenity that go from your heart into infinity.

At this point there is only love, only harmony and peace. As you follow this love, harmony, and peace in and out of your heart, you are ready to relax into a deep, restful sleep where you regenerate and renew yourself.

Here are twelve other meditations compiled by our HuffPost senior health and science writer, Carolyn Gregoire. To avoid the temptations of having your smartphone by your bed, I recommend putting these meditations on an iPod. But if you're one of those strong enough to resist the texting and social-media temptations of your phone, there are four meditation apps at the end of the list.

1. Body-Scan Meditation from *Mindfulness: Finding Peace in a Frantic World* by Dr. Mark Williams and Dr. Danny Penmar

Allow yourself to move into a state of relaxation with a fourteen-minute body-scan meditation recommended for sleep.

This meditation guides you to gently focus on your breathing and then to redirect your attention from your overcrowded mind by releasing lingering tensions from the day.

Available for free download at www.franticworld.com.

2. "Tuck Me In: Relaxing Yourself to Sleep" by Martha Ringer

Martha Ringer, a productivity consultant, created this soothing eight-minute meditation to recapture the feeling of comfort and safety we felt as children being tucked in to bed.

Available for $0.99 on Amazon.com, Google Play, and iTunes.

3. *Deep Calm* by Dr. Andrew Weil and Joshua Leeds

Deep Calm features psychoacoustically rearranged relaxing classical melodies from composers including Schubert, Chopin, and Beethoven, selected by holistic-health expert Dr. Andrew Weil and sound researcher Joshua Leeds. A change from nature noises and synthesizer soundscapes, it helps calm the mind and prepares the body for sleep.

Available starting at $7.99 on Amazon.com, Google Play, iTunes, and Sounds True.

4. *Delta Sleep System* by Dr. Jeffrey Thompson

In two tranquil thirty-minute tracks, acoustics expert and composer Jeffrey Thompson will help prepare your mind for sleep. Sounds of wind, flowing water, and chimes are layered on tones designed to increase delta-brain-wave activity, which is associated with deep sleep.

Available starting at $7.99 on Amazon.com, Google Play, iTunes, and Sounds True.

5. "Dying Each Day" Meditation by John-Roger

Invoking the traditional biblical idea that we are born and die each day, spiritual teacher John-Roger's "Dying Each Day" meditation guides you in finding stillness at the end of the day by letting go of your attachments. As you surrender your challenges and worries, you'll experience an expanded sense of peace and love—and deeper sleep.

Free download available from the Movement of Spiritual Inner Awareness online store. Go to bit.ly/dyingeachdaymeditation and use promo code 4HUFF1.

6. "Body Balance" Meditation by John-Roger

In this meditation, John-Roger guides you to release any tensions, pains, or stuck energy from the day through an exercise in progressive relaxation. Once your body is relaxed, you'll imagine yourself being transformed by a healing white light, which will help you drift off to sleep.

Free download available from the Movement of Spiritual Inner Awareness online store. Go to bit.ly/bodybalancemeditation and use promo code 4MS1A8.

7. *The Zen Effect* by Rolfe Kent

This album from the composer Rolfe Kent uses soothing sounds aimed at stilling the mind in each twenty- to thirty-minute track.

Available starting at $5.49 on Amazon.com and iTunes.

8. *Majesty* by Aeoliah

This series of four ten-minute meditative tracks from Aeoliah is intended to lull you into a deep sleep with tranquil synthesizer music and choral voices.

Available starting at $3.97 on Amazon.com, Google Play, and iTunes.

9. Sleep Meditations from Headspace

The popular meditation app Headspace, created by the mindfulness teacher and former Buddhist monk Andy Puddicombe, features a collection of thirty short meditations designed for promoting sleep, as well as two individual ten-minute sleep meditations. Guided by Puddicombe's soothing voice, you'll begin to quiet your racing thoughts, and prepare your mind for rest.

Available for free download from the Apple App Store and Google Play; $7.99/month with a yearly subscription.

10. iSleep Easy: Meditations for Restful Sleep

Created by the founders of the popular podcast and website Meditation Oasis, iSleep Easy includes a collection of guided meditations, sleep playlists, and "wee hours rescue," which allows you to create a customized combination of voice-guided audio and relaxing background music. You may want to start with the short but sweet "Put Away the Day" meditation, which guides you in putting your concerns into a container, where they'll be waiting for you the next day!

Available for download from the Apple App Store ($4.99) and Google Play ($2.99).

11. "Fade" and "Hello" from Buddhify

Designed to "turn down the senses" so that the mind can prepare for sleep, the meditation app Buddhify's "Fade" meditation leads you through a process of "fading out" each of the five senses as you fall asleep. Another meditation, "Hello," guides you in a playful mindfulness technique of naming and saying hello to various emotions and thought patterns that might be keeping you awake.

Available for download from the Apple App Store ($4.99) and Google Play ($2.99).

12. 7 Days of Sleep by Calm.com

Calm.com, a website that offers short guided and nonguided meditations featuring beautiful nature backdrops, also offers a range of sleep meditations. Its 7 Days of Sleep program features a series of daily meditations meant to be used over the course of a week, which teach a range of techniques for better rest. The eleven-minute meditations—including "Relax the Body," "Eliminate Worry," and "Thinking like a Good Sleeper"—will help you get around the most common roadblocks to a good night's rest.

Available for free download from the Apple App Store and Google Play; $3.33/month with a yearly subscription.

APPENDIX C

THE HOTEL SLEEP REVOLUTION:
Pillow Menus, Quiet Zones, and Beds You'll Want to Take Home

"The Way Forward" highlights many of the hotels across the country and around the world taking steps to help their guests get the best sleep possible. Here are some more hotels that are tapping into the creativity of designers, engineers, and scientists for the purpose of improving guests' sleep.

CORINTHIA HOTEL LONDON (LONDON, UNITED KINGDOM)

The Corinthia Hotel London wants to make sleep the main event of your stay. If you book its "Sumptuous Sleep Retreat," you get the expertise of a sleep professional, a nutritionist, and a chef in addition to blackout curtains, a choice of pillows, and white-noise machines. The retreat also includes a 120-minute sleep ritual that includes a foot massage and hot-stone scalp massage, specifically designed to reduce stress after a day of travel and technology immersion. The spa also offers sleep acupuncture, sleep osteopathy, and a specialized Ayurvedic treatment with aromatherapy oils.

www.corinthia.com/hotels/london

CROWNE PLAZA HOTELS & RESORTS

For its Crowne Plaza Hotels, the InterContinental Hotel Group has created a Sleep Advantage program, so that guests who seek peace and quiet can be grouped together on "quiet zone" floors. In addition to like-minded sleep-loving neighbors, the zones have reduced housekeeping and engineering activity. Guests also receive sleep kits with lavender sprays and, in some rooms, special headboards that are padded and curved to significantly reduce noise.

www.crowneplaza.com

FOUR SEASONS HOTELS AND RESORTS

Four Seasons Hotels and Resorts developed its own custom heat-absorbing Simmons mattress, with a stabilizing feature to keep you still when your partner gets up or moves during the night. And if you love your bed, you can buy it! Four Seasons also soundproofs each of its rooms by placing heating and cooling systems in the ceiling to reduce noise, insulating walls and doors, and utilizing headboard-to-headboard room layouts (so TV noise does not disturb guests in the next room). It also offers a sleep-focused turndown service in which a staffer will dim the lights, adjust the temperature to a sleep-friendly zone, and put on soft music. But don't expect a chocolate on your pillow. Four Seasons has replaced the traditional treat (because of the caffeine and sugar) with herbal tea and other sleep-friendly amenities.

www.fourseasons.com

HILTON HOTELS AND RESORTS

Hilton's Canopy bed is the result of a partnership with Serta, with fabric that regulates heat flow. Given that sleeping in a cooler environment leads to better rest, the bed also incorporates memory foam infused with Serta's MicroSupport gel to reduce pressure and therefore reduce heat buildup in the body overnight. And guests can purchase the bed.

www.hilton.com

MARRIOTT INTERNATIONAL

In 2013, Marriott opened a 10,000-square-foot lab in Bethesda, Maryland, where the hotel chain can try out various room and bed layouts. Guests who stay at the company's JW Marriott properties can select the Nightly Refresh Program. The "curated turndown service" includes Revive Oil, an essential oil that JW Marriott provides in partnership with Aromatherapy Associates.

www.marriott.com

MGM GRAND LAS VEGAS HOTEL & CASINO (LAS VEGAS, NEVADA)

At the MGM Grand Las Vegas Hotel & Casino, Delos, a wellness real estate company, collaborated with the Cleveland Clinic and Dr. Deepak Chopra to pioneer Stay Well hotel rooms, which feature air purification, vitamin C–infused showers, aromatherapy, a healthy menu, and special lighting timed to circadian rhythms. "Light levels," Paul Scialla, the founder of Delos, says, "constitute one of the most powerful external cues the body uses to align its circadian rhythms with the solar day." So Stay Well rooms feature soft, warm white lighting to minimize disruption to circadian rhythms, subtle red lighting at night that does not suppress melatonin, dawn simulators to wake guests naturally, and, in the morning, an energizing light that has the effect of sunlight.

www.mgmgrand.com

STARWOOD HOTELS & RESORTS

In 2011, Starwood, the parent company of Westin Hotels & Resorts, opened an 11,000-square-foot lab in Stamford, Connecticut, where it has tested lighting technology that could help guests sleep better. Its researchers are also testing how the feeling of natural surroundings affects our sleep. This involves walls covered with patterns that mimic a leafy forest, curtains with images of dragonfly wings, and terrariums in rooms.

Some sleep-friendly features at the Westin are already on the market, such as its Heavenly Bed, so beloved that the hotel has sold one hundred thousand of them. The Heavenly Bed features an all-white design, three-hundred-thread-count Egyptian cotton bedding, five pillows, three sheets, and a custom-designed mattress.

www.starwoodhotels.com

BIG SLEEP PERKS FOR LITTLE TRAVELERS

The new sleep consciousness, of course, extends to children. At the Hilton Waikoloa Village on the Big Island of Hawaii, there's a special kids' turndown service, which features books on Hawaiian culture and flash cards with stories about the Hawaiian goddess Pele. Great Wolf Lodge, a chain of family resorts in the

United States and Canada, offers a pajama story time in front of their fireplaces. And at the Ritz-Carlton on Amelia Island in Florida, kids can enjoy the "Pirate Tuck In," with costumed "pirates" bearing cookies and milk (hopefully the new sleep consciousness has reached the pirate community, so they know to make those cookies light on before-bedtime sugar).

www.hiltonwaikoloavillage.com
www.greatwolf.com
www.ritzcarlton.com/en/properties/ameliaisland

HOTELS THAT HELP YOU UNPLUG

With some hotels, sleep enhancement comes less from added bells and whistles and more from what's taken away. We're often our own worst enemies when it's time to shut down our devices and turn off our connection to the world. So some hotels are doing what they can to help.

FOUR SEASONS RESORT COSTA RICA AT PENINSULA PAPAGAYO (PENINSULA PAPAGAYO, COSTA RICA)

This hotel offers a Disconnect to Reconnect program, in which you surrender your smartphone for a day. For your withdrawal pains, you'll get it back, safe and sound, in a new case.

www.fourseasons.com/costarica

MOUNT SNOW RESORT (WEST DOVER, VERMONT)

To get parents and kids working together toward better sleep, this hotel offers a Family Camp package where mobile devices are highly discouraged. Wi-Fi is available only in the camp's main lodge, and most rooms are Wi-Fi-free. Camp staff encourages families to put down their devices and enjoy games, water sports, chef-made meals, and the great outdoors as they slow down and connect with one another instead of with the entire world.

www.mountsnow.com

PETIT ST. VINCENT ISLAND AND RESORT (PETIT ST. VINCENT)

All accommodations at this Grenadine island resort are free of telephones, television, and Wi-Fi. Guests use a flag system to signal for room service or any other service (including, presumably, requests for more flags?).

www.petitstvincent.com

RIVERPLACE HOTEL (PORTLAND, OREGON)

The RiverPlace Hotel in Portland offers a service where you can check your smartphones, tablets, and laptops in a safe and in exchange receive truffles, a private bath butler who personally draws a bath with amenities such as bath oil and salts, and wine (which you can use to toast being unplugged and in the moment). Sounds like a great trade!

www.riverplacehotel.com

VILLA STÉPHANIE (BADEN-BADEN, GERMANY)

Here you can choose a room that allows you to flip a switch and shut off all online connections to the room. Maybe someday this will be standard in all hotels—and homes.

www.brenners.com/eng/villa-stephanie

And here are a few other hotels that prioritize sleep, assembled by HuffPost associate lifestyle editor Suzy Strutner:

AKA (NEW YORK, NEW YORK)

If you find yourself in need of an extended stay in New York for business or pleasure, AKA's four Manhattan properties have partnered with the New York University School of Medicine Sleep Disorders Center and the New York Sleep Institute to have experts available for in-room sleep screenings. Complimentary features of the Sleep Institute include in-room light boxes, blackout curtains, and sleep seminars on topics such as bedtime routines and sleep apnea.

www.stayaka.com

THE BODYHOLIDAY (CASTRIES CITY, ST. LUCIA)

At this Caribbean island getaway, a two-day Sleep Restoration Program offers a range of massage, bodywork, aromatherapy, and nutritional counseling to send you back home with better sleep habits.

www.thebodyholiday.com

FAIRMONT VANCOUVER AIRPORT (VANCOUVER, BRITISH COLUMBIA)

Nothing quite says terrible night's sleep like an airport hotel. But this one, within the busy Vancouver International Airport and a two-minute walk from the baggage-claim carousels, has soundproofed rooms with triple-paned windows. For jet-lagged travelers, there's the Quiet Zone, with no service interruptions or knocks on the door from 8 p.m. to 8 a.m.

www.fairmont.com/vancouver-airport-richmond

GRAND RESORT BAD RAGAZ (BAD RAGAZ, SWITZERLAND)

In Switzerland, while you're at the Grand Resort Bad Ragaz, you can get a thorough sleep diagnosis that includes an EEG, respiration monitoring, and blood-oxygen-level readings, all of which its medical staff will analyze and then make recommendations for how you can improve your sleep.

www.resortragaz.ch

THE HERMITAGE HOTEL (NASHVILLE, TENNESSEE)

The pillow menu here isn't just an afterthought amenity, it's a passion. If the goose-down, buckwheat, latex-foam, and memory-foam pillows waiting in your room aren't enough, call for reinforcements: neck pillows, body pillows, water pillows, reading pillows, leg pillows, diamond-filled pillows (okay, the last one is made up). And if you develop a particularly strong pillow bond during your stay, they're all available for purchase.

www.thehermitagehotel.com

KAMALAYA KOH SAMUI (KOH SAMUI, THAILAND)

Kamalaya's Sleep Enhancement program is for guests who are serious about renewing their relationship with sleep. Since that takes time, the hotel asks for a five-night minimum commitment. Influenced by traditional Chinese medicine, the program takes you through a range of therapies and treatments—from acupuncture, yoga, and herbal foot baths to Ayurvedic massages—all designed to help you develop healthy sleep habits that will stay with you long after you head home.

www.kamalaya.com

LIBRARY HOTEL COLLECTION (NEW YORK, NEW YORK; BUDAPEST, HUNGARY; PRAGUE, CZECH REPUBLIC)

This line of four boutique hotels in Manhattan (with additional locations in Budapest and Prague) offers a carefully curated Escape to Serenity program, where you can request a range of complimentary items that help you prepare for sleep, such as fleece blankets, feather-bed mattress toppers, hypoallergenic Micro Gel fiber pillows, and headphones that emit soothing sounds as you fall asleep.

www.libraryhotel.com

LORIEN HOTEL & SPA (ALEXANDRIA, VIRGINIA)

Here guests find a "dream button" on their room phone that lets them choose from the Dream Service Menu. There are scent diffusers to relieve tension, bedtime books for a calming lullaby read, and sleep masks to block the outside world. Choose from an extensive list of pillows, including a magnetic pillow that reduces swelling. For little ones, the menu also includes children's books and special night-lights.

www.lorienhotelandspa.com

MIRAVAL RESORT & SPA (TUCSON, ARIZONA)

This property in Tucson features Definity Digital Good Night LED bulbs, which reduce blue-light exposure to better maintain your body's natural sleep cycle. The resort consulted with a sleep specialist to outfit rooms with the bulbs, which use the same light-filtering technology developed for astronauts in space.

www.miravalresorts.com

PARK HYATT BEAVER CREEK RESORT AND SPA (BEAVER CREEK, COLORADO)

Working with sleep expert Nancy Rothstein, Beaver Creek has introduced the Sound Sleep Initiatives to improve sleep for guests and employees alike. There's a TV channel dedicated to sleep (with music composed by sleep expert Jeffrey Thompson), slumber kits including eye masks and earplugs, relaxing massages, and a "sleep elixir" with chamomile and apple cider to help guests power down.

www.beavercreek.hyatt.com

PARK HYATT TOKYO (TOKYO, JAPAN)

Here guests are invited to prepare for bed with a complimentary Good Night Sleep Stretch. Guided by a physical trainer, the thirty-minute session uses stretching, essential oils, and herbal tea to help guests unwind in a scenic studio forty-seven stories above the busy city. You'll also practice breathing exercises to loosen your muscles and prepare for rest.

www.tokyo.park.hyatt.com

SIX SENSES HOTELS RESORTS SPAS

With properties all over the world, Six Senses offers a Yogic Sleep program for guests, focusing on yoga nidra, the sleeplike state that yogis enter during meditation. Rooms are set to the optimal temperature for deep sleep, and "pillow mist" aromatherapy products and relaxing music are part of the guest experience. Guests receive a sleep journal to clear the mind, prepare for the day ahead, or log thoughts on their trip, as well as a guide filled with sleep tips to take home.

www.sixsenses.com

SWISSÔTEL BERLIN (BERLIN, GERMANY)

Good sleep habits follow you throughout the day at Swissôtel Berlin, a luxury property on one of the city's most hectic streets. Book the DeepSleep Package to awaken with a "power drink" that includes maté tea and a bright-light lamp session to energize your body for the day. Aromatherapy, calming drinks, and specialized "sound pillows" with brain-wave-calming beats help you wind down.

www.swissotel.com/hotels/berlin

WESTHOUSE (NEW YORK, NEW YORK)

Through a partnership with the innovative specialty sleep retailer Sleep Studio, WestHouse lets you tailor your sleep experience with sleep masks, aromatherapy oils, and Sleep Studio's proprietary mattresses.

www.westhousehotelnewyork.com

APPENDIX D

GOING TO THE MATTRESSES

It's not really a surprise that a quality mattress is a key factor in getting a good night's sleep. And a great deal of scientific, engineering, and design skill is being poured into the mattress industry, which has become its own hub of sleep-related innovation.

This change reflects a larger shift, away from dealing with sleep as some sort of necessary evil and toward savoring it and enhancing its many benefits. That extends to the experience of buying a bed. As Michael Silverstein, a Boston Consulting Group senior partner, put it, "The market for beds is a very large one, with a high degree of dissatisfaction." So the would-be disruptors have flooded that market and injected some twenty-first-century verve into what just a few years ago was one of the most stagnant and, yes, sleepy industries out there. Not long ago, mattresses were advertised mostly in holiday weekend newspaper inserts you threw out or used to clean up spills. Now they're at the center of a start-up revolution.

CASPER

Casper offers one mattress and sells directly to consumers. It has an interesting origin story. As CEO Philip Krim said, he met his fellow cofounders while working for different companies at a shared workspace in New York City. "We noticed that everyone was drinking green juice and working at standing desks to stay healthy and increase productivity, yet sleep was something that everyone sacrificed," he said. "Even worse: they bragged about how little they slept." So they saw a business opportunity. "We realized sleep is something that you should take seriously," he said. And Casper was born. And in 2015, Casper launched Van Winkle's, a news website dedicated to all things sleep.

www.casper.com

COCO-MAT

Coco-Mat was founded in Greece and now has stores in the United States, Europe, Asia, and the Middle East. Shoppers testing the store's handmade, all-natural mattresses get free food, drinks, robes, and slippers, and they can "test-drive" the beds—that is, settle in for a real nap—in Coco-Mat's "nap chambers." After all, as Mike Efmorfidis, Coco-Mat CEO, told me, "When you buy a car, you take it out for a test drive. No reason a mattress should be any different."

www.coco-mat.com

SLEEP NUMBER

Sleep Number's smart mattress has interior sensors to track your sleep, giving you a daily SleepIQ score from 1 to 100 that includes how much restful time you spent in bed, along with your average heart and breathing rates. If a partner shares your bed, you'll get a reading of how his or her sleep affects you and vice versa—making for some fun breakfast table discussion, no doubt. For those who don't want wearable sleep trackers, Sleep Number eliminates the need by putting them into the mattress. When I met Sleep Number's CEO, Shelly Ibach, she greeted me not just by shaking hands but by giving me her SleepIQ score. Sleep transparency as an intimacy-building tool!

www.sleepnumber.com

TEMPUR-PEDIC

The mattress company Tempur-Pedic has its roots in space exploration. When NASA developed a temperature-sensitive material in the early 1970s to cushion astronauts during liftoff, a group of Swedish scientists began to test the material for use in mattresses. Today Tempur-Pedic has a number of innovative features for comfort, support, and keeping you cool at night. Its famous TV commercial, with a glass of red wine set on a Tempur-Pedic mattress and not spilling even as a woman in pajamas jumped on the bed, was a memorable way of showing that two people could sleep on the same mattress without disturbing each other, which, as we know, can be a significant problem with significant others.

www.tempurpedic.com

THE LATEST START-UPS

Other companies are also getting creative and making a difference—from Yogabed, an online mattress retailer that uses luxury foam that supports the body and reduces pressure points, to Leesa, which donates one mattress to homeless shelters for every ten sold, to Helix, which sells custom-made mattresses based on sleep preferences and body types, to Saatva, which got some enviable press in September 2015 when Pope Francis slept on a Saatva mattress (queen-size, memory-foam mattress, organic cotton covers) during his visit to Philadelphia.

www.yogabed.com
www.leesa.com
www.helixsleep.com
www.saatvamattress.com

MATTRESS TECHNOLOGY

There's also a shift toward incorporating technology into our beds and bedding. While we're sleeping, our beds can be working.

SLEEPSENSE

Samsung's SleepSense, announced in September 2015, is a gadget that goes under your mattress. It tracks your heart rate, movement, and breathing patterns and will also provide you with customized advice from Harvard Medical School professor Dr. Christos Mantzoros. SleepSense emails you a report of how you slept, and its "family care" option allows you to keep tabs on how a loved one is sleeping. You can even program it to communicate with other smart devices in your home—for instance, tell your television to turn itself off when you've fallen asleep.

www.sleepsense.com

LUNA

In 2015, San Francisco–based Matteo Franceschetti set out to create a smart mattress cover. His goal on Indiegogo was to raise $100,000; he raised nearly $1 million. Using several layers, each with a different purpose, Luna's Wi-Fi-enabled mattress cover promises not only to track your sleep—by monitoring respiration and heart rate—but also to learn and adapt to your sleep patterns and preferences. For instance, it can automatically adjust the temperature on each half of the bed separately, adjust the temperature in the room, put on relaxing music, and, if it makes you feel less anxious, lock your bedroom door for you. It can even start your coffee pot in the morning so you don't have to wait for that first cup (though if you've slept well, you shouldn't be as desperate for it). A future version will even get up and take your kids to school (I'm kidding, but this is one full-featured mattress cover).

www.lunasleep.com

BEDDIT

Beddit, another Indiegogo success, monitors sleep, via heart rate and breathing, by using a sensor that you put underneath the sheets. When you wake up, you find a sleep report waiting for you. The data include noise and light levels as well as a record of your snoring. You'll also get suggestions for improvement.

www.beddit.com

ACKNOWLEDGMENTS

From the start, I wanted *The Sleep Revolution* to include both the most important recent scientific discoveries on sleep and a wide range of human stories and experiences. And, as I kept going, I kept finding more voices to include. So in many ways it became the book equivalent of co-sleeping—with more and more people and ideas crawling in. The book is all the richer for it, and I'm tremendously grateful to everyone who has helped make it what it is.

Sleep has been one of my passions for years, but it was my great friend and literary agent Jennifer Rudolph Walsh who saw the potential for a book all about sleep. She sent me on this amazing journey and has been with me every step of the way, giving me feedback, guidance, and wisdom.

The Sleep Revolution is built on a mountain of scientific research, and there was nothing I cared about more than establishing the importance of sleep in our lives in a scientifically rigorous way. My profound thanks to Brian Levin, Anna McGrady, Margaux McGrath, Marcos Saldivar, and David Sze for their skill and commitment in researching, organizing, and fact-checking every last detail—including the 1,200 endnotes—as the book expanded and evolved over time.

I'm deeply grateful to my editor, Roger Scholl, for his masterful editing of the book and for encouraging me to add more anecdotes from my own family as well as from people I've met and from HuffPost readers around the world. This is our third book together and it gets better and better every time! Thank you also to Ed Faulkner, my UK editor at Random House, for all his insightful edits, including his guidance on how to give the book a global resonance. I'm so lucky to work with the amazing team at the Crown Publishing Group: president Maya Mavjee; Aaron Wehner, publisher of the Harmony imprint; and editorial director of Harmony, Diana Baroni. Also production editor Patricia Shaw, the guardian of the process that turned the manuscript into a book; Chris Brand for the book's inspired jacket design, and Elizabeth Rendfleisch for her smart and accessible book design; Dannalie Diaz, editorial assistant to Roger Scholl; and the entire Crown sales force for all they've done to ensure that the book and its message get out into the world. And a special shout-out to Crown's director of marketing, Julie Cepler, and senior marketing manager Christina Foxley for all the imagination they have brought to the book's rollout, and to executive publicist Penny Simon and senior publicist Rebecca Marsh for all their work and commitment to making sure people actually, you know, read it.

Then there's Stephen Sherrill and Greg Beyer, who edited countless drafts, greatly improving all of them. And deep thanks to Roy Sekoff—this is my eighth book he has edited through our sixteen years of working together. Also many thanks to Carolyn Gregoire, Suzy Strutner, Damon Beres, Tyler Kingkade, and Krithika Varagur, who have written about sleep and meditations, sleep and hotels, sleep and colleges, and sleep and technology on *The Huffington Post* and whose research has been invaluable.

I reached out to many scientists, doctors, and historians—studying everything from REM sleep and chronobiology to dream incubation and segmented sleep—and was awed by the generosity of their responses, which have enriched every aspect of the book. So my profound gratitude to Jennifer Ailshire, M. Safwan Badr, John Bargh, Mathias Basner, Christian Benedict, Rakesh Bhattacharjee, Michael Breus, Kelly Bulkeley, Victor Carrion, Mary Carskadon, Anjan Chatterjee, Christopher Colwell, Elizabeth Damato, Richard Davidson, Horacio de la Iglesia, Michael Decker, William Dement, David Dinges, Murali Doraiswamy, Helene Ensellem, Russell Foster, Indira Gurubhagavatula, Gregg Jacobs, Harvey Karp, Paul Kelley, Kristen Knutson, Frank Lipman, Cheri Mah, Pittman McGehee, James McKenna, Emmanuel Mignot, Rubin Naiman, Maiken Nedergaard, Matthieu Ricard, Rebecca Robbins, Till Roenneberg, Michael Roizen, Clifford Saper, Clare Sauro, Richard Schwab, Claire Sexton, Jerome Siegel, John Timmerman, Wendy Troxel, Eus van Someren, Joan Williams, Chris Winter, Heather Cleland Woods, Carol Worthman, Duncan Young, and Janet Zand.

Patrick Fuller generously read the entire manuscript and helped translate complex scientific findings into layman's terms, and Colin Espie created the sleep questionnaire in the appendix. And my deep thanks go to Alan Derickson, Kat Duff, and Roger Ekirch for their work on the history of sleep, which has informed and broadened my understanding, and for taking the time to read the manuscript and send suggestions.

I'm deeply grateful to Sheryl Sandberg for reading an early draft of the manuscript and not only identifying missed opportunities but actually sending me line-by-line edits and requests for more humor in the middle of all the science! And also to Sherry Turkle for her thorough edits that vastly improved the structure of the book and for reminding me that I didn't need to include every single scientific study.

Special thanks to Paul Kaye, whose wisdom and unwavering support have helped me both in writing the book and on my own journey to prioritizing sleep in my life, and to Patricia Fitzgerald, our HuffPost wellness editor, for sharing her insights about acupuncture, herbs, homeopathy, and all sorts of natural ways to improve our sleep.

To Patty Gift, John Montorio, Elaine Lipworth, Faith Bethelard, Shelley Reid, Fran Lasker, Jan Shepherd, Timothea Stewart, and Joan Witkowski, many thanks for all the thoughtful edits.

Thank you to Dan Katz, Jeff Swafford, Katie Spear, and Horacio Fabiano for all their support, and also to the great team that was responsible for bringing the book to many countries around the world: Monica Lee, Lena Auerbuch, Tracy Fisher, Rafaella De Angelis, Elizabeth Sheinkman, Eric Zohn, Katie Giarla, and Elizabeth Goodstein.

And finally, I want to thank my sister, Agapi, who has walked alongside me since childhood in our shared quest for better sleep. She read every draft multiple times, reminded me of stories I had forgotten, and made it better in so many ways. And my daughters, Christina and Isabella, who I'm happy to say were converts to sleep at an early age, and who are actually now checking up on me to make sure I'm getting all the sleep I need when I'm traveling. One great unintended consequence of Isabella reading the Dreams chapter is that she now pays much more attention to her dreams and shares them with me, which has led to some fascinating conversations.

I dedicated this book to all the millions of people around the world who are sick and tired of being sick and tired, and longing for a good night's sleep. I hope that *The Sleep Revolution* will help them get it.

NOTES

INTRODUCTION

5 **Adam Mansbach's 2011 book *Go the F**k to Sleep*:** Andy Lewis, "'Go the F—k to Sleep' Debuts at No. 1 on NYT Bestseller List," *The Hollywood Reporter*, June 15, 2011, www.hollywoodreporter.com.

7 **"The train is easy to board":** Milan Kundera, *The Art of the Novel*, trans. Linda Asher (New York: Perennial Classics, 2003), 8.

8 **"civilization's disease":** Pascal Chabot, "Le Burn-Out Est Global [Burn-Out Is Global]," *Le Huffington Post*, January 20, 2013, www.huffingtonpost.fr.

8 **"What is more gentle":** John Keats, *The Complete Poetical Works of Keats*, ed. Horace E. Scudder (Boston and New York: Houghton, Mifflin and Co., 1899), 18.

9 **"Dreams give information":** Carl Jung, *Modern Man in Search of a Soul*, trans. Cary F. Baynes (Oxon: Routledge Classics, 2001), 16.

9 **In the 1970s:** Matthew J. Wolf-Meyer, *The Slumbering Masses: Sleep, Medicine, and Modern American Life* (Minneapolis: University Press of Minnesota, 2012), Kindle edition.

10 **more than 2,500 accredited sleep centers:** Lynn Celmer (communications coordinator, American Academy of Sleep Medicine), email to the author, March 19, 2015.

10 **"Learning to let go":** Ray Bradbury, *Farewell Summer* (New York: William Morrow, 2007), Kindle edition.

11 **More than 40 percent of Americans:** Jeffrey M. Jones, "In U.S., 40% Get Less Than Recommended Amount of Sleep," *Gallup*, December 19, 2013, www.gallup.com.

11 **Industrial Revolution:** Alan Derickson, *Dangerously Sleepy: Overworked Americans and the Cult of Manly Wakefulness* (Philadelphia: University of Pennsylvania Press, 2013), Kindle edition.

11 **the labor movement:** "Troopers Stop Meetings: Arrest 19 Men Including Labor Union Organizers," *The New York Times*, September 22, 1919, www.nytimes.com.

11 **birth of the new science of sleep:** Lynne Lamberg, "The Student, the Professor and the Birth of Modern Sleep Research," *Medicine on the Midway*, Spring 2014, 16–25.

11 **diabetes:** Denise Mann, "The Sleep-Diabetes Connection," *WebMD*, January 19, 2010, www.webmd.com.

11 **heart attack:** "How Sleep Deprivation Affects Your Heart," National Sleep Foundation, www.sleepfoundation.org.

11 **stroke:** Janice Lloyd, "Lack of Sleep Increases Stroke Risk," *USA TODAY*, June 11, 2012, www.usatoday.com.

11 **cancer:** John Easton, "Fragmented Sleep Accelerates Cancer Growth," *UChicago News*, January 27, 2014, news.uchicago.edu.

11 **obesity:** "Sleep Deprivation and Obesity," Harvard T. H. Chan School of Public Health, www.hsph.harvard.edu.

11 **Alzheimer's disease:** Yasmin Anwar, "Poor Sleep Linked to Toxic Buildup of Alzheimer's Protein, Memory Loss," *Berkeley News*, June 1, 2015, vcresearch.berkeley.edu.

1. OUR CURRENT SLEEP CRISIS

17 **Sarvshreshth Gupta:** Andrew Ross Sorkin, "Reflections on Stress and Long Hours on Wall Street," *The New York Times*, June 1, 2015, www.nytimes.com.

17 **He had jumped:** Julia La Roche, "A 22-Year-Old Goldman Sachs Analyst's Death Has Been Ruled a Suicide," *Business Insider*, June 10, 2015, www.businessinsider.com.

17 ***karoshi*:** "Are the Japanese Worked to Death?," *Science from Virginia Tech*, 1995, www.research.vt.edu.

17 ***guolaosi*:** Shai Oster, "In China, 1,600 People Die Every Day from Working Too Hard," *Bloomberg Business*, July 3, 2014, www.bloomberg.com.

17 ***gwarosa*:** John W. Budd, *The Thought of Work* (Ithaca: Cornell University Press, 2011), 108.

18 **hit Bon Jovi song:** Jon Bon Jovi, Richie Sambora, and Desmond Child, "I'll Sleep When I'm Dead," *Keep the Faith*, Mercury Records, 1992.

18 **album by the late rocker Warren Zevon:** Warren Zevon, *I'll Sleep When I'm Dead (An Anthology)*, Rhino Entertainment, 1996.

18 **crime film starring Clive Owen:** *I'll Sleep When I'm Dead*, directed by Mike Hodges (2004; Hollywood: Paramount Pictures, 2004), DVD.

19 **Rajiv Joshi:** Rajiv Joshi, email to the author, September 2, 2015.

19 **According to a recent Gallup poll:** Jones, "In U.S., 40% Get Less Than Recommended Amount of Sleep."

19 **"just as important":** *Sleepless in America*, directed by John Hoffman (Washington, D.C.: National Geographic Channel, 2014), Television Documentary.

19 **"is our most underrated":** "GO! to Sleep," Cleveland Clinic Wellness, www.clevelandclinicwellness.com.

19 **A National Sleep Foundation report:** "Annual Sleep in America Poll Exploring Connections with Communications Technology Use and Sleep," National Sleep Foundation press release, March 7, 2011, www.sleepfoundation.org.

20 **In 2011, 32 percent of people:** Paul Rodgers, "The Sleep Deprivation Epidemic," *Forbes*, September 9, 2014, www.forbes.com.

20 **In 2013 more than a third of Germans:** "National Sleep Foundation 2013 International Bedroom Poll First to Explore Sleep Differences Among Six Countries," National Sleep Foundation press release, September 3, 2013, www.sleepfoundation.org.

20 ***inemuri*:** Brigitte Stegar, "Getting Away with Sleep—Social and Cultural Aspects of Dozing in Parliament," *Social Science Japan Journal* 6 (2003): 181–97.

20 **Jawbone:** Jim Godfrey (vice president of global communications, Jawbone), email to the author, September 25, 2015.

21 **"Sleep deprivation now resides":** Derickson, *Dangerously Sleepy*.

21 **From 1990 to 2000:** "New ILO Study Shows U.S. Workers Are Spending an Extra Week on the Job Each Year," International Labor Organization press release, August 31, 2001, www.prnewswire.com.

21 **A 2014 survey by Skift:** Rafat Ali, "Travel Habits of Americans: 42 Percent Didn't Take Any Vacation Days in 2014," *Skift*, January 5, 2015, www.skift.com.

21 **Dr. Charles Czeisler:** Maria Konnikova, "Why Can't We Fall Asleep?," *The New Yorker*, July 7, 2015, www.newyorker.com.

21 **Thirty percent of employed Americans:** "Short Sleep Duration Among Workers—United States, 2010," *Morbidity and Mortality Weekly Report*, April 27, 2012, www.cdc.gov.

22 **Getting by on less than six hours:** Marie Söderström, Kerstin Jeding, Mirjam Ekstedt, Aleksander Perski, and Torbjörn Åkerstedt, "Insufficient Sleep Predicts Clinical Burnout," *Journal of Occupational Health Psychology* 17 (2012): 175–83.

22 **"lower socio-economic position":** Kristen L. Knutson, "Sociodemographic and Cultural Determinants of Sleep Deficiency: Implications for Cardiometabolic Disease Risk," *Social Science & Medicine* 79 (2013): 7–15.

22 **"I have never seen a study":** Brian Resnick, "The Black-White Sleep Gap," *National Journal*, October 23, 2015, www.nationaljournal.com.

23 **We sacrifice sleep:** Ronald C. Kessler, Patricia A. Berglund, Catherine Coulouvrat, Goeran Hajak, Thomas Roth, Victoria Shahly, Alicia C. Shillington, Judith J. Stephenson, and James K. Walsh, "Insomnia and the Performance of US Workers: Results from the America Insomnia Survey," *SLEEP* 34 (2011): 1161–71.

23 **annual cost of sleep deprivation:** Ibid.

23 **"Americans are not missing work":** Tom Rath, *Eat Move Sleep: How Small Choices Lead to Big Changes* (Arlington: Missionday, 2013), Kindle edition.

23 **Sleep disorders cost Australia:** "Re-Awakening Australia: The Economic Cost of Sleep Disorders in Australia, 2010," Sleep Health Foundation report, October 2011, www.sleephealthfoundation.org.au.

23 **In the United Kingdom:** Becky Frith, "Fatigued Employees Costing UK Businesses," *HR Magazine*, July 20, 2015, www.hrmagazine.co.uk.

23 **The researchers estimated:** Ibid.

23 **In Canada, 26 percent:** "Sleep Centre Study Says One in Four Canadians Call in Sick to Catch Up on Sleep," IPG Mediabrands press release, June 8, 2015, www.marketwired.com.

23 **nearly two-thirds of Canadian adults:** "Lack of Sleep Called 'Global Epidemic,'" *CBC News*, March 18, 2011, www.cbc.ca.

23 **women need more sleep than men:** Edward C. Suarez, "Self-Reported Symptoms of Sleep Disturbance and Inflammation, Coagulation, Insulin Resistance and Psychosocial Distress: Evidence for Gender Disparity," *Brain, Behavior and Immunity* 22 (2008): 960–68.

24 **"We found that for women":** "Wake-Up Call on Sleep," *Duke Magazine*, June 1, 2008, www.dukemagazine.duke.edu.

24 **"They have so many commitments":** Michael J. Breus, January 20, 2010 (12:51 p.m.), comment on "Sleep Challenge 2010: Perchance to Dream," *The Huffington Post*, January 19, 2010, www.huffingtonpost.com.

24 **According to Dr. William Dement:** James B. Maas, *Power Sleep: The Revolutionary Program That Prepares Your Mind for Peak Performance* (New York: Villard Books, 1998), Kindle edition.

24 **"Do you ever have":** Sarah Bunton, "Mommy Needs a Nap," *The Huffington Post*, May 18, 2015, www.huffingtonpost.com.

25 **"Let's face it, women today are tired":** Karen Brody, "Women: Time to Tell a New Story on Exhaustion," *The Huffington Post*, February 23, 2015, www.huffingtonpost.com.

25 **"I started calling":** Frank Lipman, manuscript of *10 Reasons You Feel Old and Get Fat . . . And How YOU Can Stay Young, Slim, and Happy!*, email to the author, March 23, 2015.

25 **"The world is too much":** William Wordsworth, *William Wordsworth: Selected Poems*, ed. John O. Hayden (London: Penguin, 1994), 166.

25 **"I felt like I earned":** Sherry Turkle, conversation with the author, October 4, 2015.

26 **The incidence of death:** "Sleep and Disease Risk," Healthy Sleep, www.healthysleep.med.harvard.edu.

26 **A 2015 CNN.com article:** Carina Storrs, "Sleep or Die: Growing Body of Research Warns of Heart Attacks, Strokes," *CNN*, June 19, 2015, www.cnn.com.

26 **even losing an hour of sleep:** Carol Ash, interview with Gayle King, Charlie Rose, and Norah O'Donnell, "Resting Easier," *CBS This Morning*, January 26, 2015, www.cbsnews.com.

26 **A Russian study found:** "Poor Sleep Associated with Increased Risk of Heart Attack and Stroke," European Society of Cardiology press release, June 15, 2015, www.escardio.org.

26 **A Norwegian study:** Lars Erik Laugsand, Linn B. Strand, Lars J. Vatten, Imre Janszky, and Johan Håkon Bjørngaard, "Insomnia Symptoms and Risk for Unintentional Fatal Injuries—The HUNT Study," *SLEEP* 37 (2014): 1777–86.

26 **A lack of melatonin:** Martin Alpert, Edward Carome, Vilnis Kubulins,

and Richard Hansler, "Nighttime Use of Special Spectacles or Light Bulbs That Block Blue Light May Reduce the Risk of Cancer," *Medical Hypothesis* 73 (2009): 324–25.

27 **like the common cold:** Sheldon Cohen, William J. Doyle, Cuneyt M. Alper, Denise Janicki-Deverts, and Ronald B. Turner, "Sleep Habits and Susceptibility to the Common Cold," *Archives of Internal Medicine* 169 (2009): 62–67.

27 **In a study by the Mayo Clinic:** Andrew D. Calvin, Rickey E. Carter, Taro Adachi, Paula G. Macedo, Felipe N. Albuquerque, Christelle van der Walt, Jan Bukartyk, Diane E. Davison, James A. Levine, and Virend K. Somers, "Effects of Experimental Sleep Restriction on Caloric Intake and Activity Energy Expenditure," *Chest* 144 (2013): 79–86.

27 **six hours of sleep:** Christine Lagorio, "Can You Sleep Off Fat?," *CBS News*, November 16, 2004, www.cbsnews.com; James E. Gangwisch, Dolores Malaspina, Bernadette Boden-Albala, and Steven B. Heymsfield, "Inadequate Sleep as a Risk Factor for Obesity: Analyses of the NHANES I," *SLEEP* 28 (2005): 1289–96.

27 **role of sleep in the production of orexin:** Danielle DePorter, Jamie Coborn, Sairam Parthasarathy, and Jennifer Teske, "Sleep Deprivation Reduces the Effectiveness of Orexin-A to Stimulate Physical Activity and Energy Expenditure," *SLEEP* Abstract Supplement 38 (2015): A113.

27 **In a Swedish study:** John Axelsson, Tina Sundelin, Michael Ingre, Eus J. W. van Someren, Andreas Olsson, and Mats Lekander, "Beauty Sleep: Experimental Study on the Perceived Health and Attractiveness of Sleep Deprived People," *BMJ* 341 (2010): doi: 10.1136/bmj.c6614.

28 **An experiment in the United Kingdom:** Guy Meadows, "Does Sleep Deprivation Have Any Impact on Our Appearance?," Bensons for Beds press release, May 18, 2015, www.bensonsforbeds.co.uk.

28 **get rid of toxins:** Maiken Nedergaard, interview with Jon Hamilton, "Brains Sweep Themselves Clean of Toxins During Sleep," *All Things Considered*, NPR, October 17, 2013, www.npr.org.

28 **"When you find depression":** Justin Pope, "Colleges Find Sleep Is Key to Grade Average," *The Associated Press*, September 4, 2012, www.college basketball.ap.org.

28 **In the Great British Sleep Survey:** "The Great British Sleep Survey 2012," Sleepio, www.sleepio.com.

28 **"When I was short on sleep":** Nancy Fox, "Sleep Is the Key to Life," *The Huffington Post*, August 6, 2014, www.huffingtonpost.com.

29 **"Your cognitive performance":** Margaux McGrath, "Unlocking the Science of Social Jet Lag and Sleep: An Interview with Till Roenneberg," *The Huffington Post*, July 21, 2015, www.huffingtonpost.com.

29 **When Golden State Warriors player:** Shannon Sweetser, "How MVP Andre Iguodala Improved His Game with UP," *The Jawbone Blog*, September 24, 2015, https://jawbone.com/blog.

29 **In just two weeks:** Hans P. A. Van Dongen, Greg Maislin, Janet M. Mullington, and David F. Dinges, "The Cumulative Cost of Additional Wakefulness: Dose-Response Effects on Neurobehavioral Functions

and Sleep Physiology from Chronic Sleep Restriction and Total Sleep Deprivation," *SLEEP* 26 (2003): 117–26.

29 **According to a *Today* show survey:** Meghan Holohan, "Why Can't We Sleep? *TODAY* 'Snooze or Lose' Survey Results May Surprise You," *Today Health & Wellness*, November 9, 2014, www.today.com.

30 **"I walked into my home":** Nalini Mani, "When My Body Shut Down, I Knew I Needed a Change," *The Huffington Post*, March 5, 2014, www.huffingtonpost.com.

30 **An Australian study found:** A. M. Williamson and Anne-Marie Feyer, "Moderate Sleep Deprivation Produces Impairments in Cognitive and Motor Performance Equivalent to Legally Prescribed Levels of Alcohol Intoxication," *Occupational & Environmental Medicine* 57 (2000): 649–55.

31 **Nearly 60 percent of train operators:** "National Sleep Foundation Annual Poll Explores Transportation Workers' Sleep," National Sleep Foundation press release, March 3, 2012, www.prnewswire.com.

31 **"Every aspect of who you are":** *Sleepless in America*, directed by Hoffman.

31 **21,113 deaths due to drunk driving:** "Board Meeting: Safety Report on Eliminating Impaired Driving," National Transportation Safety Board, May 14, 2013, www.ntsb.gov.

31 **By 2013:** "Traffic Safety Facts 2013," National Highway Traffic Safety Administration, December 2014, www.nhtsa.gov.

31 **"Sleepiness-related motor vehicle crashes":** Namni Goel, Hengyi Rao, Jeffrey S. Durmer, and David F. Dinges, "Neurocognitive Consequences of Sleep Deprivation," *Seminars in Neurology* 29 (2009): 320–99.

32 **A report from the Centers for Disease Control and Prevention:** "Unhealthy Sleep-Related Behaviors," *Morbidity and Mortality Weekly Report*, March 4, 2011, www.cdc.gov.

32 **And in a National Sleep Foundation poll:** "2005 Sleep in America Poll: Summary of Findings," National Sleep Foundation, March 2005, www.sleepfoundation.org

32 **"Dazed and confused"**: Carin Kilby Clark, "How Are You Going to Thrive?," *The Huffington Post*, May 5, 2014, www.huffingtonpost.com.

32 **328,000 accidents each year:** "Prevalence of Motor Vehicle Crashes Involving Drowsy Drivers, United States, 2009–2013," AAA Foundation for Traffic Safety, November 2014, www.aaafoundation.org.

32 **"microsleep":** "Brain Regions Can Take Short Naps During Wakefulness, Leading to Errors," University of Wisconsin–Madison School of Medicine and Public Health press release, April 27, 2011, www.eurekaalert.org.

32 **Men are 11 percent more likely:** "2002 'Sleep in America' Poll," National Sleep Foundation, March 2002, www.sleepfoundation.org.

33 **"The men engaged in long-haul trucking":** Derickson, *Dangerously Sleepy*, Kindle edition.

33 **2 million truckers:** David Voreacos and Jeff Plungis, "Trucker in Massive Rig Destroys Two Families in His Sleep," *Bloomberg Business*, September 30, 2014, www.bloomberg.com.

33 **accidents involving trucks:** "Statement of FMCSA Administrator Anne S. Ferro Before the House Transportation and Infrastructure Subcommittee on Highways and Transit on the Hearing 'Compliance, Safety, Accountability Program,'" Federal Motor Carrier Safety Administration, September 13, 2012, www.fmcsa.dot.gov.

33 **More than 60 percent:** Troy Green (National Highway Traffic Safety Administration Office of Communications and Consumer Information), email to the author, April 9, 2015.

33 **nearly half of all truckers:** Federal Motor Carrier Administration, Proposed Rule, "Hours of Service of Drivers," *Federal Register* 75, no. 249 (December 29, 2010): 82170, www.gpo.gov.

33 **In 2014 alone, 725 truckers:** "National Census of Fatal Occupational Injuries in 2014 (Preliminary Results)," Bureau of Labor Statistics, September 17, 2015, www.bls.gov.

33 **a Walmart truck:** Jason Hanna and Rene Marsh, "Trucker in Tracy Morgan Crash Hadn't Slept for 28 Hours, NTSB Says," *CNN*, August 12, 2015, www.cnn.com.

34 **"My response to":** Pete Bigelow, "Tracy Morgan Crash Sparks Another Debate over Tired Truckers," *Autoblog*, June 9, 2014, www.autoblog.com.

34 **Arkansas and New Jersey:** Jon Hilkevitch, "Federal Traffic Agency Targets Drowsy Driving," *Chicago Tribune*, March 16, 2015, www.chicagotribune.com.

34 **Senator Susan Collins:** "Sen. Collins Secures Critical Investments in Transportation Infrastructure and Housing," Susan Collins, United States Senator for Maine, press release, December 10, 2014, www.collins.senate.gov.

34 **"With one amendment":** Bigelow, "Tracy Morgan Crash Sparks Another Debate."

34 **Current regulations:** "Interstate Truck Driver's Guide to Hours of Service," Federal Motor Carrier Safety Administration, March 2015, www.fmcsa.dot.gov.

34 **much stricter standards:** "FAA Issues Final Rule on Pilot Fatigue," Federal Aviation Administration, December 21, 2011, www.faa.gov.

35 **A study by the National Transportation Safety Board:** Stephen Pope, "Fighting Pilot Fatigue: New Views on Staying Alert," *Flying Magazine*, November 26, 2014, www.flyingmag.com.

35 **Air India crash:** Government of India, Ministry of Civil Aviation, *Report on Accident to Air India Express Boeing 737–800 Aircraft VT-AXV on 22nd May 2010 at Mangalore* (New Delhi: October 31, 2010), www.skybrary.aero.

35 **"It is not unusual":** *Sleep Alert*, produced by James B. Maas (Ithaca: Cornell University Film Unit, 1990), PBS television special.

35 **In April 2014:** Sabina Gherbremedhin, "Sleeping Baggage Handler Says He Expected to Die After Waking Inside Cargo Hold: Exclusive," *ABC News*, April 23, 2015, www.abcnews.go.com.

35 **this problem extends to luggage screeners:** Mathias Basner, Joshua

Rubinstein, Kenneth M. Fomberstein, Matthew C. Coble, Adrian Ecker, Deepa Avinash, and David F. Dinges, "Effects of Night Work, Sleep Loss and Time on Task on Simulated Threat Detection Performance," *SLEEP* 31 (2008): 1251–59.

35 **federal air marshals:** Nelli Black, Curt Devine, and Drew Griffin, "Sleep-Deprived, Medicated, Suicidal and Armed: Federal Air Marshals in Disarray," *CNN Investigations*, August 14, 2015, www.cnn.com.

35 **a study by NASA:** Judith Orasanu, Bonny Parke, Norbert Kraft, Yuri Tada, Alan Hobbs, Barrett Anderson, Lori McDonnell, and Vicki Dulchinos, "Evaluating the Effectiveness of Schedule Changes for Air Traffic Service (ATS) Providers: Controller Alertness and Fatigue Monitoring Study," DOT/FAA/HFD-13/001, December 2012, www.faa.gov.

36 **new rules went into effect:** Susan Carey and Andy Pasztor, "Airlines Brace for Big Wake-up Call," *The Wall Street Journal*, January 2, 2014, www.wsj.com.

36 **William Rockefeller:** Murray Weiss, "William Rockefeller, Metro-North Engineer, Fell Asleep Before Fatal Train Derailment: Report," *The Huffington Post*, December 3, 2013, www.huffingtonpost.com.

36 **"We feel 100 percent confident":** Lydia DePillis, "Was the Engineer on Amtrak 188 Too Tired to Drive?," *The Washington Post*, May 15, 2015, www.washingtonpost.com.

36 **"Health is deeply intertwined":** Sam Stein, "The Surgeon General Wants You, America, to Sleep More," *The Huffington Post*, October 6, 2015, www.huffingtonpost.com.

37 **"part martyr and part hero":** Brian Goldman, "It's Time for Doctors to Admit That Our Lack of Sleep Is Killing Patients," *Quartz*, May 5, 2015, www.qz.com.

37 **Researchers from Harvard Medical School:** Laura K. Barger, Najib T. Ayas, Brian E. Cade, John W. Cronin, Bernard Rosner, Frank E. Speizer, and Charles A. Czeisler, "Impact of Extended-Duration Shifts on Medical Errors, Adverse Events, and Attentional Failures," *PLoS Medicine* 3 (2006): e487.

37 **In a Pennsylvania hospital in 2015:** "Newborn Dropped by Nurse Has Been Released from Hospital," *WPXI News*, July 8, 2015, www.wpxi.com.

37 **Sleep-deprived health-care workers:** Venkatesh Krishnamurthy, Luisa Bazan, Thomas Roth, and Christopher L. Drake, "Insomnia Affects Empathy in Health Care Workers," *SLEEP* Abstract Supplement 38 (2015): A241.

37 **James Reason:** Darshak Sanghavi, "The Phantom Menace of Sleep-Deprived Doctors," *The New York Times*, August 5, 2011, www.nytimes.com.

38 **The brains of young children:** Nandini Mundkur, "Neuroplasticity in Children," *Indian Journal of Pediatrics* 72 (2005): 855–57.

38 **"REM sleep":** Rebecca Phillips, "REM Sleep Critical for Young Brains; Medication Interferes," *WSU News*, July 3, 2015, www.news.wsu.edu.

38 **Dr. Aneesa Das:** "How Lack of Sleep Impacts Different Age Groups,"

The Ohio State University Wexner Medical Center press release, November 2013, www.osuwmc.multimedianewsroom.tv.

38 **diagnosis of ADHD:** "ADHD and Sleep," National Sleep Foundation, www.sleepfoundation.org.

38 **observed more than eleven thousand British children:** Karen Bonuck, Katherine Freeman, Ronald D. Chervin, and Linzhi Xu, "Sleep-Disordered Breathing in a Population-Based Cohort: Behavioral Outcomes at 4 and 7 Years," *Pediatrics* 129 (2012): e857–65.

39 **Researchers from the University of Hong Kong:** Ka-Fai Chung and Miao-Miao Cheung, "Sleep-Wake Patterns and Sleep Disturbance Among Hong Kong Chinese Adolescents," *SLEEP* 31 (2008): 185–94.

39 **Mary Carskadon:** Mary Carskadon, email to the author, March 26, 2015.

40 **"Asking a teenager":** Meeri Kim, "Blue Light from Electronics Disturbs Sleep, Especially for Teenagers," *The Washington Post*, September 1, 2014, www.washingtonpost.com.

40 **"Television, video games, smartphones":** Rakesh Bhattacharjee, email to the author, February 24, 2015.

40 **light from those devices:** Kim, "Blue Light from Electronics Disturbs Sleep, Especially for Teenagers."

40 **Uppsala University in Sweden:** Olga E. Titova, Pleunie S. Hogenkamp, Josefin A. Jacobsson, Inna Feldman, Helgi B. Schiöth, and Christian Benedict, "Associations of Self-Reported Sleep Disturbance and Duration with Academic Failure in Community-Dwelling Swedish Adolescents: Sleep and Academic Performance at School," *Sleep Medicine* 16 (2015): 87–93.

40 **poor sleep, grades, and dropout rates:** Skye Allan, "Undiagnosed Sleep Disorders May Damage College Students' Academic Success," *Inside UNC Charlotte*, August 7, 2015, www.inside.uncc.edu.

40 **A 2014 study by the University of Sydney:** Nicholas Glozier, Alexandra Martiniuk, George Patton, Rebecca Ivers, Qiang Li, Ian Hickie, Teresa Senserrick, Mark Woodward, Robyn Norton, and Mark Stevenson, "Short Sleep Duration in Prevalent and Persistent Psychological Distress in Young Adults: The DRIVE Study," *SLEEP* 33 (2010): 1139–45.

40 **A 2015 survey by the Sleep Council:** Lisa Artis, "Revision Robs Teens of Sleep," The Sleep Council press release, March 27, 2015, www.sleepcouncil.org.uk.

40 **death of Marina Keegan:** Jocelyn Richards, "Marina Keegan Dead: Yale Student, 22, Dies in Car Crash Days After Graduation," *The Huffington Post*, May 28, 2012, www.huffingtonpost.com.

41 **"No politician would smoke":** McGrath, "Unlocking the Science of Social Jet Lag and Sleep."

41 **Scott Walker's presidential campaign:** Patrick Healy, "A Sleep-Deprived Scott Walker Barnstorms Through South Carolina," *The New York Times*, July 15, 2015, www.nytimes.com.

41 **As former President Bill Clinton once said:** Weston Kosova, "Running on Fumes: Pulling All-Nighters, Bill Clinton Spent His Last Days

Obsessing over Details and Pardons," *Newsweek*, February 26, 2001, www.newsweek.com.

41 **David Gergen went deeper on Clinton's sleep habits:** David Gergen, *Eyewitness to Power: The Essence of Leadership Nixon to Clinton* (New York: Simon & Schuster, 2001), Kindle edition.

42 **Ted Cruz:** "Skimm Your Candidate: Sen. Ted Cruz (TX), Republican," *theSkimm* email newsletter, August 4, 2015.

42 **Carly Fiorina:** "Skimm Your Candidate: Carly Fiorina, Former CEO of Hewlett-Packard (R)," *theSkimm* email newsletter, May 5, 2015.

42 **Hillary Clinton:** "Skimm Your Candidate: Fmr. US Sec. of State Hillary Clinton, Democrat," *theSkimm* email newsletter, July 30, 2015.

43 **Supreme Court Justice Ruth Bader Ginsburg:** Al Kamen and Emily Heil, "Obama's Speech Didn't Excite Justice Ginsburg," *The Washington Post*, February 13, 2013, www.washingtonpost.com; Richard Wolf, "Justice Ginsburg: Not '100% Sober' at State of the Union," *USA TODAY*, February 13, 2015, www.usatoday.com.

43 **Secretary of Homeland Security Janet Napolitano:** Jamie Fuller, "Who Will Fall Asleep During the State of the Union Address Tonight?," *The Washington Post*, January 20, 2015, www.washingtonpost.com.

43 **Vice President Joe Biden:** Ryan Haggerty, "Joe Biden Falls Asleep During Speech," *Chicago Tribune*, April 15, 2011, www.chicagotribune.com.

43 **Former President Bill Clinton:** Post Staff Report, "Bill Has a 'Dream,'" *New York Post*, January 21, 2008, www.nypost.com.

43 **Larry Summers:** Ryan Lizza, "Inside the Crisis: Larry Summers and the White House Economic Team," *The New Yorker*, October 12, 2009, www.newyorker.com.

43 **Gordon Brown:** "In Praise of Nap Time: Politicians Caught with Their Eyes Closed," *The Telegraph*, www.telegraph.co.uk.

43 **Members of Parliament in Japan:** "Tuesday, August 24: Prime Minister Chats with School Pupils," What's Up Around the Prime Minister, August 24, 1999, www.japan.kantei.go.jp/diary.

43 **In Uganda:** Eriasa Mukiibi Sserunjogi, "Ugandans Baffled by Sleeping Ministers," *Al Jazeera*, August 6, 2014, www.aljazeera.com.

44 **one marathon session:** Mehreen Khan and Ben Wright, "'Crucified' Tsipras Capitulates to Draconian Measures After 17 Hours of Late Night Talks: As It Happened," *The Telegraph*, July 13, 2015, www.telegraph.co.uk.

44 **Jean-Claude Juncker:** Katerina Nanopoulou, "When Tired Politicians Are Called On to Make Important Decisions," *The Huffington Post*, July 9, 2015, www.huffingtonpost.com.

44 **"Clearly it is a very suboptimal":** Matthew Weaver, "Greece Crisis: What Are the Effects of Sleep Deprivation on Decision-Making?," *The Guardian*, July 13, 2015, www.theguardian.com.

44 **Eric Fehrnstrom:** Arianna Huffington, "Is Sleep Deprivation the Reason the Romney Campaign Is Blowing It?," *The Huffington Post*, September 19, 2012, www.huffingtonpost.com.

45 **a 2015 report by the RAND Corporation:** Wendy M. Troxel, Regina A. Shih, Eric R. Pedersen, Lily Geyer, Michael P. Fisher, Beth Ann Griffin, Ann C. Haas, Jeremy Kurz, and Paul S. Steinberg, *Sleep in the Military Promoting Healthy Sleep Among U.S. Servicemembers* (Santa Monica: RAND Corporation, 2015), www.rand.org.

45 **Lieutenant Colonel Kate Van Arman:** David Vergun, "Sleep Issues Bedeviling Soldiers' Health," *U.S. Army*, September 10, 2015, www.army.mil.

45 **study of almost five thousand police officers:** Shantha M. W. Rajaratnam, Laura K. Barger, Steven W. Lockley, Steven A. Shea, Wei Wang, Christopher P. Landrigan, Conor S. O'Brien, Salim Qadri, Jason P. Sullivan, Brian E. Cade, Lawrence J. Epstein, David P. White, and Charles A. Czeisler, "Sleep Disorders, Health, and Safety in Police Officers," *The Journal of the American Medical Association* 306 (2011): 2567–78.

2. THE SLEEP INDUSTRY

46 **Lifehacker even published an article:** Thorin Klosowski, "Build an Insanely Loud Alarm to Get Yourself Out of Bed No Matter What," *Lifehacker*, August 11, 2015, www.lifehacker.com.

46 **"a sudden fear or distressing suspense":** "alarm," Dictionary.com, www.dictionary.reference.com.

47 **American Academy of Sleep Medicine:** "Publication of Sleep Medicine Quality Measures Promotes Value-Based Care," American Academy of Sleep Medicine, March 13, 2015, www.aasmnet.org.

47 **more than 55 million prescriptions:** Nina Gill (account director, MSL Boston), IMS Health data set, email to the author, July 15, 2015.

47 **2013 Centers for Disease Control report:** Yinong Chong and Qiuping Gu, "Prescription Sleep Aid Use Among Adults: United States, 2005–2010," *NCHS Data Brief*, no. 127, August 2013, www.cdc.gov.

47 **A National Sleep Foundation poll:** "Stressed-Out American Women Have No Time for Sleep," National Sleep Foundation, March 6, 2007, www.sleepfoundation.org.

47 **survey by *Parade:*** "Pillow Talk," Athlon Media Group/Parade.com survey results infographic, email to the author, July 16, 2015.

47 **$58 billion on sleep-aid products:** "Sleep Aids: Technologies and Global Markets," BCC Research report, June 2014, www.bccresearch.com.

47 **use of sleeping pills is highest:** Chong and Gu, "Prescription Sleep Aid Use Among Adults."

48 **"In twenty years":** Jerome Siegel, email to the author, November 3, 2015.

49 **"empowering medical practitioners":** Wolf-Meyer, *The Slumbering Masses.*

49 **the drug zolpidem:** Gill, IMS Health data set.

50 **"At the end of the test":** Mohamed El-Erian, conversation with the author, September 26, 2015.

50 **"necessarily produces an imbalance":** Patrick Fuller, email to the author, May 11, 2015.

51 **November 2014 appearance on *The Late Show*:** Allison Takeda, "Anna Kendrick Talks Dildos, Sleepwalking on Ambien with David Letterman: 'I Wake Up to a Surprise Every Time,'" *Us Weekly*, December 17, 2014, www.usmagazine.com.

51 **The *Today* show's Julia Sommerfeld:** Julia Sommerfeld, "While I Was Sleeping: Shopping Sprees, Sugar Binges and Other Confessions of an Ambien Zombie," *TODAY*, November 13, 2014, www.today.com.

52 **"I simply do not remember":** Robert Pear and Carl Hulse, "Patrick Kennedy Says He'll Seek Help for Addiction," *The New York Times*, May 5, 2006, www.nytimes.com.

52 **University of Washington study:** Ryan N. Hansen, Denise M. Boudreau, Beth E. Ebel, David C. Grossman, and Sean D. Sullivan, "Sedative Hypnotic Medication Use and the Risk of Motor Vehicle Crash," *American Journal of Public Health* 105 (2015): e64–69.

52 **the FDA in 2013:** "FDA Drug Safety Communication: FDA Approves New Label Changes and Dosing for Zolpidem Products and a Recommendation to Avoid Driving the Day After Using Ambien CR," U.S. Food and Drug Administration, May 14, 2013, www.fda.gov.

52 **Allison McCabe told:** Allison McCabe, "Ambien Zombies, Murder, and Other Disturbing Behavior," *The Fix*, Jan 10, 2014, www.thefix.com.

54 **"Criminal laws are not well suited":** Ted Olson, email to the author, July 14, 2015.

54 **In 2009, Julie Ann Bronson:** Craig Kapitan, "Jury Grants Probation for Drunken Ambien Wreck," *San Antonio Express-News*, May 16, 2012, www.mysanantonio.com.

55 **Human-rights activist Kerry Kennedy:** Colleen Curry and Aaron Katersky, "Kerry Kennedy Says Ambien 'Overtook' Her, Causing Car Crash," *ABC News*, February 26, 2014, www.abcnews.go.com.

55 **Lunesta has many of the same dangers:** "FDA Requiring Lower Starting Dose for Sleep Drug Lunesta," U.S. Food and Drug Administration, May 15, 2014, www.fda.gov.

55 **outlined clearly in the drug warning:** "Possible Side Effects," Lunesta, www.lunesta.com.

56 **Belsomra:** "FDA Approves New Type of Sleep Drug, Belsomra," U.S. Food and Drug Administration, August 13, 2014, www.fda.gov.

56 **hailed in the press as "groundbreaking":** Darian Lusk, "Groundbreaking Sleeping Pill May Put Insomnia Issues to Bed," *CBS News*, August 14, 2014, www.cbsnews.com.

56 **"Walking, eating, driving":** Belsomra, "Belsomra Commercial: Furry Sleep/Wake Creatures," YouTube video, August 9, 2015, www.youtube.com.

56 **increases the risk of developing Alzheimer's:** Sophie Billioti de Gage, Yola Moride, Thierry Ducruet, Tobias Kurth, Hélène Verdoux, Marie

Tournier, Antoine Pariente, and Bernard Bégaud, "Benzodiazepine Use and Risk of Alzheimer's Disease: Case-Control Study," *BMJ* 349 (2014): g5205.

57 **Sleeping pills carry major health risks:** Daniel F. Kripke, Robert D. Langer, and Lawrence E. Kline, "Hypnotics' Association with Mortality or Cancer: A Matched Cohort Study," *BMJ* Open 2 (2012): doi: 10.1136/bmjopen-2012-000850.

57 **In 2015, Kripke:** Daniel Kripke, "Petition to the FDA Regarding Hypnotic Drugs," CBT for Insomnia, www.cbtforinsomnia.com.

58 **In 2015, *Consumer Reports*:** "The Truth About Sleeping Pills," *Consumer Reports*, March 2015, www.consumerreports.org.

58 **Procter & Gamble, the maker of ZzzQuil:** John Bussey, "The Innovator's Enigma," *The Wall Street Journal*, October 4, 2012, www.wsj.com.

58 **active ingredient diphenhydramine:** "ZzzQuil Liquicaps—Package Information," ZzzQuil, www.vicks.com.

58 **also found in Benadryl:** "Diphenhydramine," U.S. National Library of Medicine MedlinePlus, www.nlm.nih.gov.

58 **Dr. Shalini Paruthi:** Alena Hall, "The Truth About Over-the-Counter Sleep Aids," *The Huffington Post*, March 23, 2015, www.huffingtonpost .com.

58 **ZzzQuil may also cause headaches:** "Vicks ZzzQuil Nighttime Sleep-Aid: Oral Capsule, Liquid Filled," CVS Pharmacy, www.cvs.com.

58 **a 2016 *Consumer Reports* survey:** "Why Americans Can't Sleep," *Consumer Reports*, January 14, 2016, www.consumerreports.org.

58 **2015 study from the University of Washington:** Shelly L. Gray, Melissa L. Anderson, Sascha Dublin, Joseph T. Hanlon, Rebecca Hubbard, Rod Walker, Onchee Yu, Paul K. Crane, and Eric B. Larson, "Cumulative Use of Strong Anticholinergics and Incident Dementia," *The Journal of the American Medical Association* 175 (2015): 401–7.

59 **Researchers at the University of Michigan:** Carol J. Boyd, Elizabeth Austic, Quyen Epstein-Ngo, Philip T. Veliz, and Sean Esteban McCabe, "A Prospective Study of Adolescents' Nonmedical Use of Anxiolytic and Sleep Medication," *Psychology of Addictive Behaviors* 29 (2015): 184–91.

60 **as Oprah puts it:** "Steep Your Soul," *Oprah.com*, www.oprah.com.

60 **"I could lay my head":** Cat Stevens, "I'm So Sleepy," *New Masters*, Dream Records, 1967.

61 **"factory workers had to function":** Tom Standage, *A History of the World in 6 Glasses* (New York: Walker Books Company, 2005), 200.

61 **traced increasing coffee consumption:** Mark Pendergrast, *Uncommon Grounds: The History of Coffee and How It Transformed Our World*, 2nd ed. (New York: Basic Books, 2010).

61 **Coffee consumption in the United States:** Jeremy Olshan, "America's Coffee Cup Is Half Full," *Market Watch*, February 20, 2013, www .marketwatch.com.

61 **Annual US sales of carbonated sodas:** Murray Carpenter, *Caffeinated: How Our Daily Habit Helps, Hurts, and Hooks Us* (New York: Hudson Street Press, 2014), 76.

61 **six times the annual sales of coffee:** "Coffee Production in the US: Market Research Report," IBISWorld, September 2015, www.ibisworld.com.

61 **eight out of the top ten best-selling soft drinks:** Carpenter, *Caffeinated*, 120.

61 **U.S. Department of Agriculture's Bureau of Chemistry:** Ibid., 80.

61 **"Why should the people":** Ibid., 86.

62 **caffeine has spilled out of beverages and into products:** Betsy Isaacson, "Our Sleep Problem and What to Do About It," *Newsweek*, January 22, 2015, www.newsweek.com; Sarah Klein, "12 Surprising Sources of Caffeine," *Health*, www.health.com; Tuck Danbridge, "30 Bizarre/Delicious Ways to Get Your Caffeine Buzz On," *Thrillist*, November 26, 2012, www.thrillist.com.

62 **Swedish condom company:** "Caffeinated Condoms Keep Guys Up," *Flash News*, flashnews.com.

62 **Mintel Group:** Marilyn Alva, "Energy Drinks Fuel Monster Beverage; Coke Jolt Next," *Investors*, April 23, 2015, www.investors.com.

62 **Red Bull sold more than 5.6 billion cans:** "The Company Behind the Can," Red Bull, energydrink-us.redbull.com.

62 **Monster Beverage:** Alva, "Energy Drinks Fuel Monster Beverage."

62 **laundry list of side effects:** "Energy Drinks," American Association of Poison Control Centers, www.aapcc.org.

62 **Emergency-room visits:** "THE DAWN REPORT: Update on Emergency Department Visits Involving Energy Drinks: A Continuing Public Health Concern," Substance Abuse and Mental Health Services Administration report, January 10, 2013, www.samhsa.gov.

63 **Provigil:** Amanda L. Chan, "Provigil: Narcolepsy Drug Being Taken by People Without the Sleep Disorder," *The Huffington Post*, July 18, 2012, www.huffingtonpost.com.

63 **smart drugs:** Carole Cadwalladr, "Students Used to Take Drugs to Get High. Now They Take Them to Get Higher Grades," *The Guardian*, February 14, 2015, www.theguardian.com.

63 **a 2014 study found:** Isaacson, "Our Sleep Problem and What to Do About It."

63 **Partnership for Drug-Free Kids:** Tara Haelle, "ADHD Stimulant Drug Abuse Common Among Young Adults: Survey," *U.S. News & World Report*, November 13, 2014, www.health.usnews.com.

63 **Among Ivy League students:** Isaacson, "Our Sleep Problem and What to Do About It."

63 **2014 report by the American Psychological Association:** "Stress in America: Are Teens Adopting Adults' Stress Habits?" American Psychological Association press release, February 11, 2014, www.apa.org.

64 **an ad for Red Bull:** Jenna Johnson, "Energy Drink Popularity Booms at College Despite Health Concerns," *The Washington Post*, December 18, 2012, www.washingtonpost.com.

64 **As an advertisement for Spotify says:** Spotify advertisement, heard by author on Spotify, September 12, 2015.

64 **Sarah Hedgecock:** Sarah Hedgecock, "The Ivy League's Insomnia Problem: When Lack of Sleep Is a Competition," *Bustle*, March 7, 2014, www.bustle.com.

64 **Angela Della Croce observed:** Angella Della Croce, "Sleep Hard to Come By in the Typical College Life," *The Miscellany News*, April 24, 2013, www.miscellanynews.org.

65 **"I get this notion that":** Fernando Hurtado, email to Jessica Kane (director of millennial outreach, *The Huffington Post*), August 18, 2015.

65 **"Catching up on sleep":** Hannah Tattersall, email to Jessica Kane (director of millennial outreach, *The Huffington Post*), August 18, 2015.

65 **"People don't really prioritize sleep":** Luis Ruuska, email to Jessica Kane (director of millennial outreach, *The Huffington Post*), August 18, 2015.

65 **"Who needs sleep":** Kenza Kamal, email to Jessica Kane (director of millennial outreach, *The Huffington Post*), August 18, 2015.

65 **"I'll get Snapchats during finals week":** Madeline Diamond, email to Jessica Kane (director of millennial outreach, *The Huffington Post*), August 18, 2015.

66 **a 2014 study:** "Poor Sleep Equal to Binge Drinking, Marijuana Use in Predicting Academic Problems," American Academy of Sleep Medicine press release, June 1, 2014, www.aasmnet.org.

66 **"I don't think":** Sarah Klein, "Sleep Problems Equal to Binge Drinking, Marijuana Use in Predicting Poor Academic Performance," *The Huffington Post*, June 3, 2014, www.huffingtonpost.com.

66 **Researchers at California State University:** Larry Rosen, "Relax, Turn Off Your Phone, and Go to Sleep," *Harvard Business Review*, August 31, 2015, www.hbr.org.

66 **2015 study from Idaho State University:** Maria M. Wong, Gail C. Robertson, and Rachel B. Dyson, "Prospective Relationship Between Poor Sleep and Substance-Related Problems in a National Sample of Adolescents," *Alcoholism: Clinical and Experimental Research* 39 (2015): 355–62.

67 **sleep-deprived students turn to stimulants:** Haelle, "ADHD Stimulant Drug Abuse Common Among Young Adults: Survey."

67 **The University of Florida found:** "UF Study: Majority of Teens Think Prescription Stimulant Use Is a Problem Among Peers," University of Florida press release, September 4, 2013, www.news.ufl.edu.

67 **Partnership for Drug-Free Kids study:** Haelle, "ADHD Stimulant Drug Abuse Common Among Young Adults: Survey."

67 **billions of dollars:** Maureen Mackey, "Sleepless in America: A $32.4 Billion Business," *The Fiscal Times*, July 23, 2012, www.thefiscaltimes.com.

3. SLEEP THROUGHOUT HISTORY

69 **"People sought peaceful sleep":** Kat Duff, *The Secret Life of Sleep* (New York: Atria Books/Beyond Words, 2014), Kindle edition.

69 **In both ancient Egypt and ancient Greece:** Ana Ruiz, *The Spirit of Ancient Egypt* (New York: Algora Publishing, 2001), 171–72; Robert Garland, *The Daily Life of Ancient Greeks, 2nd Edition* (Westport: Greenwood Publishing Group, 2009), 77.
69 **"The Golden God":** Stephen Mitchell, email to the author, December 21, 2014.
70 **"Since God has shown you":** Genesis 41:37–40, ESV.
70 **"Even a soul submerged in sleep":** Heraclitus, *Fragments: The Collected Wisdom of Heraclitus*, trans. Brooks Haxton (New York: Viking, 2001), Kindle edition.
70 **The Greeks and the Romans:** David Randall, *Dreamland: Adventures in the Strange Science of Sleep* (New York: W. W. Norton & Company, 2012), Kindle edition; Mary Ann Dwight, *Grecian and Roman Mythology* (New York: George P. Putnam, 1849), 72.
70 **As David Randall writes:** Randall, *Dreamland.*
70 **Lethe, the river of forgetfulness:** Duff, *The Secret Life of Sleep.*
70 **As Heraclitus:** Ibid.
70 **Around the same time:** "Sleep: A Historical Perspective," Healthy Sleep, www.healthysleep.med.harvard.edu.
70 **Aristotle defined sleep:** Aristotle, *On Sleep and Sleeplessness*, trans. J. I. Beare, MIT Internet Classics Archive, www.classics.mit.edu.
71 **Ancient Chinese literature:** Duff, *The Secret Life of Sleep.*
71 **In Islam the existence of sleep:** Ahmed S. BaHammam, "Sleep from an Islamic Perspective," *Annals of Thoracic Medicine* 6 (2011): 187–92.
71 **"During sleep":** René Descartes, *Treatise of Man* (Amherst: Prometheus Books, 2003), Kindle edition.
71 **One of the earliest references:** Homer, *The Odyssey*, trans. George Chapman (Hertfordshire: Wordsworth Editions, 2002), 82.
72 **"This non-continuous sleep pattern":** Gregg Jacobs, email to the author, March 11, 2015.
72 **"Fires needed to be tended":** A. Roger Ekirch, email to the author, March 16, 2015.
72 **"When you awake in the night":** Richard Allestree, *The Whole Duty of Prayer Containing Devotions for Every Day in the Week, and for Several Occasions, Ordinary and Extraordinary* (Ann Arbor: Text Creation Partnership), quod.lib.umich.edu.
72 **"A sixteenth-century French physician":** Ekirch, email to the author.
72 **"The influence dreams had":** A. Roger Ekirch, *At Day's Close: Night in Times Past* (New York: W. W. Norton & Company, 2005), Kindle edition.
73 **"a class of fancies":** Edgar Allan Poe, "Marginalia [part V]," *Graham's Magazine* 28 (1846): 116–18, www.eapoe.org.
73 **"It seemed to me":** Robert Louis Stevenson, *The Cevennes Journal: Notes on a Journey Through the French Highlands* (Edinburgh: Mainstream Publishing, 1978), 115.
73 **"Within some homes":** Ekirch, *At Day's Close.*

74 **communal sleeping:** Jean-Louis Flandrin, *Families in Former Times: Kinship, Household and Sexuality* (Cambridge, Eng.: Cambridge University Press, 1979), 101.

74 **"Sleeping with others":** Carol Worthman, email to the author, July 8, 2015.

74 **Benjamin Franklin and John Adams had to share a bed:** James Parton, *Life and Times of Benjamin Franklin, vol.* 2 (New York: Mason Brothers, 1864), 143.

74 **In a National Institute of Mental Health study:** Thomas A. Wehr, "In Short Photo Periods, Human Sleep Is Biphasic," *Journal of Sleep Research* 1 (1992): 103–7.

75 **"It's the seamless sleep":** Jon Mooallem, "The Sleep-Industrial Complex," *The New York Times*, November 18, 2007, www.nytimes.com.

75 **"regard themselves as abnormal":** Ekirch, email to the author.

75 **The first public lamp:** "History of the Public Lighting of Paris," *Nature* 132 (1933): 888–89.

75 **In 1667:** Doug Peterson, "Who's Afraid of the Dark?," *LASNews*, Summer 2013, www.las.illinois.edu.

75 **Other cities soon followed:** Stephanie Hegarty, "The Myth of the Eight-Hour Sleep," *BBC News*, February 22, 2012, www.bbc.com.

75 **early movement to light up the night:** Ibid.

75 **History professor Craig Koslofsky:** Peterson, "Who's Afraid of the Dark?"

75 **more than fifty cities:** Hegarty, "The Myth of the Eight-Hour Sleep."

75 **In 1807, London's Pall Mall:** Christopher Winn, *I Never Knew That About London* (New York: St. Martin's Press, 2007), Kindle edition.

75 **By the dawn of the twentieth century:** "History of the Public Lighting of Paris."

75 **Across the pond, Baltimore:** James G. Speight, *Natural Gas: A Basic Handbook* (Houston: Gulf Publishing Company, 2007), 22.

76 **In Southeast Asia:** Nor-Afidah Abd Rahman, "Street Lighting," *Singapore Infopedia*, 1998, www.eresources.nlb.gov.sg.

76 **"owners and managers treated":** Kevin Hillstrom and Laurie Collier Hillstrom, *The Industrial Revolution in America: Iron and Steel* (Santa Barbara: ABC-CLIO, 2005), 107.

76 **an act of masculinity:** Derickson, *Dangerously Sleepy.*

77 **"Extreme hours become a way men compete":** Joan Williams, email to the author, March 15, 2015.

77 **Women particularly suffered:** Derickson, *Dangerously Sleepy.*

77 **mounting consensus from courts:** Ibid.

77 **Louis Brandeis:** United States, Supreme Court, *Women in Industry: Decision of the United States Supreme Court in Curt Muller Vs. State of Oregon, Upholding the Constitutionality of the Oregon Ten-Hour Law for Women and Brief for the State of Oregon*, 1908, https://fraser.stlouisfed.org.

77 **"Places that clung to their traditional":** Randall, *Dreamland.*

78 **Steelworkers across America:** "Special Reports: A Pittsburgh Cen-

tury," *Pittsburgh Post-Gazette*, www.post-gazette.com; "TROOPERS STOP MEETINGS: Arrest 19 Men Including Labor Union Organizers."

78 **Throughout the early 1920s:** Hillstrom and Hillstrom, *The Industrial Revolution in America*, 103–7.

78 **"The twelve-hour day":** Charles Rumford Walker, *Steel: The Diary of a Furnace Worker* (Boston: The Atlantic Monthly Press, 1923), 156.

78 **"Workers regularly crawled":** John Hinshaw and Peter N. Stearns, *Industrialization in the Modern World: From the Industrial Revolution to the Internet*, vol. 1, A–L (Santa Barbara: ABC-CLIO, 2014), 4.

78 **"I often grieved when I saw":** Derickson, *Dangerously Sleepy.*

79 **Trade unionists had marched:** Roy Rosenzweig, *Eight Hours for What We Will: Workers & Leisure in an Industrial City, 1870–1920* (Cambridge, Eng.: Cambridge University Press, 1983), 1.

79 **But it was not until 1926:** Douglas Brinkley, "The 40-Hour Revolution," *TIME*, March 31, 2003, https://content.time.com.

79 **The idea of sleep as a labor issue:** "The Evolution and History of the Union," National A. Philip Randolph Pullman Porter Museum, www.aphiliprandolphmuseum.com.

79 **"The Pullman porter":** Edward Burman, "The Pullman Porters Win," *The Nation*, August 21, 1935, www.socialwelfarehistory.com.

79 **At the turn of the century, Edward Moseley:** Edward Moseley, *The American Monthly Review of Reviews* (New York: The Review of Reviews, 1904), 595.

80 **"The truly moral man":** Daniel T. Rodgers, *The Work Ethic in Industrial America, 1850–1920*, 2nd ed. (Chicago: University of Chicago Press, 2014), Kindle edition.

80 **young Benjamin Franklin:** Benjamin Franklin, *Poor Richard's Almanack* (Waterloo, Iowa: U.S.C. Publishing Co., 1914), 56.

80 **It was certainly a way of thinking:** Roberto De Vogli, *Progress or Collapse: The Crises of Market Greed* (Abingdon, Eng.: Routledge, 2013), 99.

80 **Horace G. Burt:** Rodgers, *The Work Ethic in Industrial America, 1850–1920.*

81 **He bragged that he never:** Olga Khazan, "Thomas Edison and the Cult of Sleep Deprivation," *The Atlantic*, May 14, 2014, www.theatlantic.com.

81 **The *Chicago Tribune* lauded:** Derickson, *Dangerously Sleepy.*

81 **"THE FUTURE MAN":** Edward Marshall, "The Future Man Will Spend Less Time in Bed," *The New York Times*, October 11, 1914, www.nytimes.com.

82 **"Seeing everybody so up":** Andy Warhol and Pat Hackett, *POPism: The Warhol Sixties* (Boston: Houghton Mifflin Harcourt, 2015), 42.

82 **"I simply can't think of sleep":** Charles A. Lindbergh, *The Spirit of St. Louis* (New York: Charles Scribner's Sons, 1953), 234.

83 **praised by President Calvin Coolidge:** Calvin Coolidge, "Address Bestowing Upon Colonel Charles A. Lindbergh the Distinguished Fly-

ing Cross, Washington, D.C.," The American Presidency Project, www.presidency.ucsb.edu.

83 **"Rip Van Winkle":** Washington Irving, "Rip Van Winkle," in *The Literary World Seventh Reader*, eds. John Calvin Metcalf, Sarah Withers, and Hetty S. Browne (Richmond: B.F. Johnson Publishing Company, 1919), 9–30.

83 **Paul Revere, the American Revolutionary hero:** "The Real Story of Revere's Ride," The Paul Revere House, www.paulreverehouse.org.

84 **Vladimir Nabokov:** Vladimir Nabokov, *Speak, Memory: An Autobiography Revisited* (New York: Vintage International, 1989), 108.

84 **When Napoleon was asked:** Till Roenneberg, "Five Myths About Sleep," *The Washington Post*, November 21, 2012, www.washingtonpost.com.

84 **William Henry Hudson explains:** William Henry Hudson, *The Man Napoleon* (New York: Thomas Y. Crowell Company, 1915), 215.

85 **"Napoleon always talked about":** David Dinges and Aaron Levy, "Sleep Like Napoleon: An Interview with David Dinges," *Cabinet Magazine*, Fall 2008, www.cabinetmagazine.org.

85 **Napoleon's sleep regimen:** Ibid.

85 **During the nineteenth century:** "Historical and Cultural Perspectives of Sleep," Healthy Sleep, www.healthysleep.med.harvard.edu.

85 **King Louis XIV was known:** Charles Pollak, Michael J. Thorpy, and Jan Yager, *The Encyclopedia of Sleep and Sleep Disorders, 3rd ed.* (New York: Facts on File, 2010), 33.

86 **by the Victorian era:** Lucy Worsely (author, *If Walls Could Talk*), interview with Terry Gross, "'If Walls Could Talk': A History of the Home," *Fresh Air*, NPR, March 13, 2012, www.npr.org.

86 **Scottish doctor Robert Macnish:** Don Todman, "A History of Sleep Medicine," *The Internet Journal of Neurology* 9 (2007): https://ispub.com.

86 **In 1869, William Hammond:** William Hammond, *Sleep and Its Derangements* (Philadelphia: J. B. Lippencott & Co., 1869).

86 **In 1885, Henry Lyman:** Henry M. Lyman, *Insomnia, and Other Disorders of Sleep* (Chicago: W. T. Keener, 1885).

86 **In 1903, the first sleeping pill:** Francisco López-Muñoz, Ronaldo Ucha-Udabe, and Cecilio Alamo, "The History of Barbiturates a Century After Their Clinical Introduction," *Neuropsychiatric Disease and Treatment* 1 (2005): 329.

86 **Other sleeping pills hit the market:** Edward Brecher and the Editors of *Consumer Reports*, *Licit and Illicit Drugs: The Consumers Union Report on Narcotics, Stimulants, Depressants, Inhalants, Hallucinogens, and Marijuana—Including Caffeine* (New York: Little Brown & Co, 1973), 429.

86 **An important milestone:** Henri Piéron, "Le Problème Physiologique du Sommeil," *Science* 37 (1915): 525–26.

86 **In Germany, a psychiatrist, Hans Berger:** Todman, "A History of Sleep Medicine."

87 **biologist and botanist Erwin Bünning:** Pollak et al., *The Encyclopedia of Sleep and Sleep Disorders*, xxxv.

87 **sleep researcher Nathaniel Kleitman:** Lamberg, "The Student, the Professor and the Birth of Modern Sleep Research."

87 **He published his seminal work:** "Kleitman, Father of Sleep Research," *The University of Chicago Chronicle* 19 (1999): chronicle.uchicago.edu.

87 **The Association of Sleep Disorders Centers:** John W. Shepard Jr., Daniel J. Buysse, Andrew L. Chesson Jr., William C. Dement, Rochelle Goldberg, Christian Guilleminault, Cameron D. Harris, Conrad Iber, Emmanuel Mignot, Merrill M. Mitler, Kent E. Moore, Barbara A. Phillips, Stuart F. Quan, Richard S. Rosenberg, Thomas Roth, Helmut S. Schmidt, Michael H. Silber, James K. Walsh, and David P. White, "History of the Development of Sleep Medicine in the United States," *Journal of Clinical Sleep Medicine* 1 (2005): 61–82; Celmer, email to the author.

87 **Three years later:** Shepard et al., "History of the Development of Sleep Medicine in the United States."

87 **cognitive scientist Carlyle Smith:** Carlyle Smith and Stephen Butler, "Paradoxical Sleep at Selective Times Following Training Is Necessary for Learning," *Physiology & Behavior* 29 (1982): 469–73.

87 **Allan Rechtschaffen:** A. Rechtschaffen, M. A. Gilliland, B. M. Bergmann, and J. B. Winter, "Physiological Correlates of Prolonged Sleep Deprivation in Rats," *Science* 221 (1983): 182–84.

88 **Cold War:** David R. Roediger and Philip S. Foner, *Our Own Time: A History of American Labor and the Working Day* (New York: Verso, 1989), 269.

88 **163 hours more per year:** Juliet Schor, *The Overworked American: The Unexpected Decline of Leisure* (New York: Basic Books, 1992), 29.

88 **"I come in every Saturday morning":** Sam Walton, *Sam Walton: Made in America* (New York: Bantam Books, 1993), Kindle edition.

88 **"The Citi Never Sleeps":** Suzanne Vranica, "Citi Awakens an Old Campaign," *The Wall Street Journal*, May 7, 2008, www.wsj.com.

89 **Gordon Gekko:** *Wall Street*, directed by Oliver Stone (1987; Los Angeles: 20th Century Fox, 2000): DVD.

89 **rise of the Japanese "salaryman":** Andrea Germer, Vera Mackie, and Ulrike Wöhr, eds., *Gender, Nation and State in Modern Japan* (London and New York: Routledge, 2014), 255.

89 **He's at his desk until his supervisor leaves:** "Sayonora, Salaryman," *The Economist*, January 3, 2008, www.economist.com.

89 **culture of the salaryman:** James Brooke, "Young Japanese Breaking Old Salaryman's Bonds," *The New York Times*, October 18, 2001, www.nytimes.com.

90 **YouTube vlogger Stu in Tokyo:** Charles Riley, "Pity Japan's Salaryman: Inside a Brutal 80-Hour Workweek," *CNN Money*, March 9, 2015, www.money.cnn.com.

90 **"Overwork has also become":** Williams, email to the author, March 15, 2015.

90 **"Women typically have a fragile hold":** Ibid.

91 **form of cultural resistance:** Jonathan Crary, *24/7: Late Capitalism and the Ends of Sleep* (London: Verso, 2013), 10.

91 ***The Wall Street Journal:*** Brett Arends, "A Full Night's Sleep Can Really Pay Off—in Salary and Investments," *The Wall Street Journal*, September 18, 2014, www.wsj.com.

91 ***The Financial Times:*** Sarah O'Connor, "Lack of Sleep Found to Lower Employees' Productivity," *The Financial Times*, May 25, 2015, www.ft .com.

91 ***The Economist:*** "To Sleep, Perchance," *The Economist*, May 16, 2015, www.economist.com.

91 ***Forbes:*** Lynda Shaw, "Important Decisions to Make? Sleep on It," *Forbes*, December 15, 2014, www.forbes.com.

91 ***Business Insider:*** Julie Bort, "I Tried a Sleep Training App and It Completely Changed How I Think About Sleep," *Business Insider*, October 29, 2015, www.businessinsider.com.

91 ***Fast Company:*** Samantha Cole, "How to Sleep in Uncomfortable, Unavoidable Situations," *Fast Company*, February 24, 2015, www.fast company.com.

4. THE SCIENCE OF SLEEP

93 **"Physics says: go to sleep":** Albert Goldbarth, "The Sciences Sing a Lullabye," *The Kitchen Sink: New and Selected Poems, 1972–2007* (St. Paul: Graywolf Press, 2007), 241.

94 **"The drive to sleep":** Adam Hadhazy, "How Long Can We Stay Awake?" *BBC News*, February 23, 2015, www.bbc.com.

94 **In 1959, New York disc jockey Peter Tripp:** Bill Jaker, Frank Sulek, and Peter Kanze, *The Airwaves of New York: Illustrated Histories of 156 AM Stations in the Metropolitan Area, 1921–1996* (Jefferson: McFarland, 1998), 126.

95 **After three days:** Simon J. Williams, *Sleep and Society* (New York: Routledge, 2005), Kindle edition.

95 **the final day:** Geoff Rolls, *Classic Case Studies in Psychology: Third Edition* (London: Routledge, 2015), 251.

95 **inactivity theory:** "Why Do We Sleep, Anyway?," Healthy Sleep, www.healthysleep.med.harvard.edu.

95 **energy conservation theory:** Ibid.

95 **restorative theory:** Ibid.

96 **brain plasticity theory:** Ibid.

96 **"sleep is for the benefit":** Patrick Fuller, email to the author, November 7, 2015.

96 **"Sleep is of the brain":** J. Allan Hobson, "Sleep Is of the Brain, by the Brain and for the Brain," *Nature* 437 (2005): 1254–56.

96 **"Now, blessings light on him":** Miguel de Cervantes, *Don Quixote* (Hertfordshire, Eng.: Wordsworth Editions, 1993), pt. 2, chap. 68.

96 **"If sleep does not serve":** Allan Rechtschaffen, "The Control of Sleep," in *Human Behavior and Its Control*, ed. William A. Hunt (Cambridge, MA: Shenkman Press, 1971), 88.
96 **Sleep and wakefulness are regulated:** Charles M. Morin and Colin A. Espie, eds., *The Oxford Handbook of Sleep and Sleep Disorders* (New York: Oxford University Press, 2012), 53.
97 **"sleep pressure":** Steven Lockley and Russell Foster, *Sleep: A Very Short Introduction* (New York: Oxford University Press, 2012), 13.
97 **circadian rhythm:** "circadian (adj.)," Online Etymology Dictionary, www.etymonline.com.
97 **governed by a small group of brain cells:** Lockley and Foster, *Sleep*, 13.
97 **a master clock:** Katia Moskvitch, "The Science of Jet Lag . . . and How Best to Beat It," *BBC Future*, November 18, 2014, www.bbc.com.
97 **dipping and rising at different times:** Lockley and Foster, *Sleep*, 19.
97 **For newborn babies:** Ibid., 58.
97 **"primary sleepiness zone":** William H. Moorcroft, *Sleep, Dreaming & Sleep Disorders: An Introduction* (Boston: University Press of America, 1993), 131.
97 **"sleep gate":** Peretz Lavie, *The Enchanted World of Sleep*, trans. Anthony Berris (New Haven: Yale University Press), 52.
98 **sleep sweet spot:** Moorcroft, *Sleep, Dreaming & Sleep Disorders*, 131.
98 **60 percent of people around the world:** "2015 Motorola Global Smartphone Relationship Survey," The Official Motorola Blog, July 28, 2015, motorola-blog.blogspot.com.
98 **four stages of sleep:** "What Is Sleep?," American Sleep Association, www.sleepassociation.org.
99 **Sleepwalking occurs in approximately:** "Sleepwalking & Sleep Talking," American Academy of Sleep Medicine, www.aasmnet.org.
99 **According to the National Sleep Foundation:** "Sleepwalking," National Sleep Foundation, https://sleepfoundation.org.
100 **sleep talking, which occurs in:** "Sleepwalking & Sleep Talking."
100 **genetic component:** "Sleep Talking," National Sleep Foundation, www.sleepfoundation.org.
100 **as Lady Macbeth discovered:** William Shakespeare, *The Tragedy of Macbeth*, ed. Nicholas Brooke (Oxford: Oxford University Press, 1990), 194–95.
100 **"I hear the secrets":** The Romantics, "Talking in Your Sleep," *In Heat*, Nemperor Records, September 1983.
100 **final phase of sleep is REM sleep:** Lockley and Foster, *Sleep*, 9.
101 **Our muscles are essentially:** "Brain Basics: Understanding Sleep," National Institute of Neurological Disorders and Stroke, www.ninds.nih.gov.
101 **wake up during this phase:** Deirdre Barrett, "What Processes in the Brain Allow You to Remember Dreams?," *Scientific American*, June 12, 2014, www.scientificamerican.com.
101 **discovery of REM sleep in 1953:** Eugene Aserinsky and Nathaniel

Kleitman, "Regularly Occurring Periods of Eye Motility, and Concomitant Phenomena, During Sleep," *Science* 118 (1953): 273–74.

101 **William Dement:** "William C. Dement," Stanford School of Medicine, www.med.stanford.edu.

101 **He told me that their team:** William C. Dement, phone conversation with the author, April 17, 2015.

101 **Kleitman hypothesized:** Ibid.

102 **link between eye movement and dreams:** Jonathan Webb, "Eye Movements 'Change Scenes' During Dreams," *BBC News*, August 12, 2015, www.bbc.com.

102 **REM stage getting longer:** Jennifer Robinson, "What Are REM and Non-REM Sleep?," *WebMD*, October 22, 2014, www.webmd.com.

102 **A study from the University of California, Berkeley:** Els van der Helm, Justin Yao, Shubir Dutt, Vikram Rao, Jared M. Saletin, and Matthew P. Walker, "REM Sleep Depotentiates Amygdala Activity to Previous Emotional Experiences," *Current Biology* 21 (2011): 2029–32.

102 **"This research shows that sleep":** Afsana Afzal, "UC Berkeley Study Shows Dream Sleep Relieves Emotional Stress," *The Daily Californian*, November 29, 2011, www.dailycal.org.

103 **results in higher levels of the stress hormone cortisol:** Rachel Leproult, Georges Copinschi, Orfeu Buxton, and Eve Van Cauter, "Sleep Loss Results in an Elevation of Cortisol Levels the Next Evening," *Sleep: Journal of Sleep Research & Sleep Medicine* 20 (1997): 865–70.

103 **gene expression:** Carla S. Möller-Levet, Simon N. Archer, Giselda Bucca, Emma E. Laing, Ana Slak, Renata Kabiljo, June C. Y. Lo, Nayantara Santhi, Malcolm von Schantz, Colin P. Smith, and Derk-Jan Dijk, "Effects of Insufficient Sleep on Circadian Rhythmicity and Expression Amplitude of the Human Blood Transcriptome," *PNAS* 110 (2013): E1132–41.

A 2015 study from Uppsala University suggested that our biological clock genes may be altered after just one night of missed sleep.

Jonathan Cedernaes, Megan E. Osler, Sarah Voisin, Jan-Erik Broman, Heike Vogel, Suzanne L. Dickson, Juleen R. Zierath, Helgi B. Schiöth, and Christian Benedict, "Acute Sleep Loss Induces Tissue-Specific Epigenetic and Transcriptional Alterations to Circadian Clock Genes in Men," *The Journal of Clinical Endocrinology & Metabolism* 100 (2015): doi: 10.1210/JC.2015–2284.

103 **"puts the body on alert":** Pallab Ghosh, "Why Do We Sleep?," *BBC News*, May 15, 2015, www.bbc.com.

103 **"It's like a dishwasher":** Nedergaard, interview with Hamilton.

104 **Nedergaard's research on mice:** Lulu Xie, Hongyi Kang, Qiwu Xu, Michael J. Chen, Yonghong Liao, Meenakshisundaram Thiyagarajan, John O'Donnell, Daniel J. Christensen, Charles Nicholson, Jeffrey J. Iliff, Takahiro Takano, Rashid Deane, and Maiken Nedergaard, "Sleep Drives Metabolite Clearance from the Adult Brain," *Science* 342 (2013): 373–77; Angela Mulholland, "Not Enough Sleep? Your Brain May Be Paying the Price: Study," *CTV News*, May 29, 2015, www.ctvnews.ca.

104 **Initial studies have shown:** "Poor Sleep Linked with Enlarged Spaces Around Brain's Blood Vessels," Sunnybrook Health Sciences Center, May 29, 2015, www.sunnybrook.ca.

104 **"The brain only has limited energy":** "To Sleep, Perchance to Clean," University of Rochester Medical Center press release, October 17, 2013, www.urmc.rochester.edu.

104 **Claire Sexton at the Oxford Centre:** Claire Sexton, email to the author, March 2, 2015.

105 **"Never waste any time":** Ben Stein, *What Would Ben Stein Do?: Applying the Wisdom of a Modern-Day Prophet to Tackle the Challenges of Work and Life* (Hoboken: Wiley, 2011), Kindle edition.

105 **University of Pennsylvania and Peking University:** Jing Zhang, Yan Zhu, Guanxia Zhan, Polina Fenik, Lori Panossian, Maxime M. Wang, Shayla Reid, David Lai, James G. Davis, Joseph A. Baur, and Sigrid Veasey, "Extended Wakefulness: Compromised Metabolics in and Degeneration of Locus Ceruleus Neurons," *The Journal of Neuroscience* 34 (2014): 4418–31.

105 **Dr. Sigrid Veasey:** "Penn Medicine Researchers Show How Lost Sleep Leads to Lost Neurons," Perelman School of Medicine/University of Pennsylvania press release, March 18, 2014, www.uphs.upenn.edu.

105 **2014 study from Duke-NUS Graduate Medical School:** June C. Lo, Kep Kee Loh, Hui Zheng, Sam K. Y. Sim, and Michael W. L. Chee, "Sleep Duration and Age-Related Changes in Brain Structure and Cognitive Performance," *SLEEP* 37 (2014): 1171–78.

106 **One study showed that:** Christian Benedict, Liisa Byberg, Jonathan Cedernaes, Pleunie S. Hogenkamp, Vilmantas Giedratis, Lena Kilander, Lars Lind, Lars Lannfelt, and Helgi B. Schiöth, "Self-Reported Sleep Disturbance Is Associated with Alzheimer's Disease Risk in Men," *Alzheimer's & Dementia* 11 (2015): 1090–97.

106 **The other revealed:** C. Benedict, J. Cedernaes, V. Giedraitis, E. K. Nilsson, P. S. Hogenkamp, E. Vågesjö, S. Massena, U. Pettersson, G. Christoffersson, M. Phillipson, J. E. Broman, L. Lannfelt, H. Zetterberg, and H. B. Schiöth, "Acute Sleep Deprivation Increases Serum Levels of Neuron-Specific Enolase (NSE) and S100 Calcium Binding Protein B (S-100B) in Healthy Young Men," *SLEEP* 37 (2014): 195–98.

106 **In the United States:** Kessler et al., "Insomnia and the Performance of US Workers."

106 **Researchers from Canada and France:** Ian D. Blum, Lei Zhu, Luc Moquin, Maia V. Kokoeva, Alain Gratton, Bruno Giros, and Kai-Florian Storch, "A Highly Tunable Dopaminergic Oscillator Generates Ultradian Rhythms of Behavioral Arousal," *eLife* 3 (2014): e05105.

106 **"Miss Susie":** Daniel Lewis and Bill Hutchinson, "Brooklyn's Susannah Mushatt Jones, the World's Oldest Person at 115, Thanks Sleep for Long Life," *Daily News*, June 23, 2015, www.nydailynews.com.

107 **recent study from the University of California:** Anwar, "Poor Sleep Linked to Toxic Buildup of Alzheimer's Protein, Memory Loss."

107 **study from the University of California, Irvine:** Steven J. Frenda,

Lawrence Patihis, Elizabeth F. Loftus, Holly C. Lewis, and Kimberly M. Fenn, "Sleep Deprivation and False Memories," *Psychological Science* 25 (2014): 1674–81.

107 **"We already know that sleep":** Anna Almendrala, "The Disturbing Link Between Sleep Deprivation and False Memories," *The Huffington Post*, July 28, 2014, www.huffingtonpost.com.

107 **researchers at Washington State University:** Paul Whitney, John M. Hinson, Melinda L. Jackson, and Hans P. A. Van Dongen, "Feedback Blunting: Total Sleep Deprivation Impairs Decision Making That Requires Updating Based on Feedback," *SLEEP* 38 (2015): 745–54.

108 **"people were slower to recover":** Maanvi Singh, "Short on Sleep? You Could Be a Disaster Waiting to Happen," *NPR*, May 12, 2015, www.npr.org.

108 **Twenty-four hours without sleep:** Bronwyn Fryer, "Sleep Deficit: The Ultimate Performance Killer," *Harvard Business Review*, October 2006, www.hbr.org.

108 **Matthew Walker:** Kenichi Kuriyama, Robert Stickgold, and Matthew P. Walker, "Sleep-Dependent Learning and Motor-Skill Complexity," *Learning & Memory* 11 (2004): 705–13.

108 **TEDx Talk:** Robert Stickgold, "Sleep, Memory and Dreams: Fitting the Pieces Together" (San Antonio: TEDxRiverCity, 2010), www.youtube.com.

109 **Demis Hassabis:** Demis Hassabis, email to the author, October 9, 2015.

109 **Stuart Russell:** Stuart Russell, email to the author, January 25, 2016.

109 **As Hassabis told me:** Hassabis, email to the author.

110 **"It is a common experience":** John Steinbeck, *Sweet Thursday* (New York: Penguin, 1979), 107.

110 **study by the University of Exeter:** Participants were told to memorize a series of made-up words. They were then tested twice—once right after memorization and again after twelve hours. The first group was allowed to sleep during the twelve-hour period, while the second group remained awake. The participants were then tested on the words that they did not remember in the first test.

"Sleep Makes Our Memories More Accessible, Study Shows," University of Exeter press release, July 27, 2015, www.exeter.ac.uk.

110 **link between sleep and memory consolidation:** Lockley and Foster, *Sleep*, 53.

A 2015 study from the Scripps Research Institute continued the exploration into sleep and memory. It's not just that more sleep helps us remember—the study found that increasing sleep decreased the dopamine neuron activity associated with forgetting. "Many scientists have tried to figure out how . . . our memories become stabilized," said Ron Davis, chair of the Scripps Research Institute Department of Neuroscience. "But far less attention has been paid to forgetting, which is a fundamental function for the brain."

Jacob A. Berry, Isaac Cervantes-Sandoval, Molee Chakraborty, and Ronald L. Davis, "Sleep Facilitates Memory by Blocking Dopamine

Neuron-Mediated Forgetting," *Cell* 161 (2015): 1498–1500; Eric Sauter and Mika Ono, "Research Paints More Complete Picture of Sleep and Memory," *The Scripps Research Institute News & Views*, June 15, 2015, www.scripps.edu.

110 **it can transform them:** Wilfredo Blanco, Catia M. Pereira, Vinicius R. Cota, Annie C. Souza1, César Rennó-Costa, Sharlene Santos, Gabriella Dias, Ana M. G. Guerreiro, Adriano B.L. Tort, Adrião D. Neto, and Sidarta Ribeiro, "Synaptic Homeostasis and Restructuring Across the Sleep-Wake Cycle," *PLOS Computational Biology* 11 (2015): doi: 10.1371/journal.pcbi.1004241.

111 **Researchers from Carnegie Mellon University:** Cohen et al., "Sleep Habits and Susceptibility to the Common Cold."

111 **And as Dr. Axel Steiger:** Katharine Gammon, "Why Sleep Soothes the Flu," *Inside Science*, January 23, 2015, www.insidescience.org.

111 **2012 study from the University of Pittsburgh:** Aric A. Prather, Martica Hall, Jacqueline M. Fury, Diana C. Ross, Matthew F. Muldoon, Sheldon Cohen, and Anna L. Marsland, "Sleep and Antibody Response to Hepatitis B Vaccination," *SLEEP* 35 (2012): 1063–69.

112 **mice injected with cancer cells:** Fahed Hakim, Yang Wang, Shelley XL Zhang, Jiamao Zheng, Esma S. Yolcu, Alba Carreras, Abdelnaby Khlayfa, Haval Shirwan, Isaac Almendros, and David Gozal, "Fragmented Sleep Accelerates Tumor Growth and Progression Through Recruitment of Tumor-Associated Macrophages and TLR4 Signaling," *Cancer Research* 74 (2014): 1329–37.

112 **"It's not the tumor":** Easton, "Fragmented Sleep Accelerates Cancer Growth."

112 **2015 study from the Fred Hutchinson Cancer Research Center:** Diane Mapes, "Good Sleep May Improve Breast Cancer Survival," *Hutch News*, June 11, 2015, www.fredhutch.org.

112 **our pain tolerance is decreased:** Robert R. Edwards, David M. Almeida, Brendan Klick, Jennifer A. Haythornthwaite, and Michael T. Smith, "Duration of Sleep Contributes to Next-Day Pain Report in the General Population," *Pain* 137 (2008): 202–7.

112 **One American falls asleep at the wheel:** Godfrey, email to the author.

113 **2013 Danish study:** Tina Kold Jensen, Anna-Maria Andersson, Niels Erik Skakkebæk, Ulla Nordstrøm Joensen, Martin Blomberg Jensen, Tina Harmer Lassen, Loa Nordkap, Inge Alhmann Olesen, Åse Marie Hansen, Naja Hulvej Rod, and Niels Jørgensen, "Association of Sleep Disturbances with Reduced Semen Quality: A Cross-Sectional Study Among 953 Healthy Young Danish Men," *American Journal of Epidemiology* 177 (2013): 1027–37.

113 **erectile dysfunction:** Lisa Shives, "How Sleep Apnea Can Wreck Your Sex Life," *The Chart*, October 12, 2011, thechart.blogs.cnn.com.

The low oxygen levels resulting from sleep apnea could also be a contributor. As Dr. Lisa Shives put it, "In some studies, the severity of the sleep apnea was the greatest predictor of erectile dysfunction while in others it was how low the oxygen went. We have known for years that chronically low oxygen levels at night adversely affect the vasculature of the heart, lungs, brain, and now we can add the penis."

113 **women who slept less than six hours:** Kathryn A. Lee and Caryl L. Gay, "Sleep in Late Pregnancy Predicts Length of Labor and Type of Delivery," *American Journal of Obstetrics & Gynecology* 191 (2004): 2041–46.

113 **2012 Harvard Medical School study:** Orfeu M. Buxton, Sean W. Cain, Shawn P. O'Connor, James H. Porter, Jeanne F. Duffy, Wei Wang, Charles A. Czeisler, and Steven A. Shea, "Adverse Metabolic Consequences in Humans of Prolonged Sleep Restriction Combined with Circadian Disruption," *Science Translational Medicine* 4 (2012): 129–43.

113 **increasing the risk of resistance to insulin:** Mann, "The Sleep-Diabetes Connection."

114 **Thomas Edison:** Edward Wirth, *Images of America: Thomas Edison in West Orange* (Charleston, SC: Arcadia Publishing, 2008), 118.

114 **University of Pennsylvania study:** Zhuo Fang, Andrea M. Spaeth, Ning Ma, Senhua Zhu, Siyuan Hu, Namni Goel, John A. Detre, David F. Dinges, and Hengyi Rao, "Altered Salience Network Connectivity Predicts Macronutrient Intake After Sleep Deprivation," *Scientific Reports* 5 (2015): doi: 10.1038/srep08215.

114 **one night of no sleep:** Alan Mozes, "Sleep Deprivation Leads to Eating More Fatty Food," *CBS News*, February 27, 2015, www.cbsnews.com.

114 **"This is thy hour O Soul":** Walt Whitman, "A Clear Midnight," in *The Chief American Poets: Selected Poems by Bryant, Poe, Emerson, Longfellow, Lowell, Whitman, and Lanier*, ed. Curtis Hidden Page (New York: Houghton Mifflin Company, 1905), 606.

114 **limited reservoir:** Roy E. Baumeister, Ellen Bratslavsky, Mark Muraven, and Dianne M. Tice, "Ego Depletion: Is the Active Self a Limited Resource?," *Journal of Personality and Social Psychology* 74 (1998): 1252–65.

114 **2015 review from Clemson University:** June J. Pilcher, Drew M. Morris, Janet Donnelly, and Hayley B. Feigl, "Interactions Between Sleep Habits and Self-Control," *Frontiers in Human Neuroscience* 9 (2015): 284.

115 **a study on smokers:** Kilian Rapp, Gisela Buechele, and Stephan K. Weiland, "Sleep Duration and Smoking Cessation in Student Nurses," *Addictive Behaviors* 32 (2007): 1505–10.

Evidence of impaired decision making was also seen in a University of Chicago study on smokers attempting to quit. The researchers determined that sleep deprivation increased smoking, because "the reward value of smoking may increase if subjects expect that the cigarette will counter their feelings of sleepiness."

Ajna Hamidovic and Harriet de Wit, "Sleep Deprivation Increases Cigarette Smoking," *Pharmacology Biochemistry and Behavior* 93 (2008): 263–69.

115 **Researchers from Chicago, Missouri, and Stanford universities:** Jen-Hao Chen, Linda Waite, Lianne M. Kurina, Ronald A. Thisted, Martha McClintock, and Diane S. Lauderdale, "Insomnia Symptoms

and Actigraph-Estimated Sleep Characteristics in a Nationally Representative Sample of Older Adults," *The Journals of Gerontology* 70 (2014): 185–92.

115 **"That time you're awake":** Paula Span, "Insomniac, but Not Sleep-Deprived," *The New York Times*, October 27, 2014, www.newoldage.blogs.nytimes.com.

115 **Michael Decker and Elizabeth Damato:** Michael Decker and Elizabeth Damato, email to the author, March 28, 2015.

116 **According to Robert Provine:** Maria Konnikova, "The Surprising Science of Yawning," *The New Yorker*, April 14, 2014, www.newyorker.com.

116 **anticipate something happening:** Ibid.

116 **Provine has broadened his theory:** Robert Provine, "Yawning," *American Scientist* 93 (2005): 532.

117 **primitive form of empathy:** M-Pierre Perriol and Christelle Monaca, "'One Person Yawning Sets Off Everyone Else,'" *Journal of Neurology, Neurosurgery, and Psychiatry* 77 (2006): 3.

117 **less than 1 percent:** Alexa Tsoulis-Reay, "What It's Like to Need Hardly Any Sleep," *New York Magazine*, March 1, 2015, www.nymag.com.

117 **result of a genetic mutation:** Harrison Wein, "Gene Regulates Sleep Length," *NIH Research Matters*, September 21, 2009, www.nih.gov.

117 **implant a short sleep gene:** Rachel E. Gross, "To Edit the Human Genome Now Would Be 'Irresponsible'," *Slate*, December 3, 2015, www.slate.com.

118 **as Till Roenneberg put it:** Till Roenneberg, "Celebrate Sleep!" (panel with Arianna Huffington, Hans Ulrich Obrist, and Miriam Meckel, Digital-Life-Design Conference, Munich, Germany, January 19, 2016).

118 **three hunter-gatherer communities:** Gandhi Yetish, Hillard Kaplan, Michael Gurven, Brian Wood, Herman Pontzer, Paul R. Manger, Charles Wilson, Ronald McGregor, and Jerome M. Siegel, "Natural Sleep and Its Seasonal Variations in Three Pre-Industrial Societies," *Current Biology* 25 (2015): 2862–68.

118 **"Some media may have emphasized":** Jerome Siegel, email to the author, November 3, 2015.

118 **"At all ages":** Kathryn Doyle, "Americans, Their Physicians Should Take Sleep Seriously: Chest Doctors," *Reuters*, June 15, 2015, www.reuters.com.

5. SLEEP DISORDERS

119 **More than 25 million American adults:** "Rising Prevalence of Sleep Apnea in U.S. Threatens Public Health," American Academy of Sleep Medicine press release, September 29, 2014, www.aasmnet.org.

119 **These apneas:** "What Is Sleep Apnea?," National Heart, Lung, and Blood Institute, www.nhlbi.nih.gov.

119 **In obstructive sleep apnea:** "Obstructive Sleep Apnea," American Sleep Association, www.sleepassociation.org.

119 **central sleep apnea:** "What Is Sleep Apnea?"

119 **may not remember waking up:** Ibid.

120 **According to Dr. M. Safwan Badr:** M. Safwan Badr, email to the author, April 8, 2015.

120 **impair cognitive function:** David J. Durgan and Robert M. Bryan Jr., "Cerebrovascular Consequences of Obstructive Sleep Apnea," *Journal of the American Heart Association* 1 (2012): e000091.

Those with severe sleep apnea have been found to have reduced white matter in the brain. The white matter is what contains the nerve fibers and the myelin that wraps around the fibers as insulation, accelerating communication among the nerve cells. Reduced white matter results in impaired cognitive function and a higher incidence of mood swings.

The good news is studies show that this damage can be reversed. A 2014 study from Vita-Salute San Raffaele University in Milan revealed that a yearlong treatment with CPAP led to a nearly full recovery of white-matter brain damage.

Vincenza Castronovo, Paola Scifo, Antonella Castellano, Mark S. Aloia, Antonella Iadanza, Sara Marelli, Stefano F. Cappa, Luigi Ferini Strambi, and Andrea Falini, "White Matter Integrity in Obstructive Sleep Apnea Before and After Treatment," *SLEEP* 37 (2014): 1465–75.

120 **linked to depression:** David T. Derrer, "Sleep Apnea," *WebMD*, 2014, www.webmd.com.

A 2015 study of almost 2,000 men conducted by the University of Adelaide and the Adelaide Institute for Sleep Health in Australia found that those with severe obstructive sleep apnea were 2.1 times more likely to be depressed. Those who had both severe obstructive sleep apnea and excessive daytime sleepiness were 4.2 times more likely to be depressed. And a 2012 study from the Centers for Disease Control and Prevention showed that women with sleep apnea were even more likely to suffer from clinical depression.

But consistent CPAP therapy may help. A study by the University of Western Australia of nearly 300 sleep apnea patients determined that more than 200 of them had significant symptoms of depression. Not only that, their depression symptoms increased with the severity of sleep apnea. But these symptoms persisted in only 9 patients after three months of consistent CPAP therapy. Furthermore, of the 41 patients who reported feelings of self-harm or thoughts of suicide at the outset of the experiment, not a single one reported them at the three-month follow-up.

Anne G. Wheaton, Geraldine S. Perry, Daniel P. Chapman, and Janet B. Croft, "Sleep Disordered Breathing and Depression Among U.S. Adults: National Health and Nutrition Examination Survey, 2005–

2008," *SLEEP* 35 (2012): 461–67; Carol Lang (Postdoctoral researcher for study), email to the author, October 28, 2015; Cass Edwards, Sutapa Mukherjee, Laila Simpson, Lyle J. Palmer, Osvaldo P. Almeida, and David R. Hillman, "Depressive Symptoms Before and After Treatment of Obstructive Sleep Apnea in Men and Women," *Journal of Clinical Sleep Medicine* (2015): doi: 10.5664/jcsm.5020.

120 **cardiac problems:** Ibid.

A 2014 study from the Penn Sleep Center at the University of Pennsylvania found that CPAP therapy drastically lowered hospital readmissions and emergency visits by cardiac patients with sleep apnea who had been discharged from the hospital in the previous thirty days.

And as a 2014 study from the UCLA School of Nursing showed, the interrupted breathing of sleep apnea also impairs blood flow to the brain and can cause cognitive damage.

Shilpa R. Kauta, Brendan T. Keenan, Lee Goldberg, and Richard J. Schwab, "Diagnosis and Treatment of Sleep Disordered Breathing in Hospitalized Cardiac Patients: A Reduction in 30-Day Hospital Readmission Rates," *Journal of Clinical Sleep Medicine* 10 (2014): 1051–59; Paul M. Macey, Rajesh Kumar, Jennifer A. Ogren, Mary A. Woo, and Ronald M. Harper, "Global Brain Blood-Oxygen Level Responses to Autonomic Challenges in Obstructive Sleep Apnea," *PLoS ONE* 9 (2014): e105261.

120 **UCLA study from 2015:** José A. Palomares, Sudhakar Tummala, Danny J. J. Wang, Bumhee Park, Mary A. Woo, Daniel W. Kang, Keith S. St. Lawrence, Ronald M. Harper, and Rajesh Kumar, "Water Exchange Across the Blood-Brain Barrier in Obstructive Sleep Apnea: An MRI Diffusion-Weighted Pseudo-Continuous Arterial Spin Labeling Study," *Journal of Neuroimaging* (2015): doi: 10.1111/jon.12288.

120 **Epilepsy, meningitis, multiple sclerosis:** Mark Wheeler, "UCLA Researchers Provide First Evidence of How Obstructive Sleep Apnea Damages the Brain," *UCLA Newsroom*, September 1, 2015, www.newsroom.ucla.edu.

120 **limited to adults:** Rakesh Bhattacharjee, email to the author, February 24, 2015.

Sleep apnea affects between 2 and 10 percent of children. "Sleep disordered breathing," Rakesh Bhattacharjee, a pediatric sleep expert at the University of Chicago, told me, "is detrimental to children's health including manifesting in neurocognitive, behavioral, inflammatory and cardiometabolic morbidity."

120 **more than 9 percent of children:** "Asthma," Centers for Disease Control and Prevention, www.cdc.gov.

120 **They found that among asthmatic children:** Rakesh Bhattacharjee, Beatrix H. Choi, David Gozal, and Babak Mokhlesi, "Association of Adenotonsillectomy with Asthma Outcomes in Children: A Longitudinal Database Analysis," *PLoS Medicine* 11 (2014): e1001753.

120 **primary treatment for sleep apnea is CPAP:** "What is CPAP?," National Heart, Lung, and Blood Institute, www.nhlbi.nih.gov.

Richard Schwab told me about developments in CPAP machines. "The machines have become 'smart'—they track how many hours you use it, how many days you use it, if it is working, if the mask leaks, etc." And for those looking for CPAP alternatives, "there are oral appliances that pull the jaw forward and open up the airways. Weight loss often helps patients, and upper-airway surgery is an option as well. The newest treatment, hypoglossal nerve stimulation, involves the hypoglossal nerve, which controls tongue movements."

Richard Schwab, conversation with the author, April 9, 2015.

120 **lighter, less cumbersome masks:** John Frank, email to the author, January 25, 2016. To address the many challenges that patients initially face when being exposed to CPAP therapy, manufacturers are offering many innovations. For instance, Philips recently launched their Dream Family of sleep therapy solutions that enables patients to initiate therapy at a lower, more comfortable pressure. As the patient acclimates to therapy, the device gradually increases pressure with automatic, personalized adjustments, until patients achieve their full therapeutic pressure.

121 **"I can't sleep; no light burns":** Alexander Pushkin, *The Bronze Horseman: Selected Poems of Alexander Pushkin*, trans. D. M. Thomas (New York: Viking Press, 1982), 79.

121 **A third of adults have a hard time:** "Insomnia—Overview and Facts," Sleep Education, www.sleepeducation.com.

121 **Music and fashion editor Sophie Eggleton:** Sophie Eggleton, "The Diary of a Hermit: Insomnia," *The Huffington Post*, November 26, 2013, www.huffingtonpost.co.uk.

122 **psychophysiological insomnia:** Duff, *The Secret Life of Sleep*.

122 **"Self-diagnosed insomnia":** Patrick Fuller and his team at Harvard conducted a study on insomnia and found that the brain stem contains neurons that trigger deep "slow wave" sleep. He explained, "We showed that we could rapidly trigger deep sleep in mice by 'remotely' activating a certain type of neuron in this brain region, as well as prevent entry into deep sleep by inhibiting these same cells." Identifying what lifestyle changes would activate or inhibit these cells would make a big difference in developing treatments for sleep disorders.

Patrick Fuller, email to the author, March 3, 2015.

122 **turning to a new source of data:** "Twitter Data May Help Shed Light on Sleep Disorders," Medical News Today press release, June 12, 2015, www.medicalnewstoday.com.

123 **Sharlene Stenseth:** Alena Hall, "26 Struggles of Exhausted Insomniacs," *The Huffington Post*, June 15, 2015, www.huffingtonpost.com.

123 **Shany Conroy:** Ibid.

123 **Amanda Guilford:** Ibid.

123 **In her 2014 memoir, *Yes Please*:** Amy Poehler, "Bad Sleeper," in *Yes Please* (New York: Dey Street Books, 2014), Kindle edition.

124 **"Although hyperaroused insomniacs":** "Chronic Insomniacs May Face Increased Risk of Hypertension," American Heart Association press release, January 26, 2015, www.newsroom.heart.org.

124 **"After a few weeks":** Jacobs, email to the author.

125 **results of cognitive behavioral therapy:** Charles M. Morin, Cheryl Colecchi, Jackie Stone, Rakesh Sood, and Douglas Brink, "Behavioral and Pharmacological Therapies for Late-Life Insomnia: A Randomized Control Trial," *The Journal of the American Medical Association* 281 (1999): 991–99.

125 **Two other trials:** Gregg D. Jacobs, Edward F. Pace-Schott, Robert Stickgold, and Michael W. Otto, "Cognitive Behavior Therapy and Pharmacotherapy for Insomnia: A Randomized Controlled Trial and Direct Comparison," *Archives of Internal Medicine* 164 (2004): 1888–96.

125 **restless legs syndrome:** The development of RLS is attributed to multiple factors. "About 50 percent of the time, it's familial," said Timothy Morgenthaler, past president of the American Academy of Sleep Medicine.

But whether you inherit it or not, alcohol and sleep deprivation can exacerbate your symptoms. RLS is also strongly associated with iron deficiency and medical conditions such as kidney failure, diabetes, and peripheral neuropathy.

So the first step is to evaluate your lifestyle in terms of sleep, caffeine intake, exercise, and nutrition. If these adjustments are made, it becomes easier to determine whether other factors—underlying disorders that cause RLS, such as iron, deficiency, diabetes, or vein diseases—are at play. Natural treatments to try at home include leg massages, ice packs, heat pads, stretching, hot baths, and relaxation techniques.

Alena Hall, "Do I Have Restless Legs Syndrome?," *The Huffington Post*, June 25, 2015, www.huffingtonpost.com; "Restless Legs Syndrome Fact Sheet," National Institute of Neurological Disorders and Stroke, www.ninds.nih.gov.

125 **sleep paralysis:** During sleep paralysis, our REM sleep spills over into waking life. During REM sleep, our muscles become paralyzed so that we don't act out our dreams. However, in sleep paralysis, the opposite happens—we become conscious and aware, but the paralysis remains. The dream-forming aspects of REM sleep can remain, too, causing hallucinations.

Sleep paralysis affects 8 percent of the general population, but that figure is much higher for students—a staggering 28 percent—which is not surprising, given that episodes tend to occur more frequently during times of sleep-schedule disruption and sleep deprivation. Fortunately, episodes of sleep paralysis are typically short and infrequent, but for the minority who suffer from frequent episodes, treating underlying conditions, such as poor sleep habits, can help.

B. A. Sharpless and J. P. Barber, "Lifetime Prevalence Rates of Sleep Paralysis: A Systematic Review," *Sleep Medicine Reviews* 15 (2011): 311–15; Melissa Dahl, "What It's Like to Have Severe Sleep Paralysis," *New York Magazine*, July 22, 2015, www.nymag.com; "Sleep Paralysis," *WebMD*, www.webmd.com.

125 **exploding head syndrome:** A Washington State University study found that out of the 211 college students surveyed, more than 16 percent had recurrent episodes of the disorder. But considering that sleep deprivation and stress can worsen the symptoms, college students might not be a representative demographic. One theory for exploding head syndrome is that as we transition between wakefulness and sleep, some parts of the brain do not transition properly. This delay is associated with a sudden burst of activity from the auditory neurons—which we register as a loud explosion. Improving sleep habits and lowering stress are, predictably, foundational steps to managing exploding head syndrome.

B. A. Sharpless, "Exploding Head Syndrome Is Common in College Students," *Journal of Sleep Research* 24 (2015): 447–49; "Exploding Head Syndrome," American Sleep Association, www.sleepassociation.org; Helen Thomson, "'I Have Exploding Head Syndrome,'" *BBC*, April 10, 2015, www.bbc.com.

6. DREAMS

126 **everything is rigged in our favor:** Daniel Ladinsky, trans., *Love Poems from God: Twelve Sacred Voices from the East and West* (New York: Penguin, 2002), 85.

127 **"Dreams are a reservoir":** Tarthang Tulku, *Openness Mind* (Cazadero: Dharma Publishing, 1978), 74.

127 **Max Planck:** J. W. N. Sullivan, "Interview with Great Scientists," *The Observer*, February 8, 1931, www.secure.pqarchiver.com.

127 **"The dream is a little door":** Carl G. Jung, *The Collected Works of C. G. Jung: Complete Digital Edition*, eds. Gerhard Adler and Michael Fordham (Princeton: Princeton University Press, 2014), 144.

128 **"Unlike the experience":** A. Roger Ekirch, "Sleep We Have Lost: Pre-Industrial Slumber in the British Isles," *The American Historical Review* 106 (2001): 385.

128 ***The Interpretation of Dreams:*** Sigmund Freud, *The Basic Writings of Sigmund Freud*, ed. and trans. A. A. Brill (New York: Random House, 1995), Kindle edition.

128 **"The dream is a psychic act":** Ibid.

129 **"The psychodynamic dream theories":** John Bargh, email to the author, August 2, 2015.

129 **"I believe":** Freud, *The Basic Writings of Sigmund Freud.*

129 **"The wishes for Freud":** Bargh, email to the author.

129 **"It is like fireworks":** Freud, *The Basic Writings of Sigmund Freud.*

130 **priestly class in ancient times:** J. Donald Hughes, "Dream Interpretation in Ancient Civilizations," *Dreaming* 10 (2000): doi: 10.1023/A:1009447606158.

130 **"If the first report":** Freud, *The Basic Writings of Sigmund Freud.*
130 **"The forgetting of dreams":** Ibid.
130 **Winston Churchill once wrote an essay:** Winston S. Churchill, *The Dream* (New York: RosettaBooks, 2014), Kindle edition.
131 **Boris Johnson wrote in *The Churchill Factor:*** Boris Johnson, *The Churchill Factor: How One Man Made History* (New York: Riverhead Books, 2014), Kindle edition.
131 **Churchill had a tumultuous relationship:** Ibid.
131 **"Carl Jung saw the unconscious as":** Pittman McGehee, email to the author, August 25, 2015.
132 **"As scientific understanding has grown":** Carl G. Jung, Marie-Louise von Franz, Joseph L. Henderson, Jolande Jacobi, and Aniela Jaffé, *Man and His Symbols* (New York: Dell Publishing, 2012), Kindle edition.
132 **A gap has opened up:** Carl G. Jung, *The Essential Jung*, ed. Anthony Storr (Princeton: Princeton University Press, 2013), 176.
132 **"In our conscious life":** Jung et al., *Man and His Symbols.*
132 **"integrally connect":** Ibid.
132 **"essential message carriers":** Ibid.
133 **"restore our psychological balance":** Ibid.
133 **"What we consciously fail to see":** Ibid.
133 **"The dream gives a true picture":** Jung, *Modern Man in Search of a Soul*, 5.
133 **"ineluctable truths":** Jung, *The Essential Jung*, 176.
133 **"Why should they mean":** Jung et al., *Man and His Symbols.*
133 **"it is plain foolishness":** Ibid.
133 **"or rather miseducated":** Jung, *Modern Man in Search of a Soul*, 12.
133 **"They wish at once":** Ibid.
133 **"God has given you dreams":** Rumi, *The Soul of Rumi: A New Collection of Ecstatic Poems*, trans. Coleman Barks (New York: HarperCollins), Kindle edition.
134 **"It is only through comparative studies":** Jung, *Modern Man in Search of a Soul*, 25.
134 **"Jung's central contribution":** Christopher Booker, *The Seven Basic Plots: Why We Tell Stories* (New York: Continuum, 2004), Kindle edition.
134 **Like Freud and Jung, Edgar Cayce:** "The Sleeping Prophet: Who Was Edgar Cayce and What Are Edgar Cayce Readings?," Edgar Cayce's A.R.E., www.edgarcayce.org.
135 **the result of the body's digesting:** Edgar Cayce, *Dreams & Visions* (Virginia Beach: A.R.E. Press, 2008), 19.
135 **most dreams meaningful on multiple levels:** "Insights from Dreams," Edgar Cayce's A.R.E., www.edgarcayce.org.
135 **two purposes of dreams:** Cayce, *Dreams & Visions*, 18.
136 **In *Hamlet*, Shakespeare plays:** William Shakespeare, *Hamlet*, eds. Barbara A. Mowat and Paul Werstine (New York: Simon & Schuster, 1992), Kindle edition.
136 **In *Julius Caesar*:** William Shakespeare, *Julius Caesar*, ed. Shane Weller (New York: Dover Publications, 1991), Kindle edition.

136 **in *The Tempest*:** William Shakespeare, *The Tempest* (New York: Dover Publications, 2012), Kindle edition.

137 **"escape from daily suffering":** Ekirch, *At Day's Close.*

137 **Jean de La Fontaine's fables:** Jean de La Fontaine, *Selected Fables*, ed. Maya Slater, trans. Christopher Wood (Oxford: Oxford University Press, 1995), 283.

137 **English novelist Emily Brontë:** Emily Brontë, *Wuthering Heights*, ed. Candace Ward (New York: Dover Publications, 2012), Kindle edition.

137 **"A Chapter on Dreams":** Robert Louis Stevenson, "A Chapter on Dreams," in *R. L. Stevenson on Fiction: An Anthology of Literary and Critical Essays*, ed. Glenda Norquay (Edinburgh: Edinburgh University Press, 1999), 136–37.

138 **The Beatles' "Let It Be":** Barry Miles, *Paul McCartney: Many Years from Now* (New York: Henry Holt and Company, 1997), 538.

138 **"hand-painted dream photographs":** "The Persistence of Memory," MoMA Learning, www.moma.org.

138 **"I am the first to be surprised":** The Museum of Modern Art press release on Dalí series, 1934, www.moma.org.

138 ***The Persistence of Memory*:** Salvador Dalí, *The Persistence of Memory*, 1931, oil on canvas, 9½ in. x 13 in., The Museum of Modern Art, New York.

138 **the 1950 animated classic:** *Cinderella*, directed by Clyde Geronimi, Wilfred Jackson, and Hamilton Luske (1950; Burbank, CA: Walt Disney Productions, 2012), DVD.

138 ***The Wizard of Oz*:** *The Wizard of Oz*, directed by Victor Fleming (1939; Beverly Hills: Metro-Goldwyn-Mayer Studios, 1999), DVD.

139 **her adventure in Wonderland:** Lewis Carroll, *Alice's Adventures in Wonderland* (Ontario: Broadview Editions, 2011), 204.

139 **Dumbledore asks Snape:** *Harry Potter and the Prisoner of Azkaban*, directed by Alfonso Cuarón (2004; Burbank, CA: Warner Bros., 2007), DVD.

139 **"It is true that dreams":** Booker, *The Seven Basic Plots.*

140 **Dr. J. Allan Hobson summed it up:** Don H. Hockenbury and Sandra E. Hockenbury, *Discovering Psychology, 5th Edition* (New York: Worth Publishers, 2011), 152.

140 **American inventor Elias Howe:** Thomas Waln-Morgan Draper, *The Bemis History and Genealogy: Being an Account, in Greater Part, of the Descendants of Joseph Bemis of Watertown, Mass.* (San Francisco: The Stanley-Taylor Co., 1900), 160.

141 **The periodic table of elements:** B. M. Kedrov, "On the Question of the Psychology of Scientific Creativity," *The Soviet Review Translations* 8 (1967): 38.

141 **Dr. Otto Loewi:** Kelly Lambert and Craig H. Kinsley, *Clinical Neuroscience: The Neurobiological Foundations of Mental Health* (New York: Worth Publishers, 2005), 51.

141 **dream about a snake eating its own tail:** Arthur Koestler, *The Act of Creation* (New York: Penguin, 1964), 118.

141 **"the most important dream":** Ibid.

141 **In the 1890s, Sarah Breedlove:** "Queen of Gotham's Colored," *The Literary Digest* 55 (1917): 76.

142 **Madam C. J. Walker's Wonderful Hair Grower:** A'Lelia Bundles, "Madam C. J. Walker: A Brief Biographical Essay," Madam C. J. Walker, www.madamcjwalker.com.

142 **made her a multimillionaire:** A'Lelia Bundles, *On Her Own Ground: The Life and Times of Madam C. J. Walker* (New York: Scribner, 2001), Kindle edition.

142 **"Yours is the truest dream":** Rumi, *The Soul of Rumi: A New Collection of Ecstatic Poems*, trans. Coleman Barks (New York: HarperCollins, 2010), Kindle edition.

142 **More recently, Google:** Larry Page, "Commencement Address," University of Michigan, May 2, 2009, www.googlepress.blogspot.com.

143 **Arthur Koestler described dreams:** Koestler, *The Act of Creation*, 210.

143 **"the displacement of attention":** Ibid., 119–20.

144 **"activation-synthesis hypothesis":** Edward F. Pace-Schott, Mark Solms, Mark Blagrove, and Stevan Harnad, eds., *Sleep and Dreaming: Scientific Advances and Reconsiderations* (Cambridge, Eng.: Cambridge University Press, 2003), 30–31.

144 **"Dreams are dripping":** J. Allan Hobson, *The Dream Drugstore: Chemically Altered States of Consciousness* (Cambridge, MA: MIT Press, 2003), 71.

144 **In 2000, the Finnish psychologist Antti Revonsuo:** Antti Revonsuo, "The Reinterpretation of Dreams: An Evolutionary Hypothesis of the Function of Dreaming," *Behavioral and Brain Sciences* 23 (2000): 877–901.

144 **scientists at Beth Israel Deaconess Medical Center:** Erin J. Wamsley, Matthew Tucker, Jessica D. Payne, Joseph A. Benavides, and Robert Stickgold, "Dreaming of a Learning Task Is Associated with Enhanced Sleep-Dependent Memory Consolidation," *Current Biology* 20 (2010): 850–55.

145 **"The subjects who dreamed":** "Dreams Tell Us That the Brain Is Hard at Work on Memory Functions," Beth Israel Deaconess Medical Center press release, April 22, 2010, www.bidmc.org.

145 **"dreams in their development":** George Noël Gordon Byron, *The Poetical Works* (London: John Dicks, 1865), 270.

145 **dreams and emotional intelligence:** Andrea N. Goldstein-Piekarski, Stephanie M. Greer, Jared M. Saletin, and Matthew P. Walker, "Sleep Deprivation Impairs the Human Central and Peripheral Nervous System Discrimination of Social Threat," *The Journal of Neuroscience* 35 (2015): 10135–45.

145 **According to Matthew Walker:** Yasmin Anwar, "The Sleep-Deprived Brain Can Mistake Friends for Foes," *Berkeley News*, July 14, 2015, www.news.berkeley.edu.

146 **"Dreams help regulate traffic":** Sander van der Linden, "The Science Behind Dreaming," *Scientific American*, July 26, 2011, www.scientificamerican.com.

146 **Rubin Naiman, a sleep and dream specialist:** Rubin Naiman, email to the author, March 1, 2015.

146 **another by Hobson:** J. Allan Hobson, "REM Sleep and Dreaming: Towards a Theory of Protoconsciousness," *Nature Reviews Neuroscience* 10 (2009): 803–13.

147 **As part of a study in the United Kingdom:** Josie E. Malinowski and Caroline L. Horton, "The Effect of Time of Night on Wake–Dream Continuity," *Dreaming* 24 (2014): 253–69.

147 **neuroscientists in Kyoto:** Tomoyasu Horkawa, Masako Tamaki, Yoichi Miyawaki, and Y. Kamitani, "Neural Decoding of Visual Imagery During Sleep," *Science* 340 (2013): 639–42.

147 **Common themes:** Michelle Carr, "Typical Dream Themes," *Psychology Today*, November 13, 2014, www.psychologytoday.com.

148 **A French study:** Isabelle Arnulf, Laure Grosliere, Thibault Le Corvec, Jean-Louis Golmard, Olivier Lascols, and Alexandre Duguet, "Will Students Pass a Competitive Exam That They Failed in Their Dreams?," *Consciousness and Cognition* 29 (2014): 36–47.

148 **"The immediate benefit of dreaming":** The British Psychological Society, "Does Dreaming of Exam Failure Affect Your Real-Life Chances of Success?," *Research Digest*, November 4, 2014, www.digest.bps.org.uk.

148 **a quarter of children aged five to twelve:** Natalie Angier, "In the Dreamscape of Nightmares, Clues to Why We Dream at All," *The New York Times*, October 23, 2007, www.nytimes.com.

149 **a study from Santiago:** Pablo E. Brockmann, Blanca Díaz, Felipe Damiani, Luis Villarroel, Felipe Núñez, and Oliviero Bruni, "Impact of Television on the Quality of Sleep in Preschool Children," *Sleep Medicine* (2015): doi: 10.1016/j.sleep.2015.06.005.

149 **"nightmares" and "night terrors":** "Nightmares and Night Terrors," Stanford Children's Health, www.stanfordchildrens.org.

149 **"Golden slumbers fill your eyes":** John Lennon and Paul McCartney, "Golden Slumbers," *Abbey Road*, Apple Records, 1969.

149 **"Nightmare rates climb":** Angier, "In the Dreamscape of Nightmares, Clues to Why We Dream at All."

149 **dates back to 1300:** Merrill Perlman, "The History of 'Nightmare,'" *Columbia Journalism Review*, January 12, 2015, www.cjr.org.

149 **"a female evil spirit":** "nightmare," *Oxford Dictionary of English* (Oxford: Oxford University Press), 1200.

150 **University of Montreal:** Geneviève Robert and Antonio Zadra, "Thematic and Content Analysis of Idiopathic Nightmares and Bad Dreams," *SLEEP* 37 (2014): 409–17.

150 **According to Patrick McNamara:** Patrick McNamara, "What a Nightmare," *Psychology Today*, May 30, 2011, www.psychologytoday.com.

151 **hit 2010 movie *Inception*:** *Inception*, directed by Christopher Nolan (2010; Burbank, CA, London, Eng., and Hollywood, CA: Legendary Pictures, Syncopy, and Warner Bros. Pictures, 2010), DVD.

151 **Freud had been exploring the phenomenon:** Freud, *The Basic Writings of Sigmund Freud.*

151 **Proponents of lucid dreaming:** "Lucid Dreaming FAQ," Lucidity Institute, www.lucidity.com.
151 **Others use their ability:** Roc Morin, "The Strange Subconscious Fantasy Worlds of Lucid Dreamers," *VICE*, January 28, 2015.
151 **going back to 1975:** Keith M. T. Hearne, *Lucid Dreams: An Electrophysiological and Psychological Study*, Ph.D. dissertation, University of Liverpool, 1978, www.keithhearne.com.
151 **Stephen LaBerge:** Stephen P. LaBerge, "Lucid Dreaming as a Learnable Skill: A Case Study," *Perceptual and Motor Skills* 53 (1980): 1039–42.
151 **LaBerge believes:** Stephen LaBerge and Howard Rheingold, *Exploring the World of Lucid Dreaming* (New York: Ballantine Books, 1991).
152 **"I have frequently wondered":** Howard P. Lovecraft, "Beyond the Wall of Sleep," The H. P. Lovecraft Archive, www.hplovecraft.com.
152 **Indian spiritual teacher Ramana Maharshi:** Stephen Mitchell, *The Second Book of the Tao* (New York: Penguin, 2009), 140.
152 **"We view dreams the way we do stars":** Naiman, email to the author.
153 **As Robert Moss writes:** Robert Moss, *The Secret History of Dreaming* (Novato, CA: New World Library, 2009), Kindle edition.
153 **"One of the great Hindu images":** *Sukhavati: A Mythic Journey*, directed by Joseph Campbell (2007; London: Acorn Media, 2007), DVD.
153 **a practice called dream incubation:** Anthony Stevens, *Private Myths: Dreams and Dreaming* (Cambridge, MA: Harvard University Press, 1997), 15.
153 **In ancient Greece:** Kelly Bulkeley, *Dreaming in the World's Religions: A Comparative History* (New York: NYU Press, 2008), 158.
154 **Kelly Bulkeley told me:** Kelly Bulkeley, email to the author, March 18, 2015.
154 **in China and in ancient Japan:** Bulkeley, *Dreaming in the World's Religions*, 73.
154 **"I have found again and again":** Jung et al., *Man and His Symbols.*
155 **Sandra Shpilberg:** Sandra Shpilberg, email to the author, August 27, 2015.
155 **Los Angeles–based writer Elizabeth Kirk:** Elizabeth Kirk, email to the author, August 26, 2015.
156 **David H. wrote that several dreams:** David H., email to the author, August 27, 2015.
156 **"Dreams, as we all know":** Fyodor Dostoyevsky, *The Dream of a Ridiculous Man* (New York: Harper Perennial Classics, 2015), 104.
157 **Linda Jacobsen:** Linda Jacobsen, email to the author, August 28, 2015.
157 **Ron Hulnick:** Ron Hulnick, email to the author, September 6, 2015.
159 **Synesius of Cyrene:** Saint Synesios, "On Dreams," trans. Isaac Myer, *The Platonist: An Exponent of the Philosophic Truth* 4 (1888): 284.
159 **the Rubin Museum:** "Dream-Over 2015: A Sleep-Over for Adults," The Rubin Museum, www.rubinmuseum.org.
159 **I asked Mary Hulnick:** Mary Hulnick, email to the author, September 6, 2015.
160 **"From breakfast on through all the day":** Robert Louis Stevenson,

"The Land of Nod," in *The Magazine of Poetry: A Monthly Review*, ed. Charles Wells Moulton (Buffalo: Charles Wells Moulton, 1894): 20-21.

7. MASTERING SLEEP

165 **"Sleep that knits up the ravell'd sleave of care":** William Shakespeare, *Macbeth*, 29.

165 **"I think that public awareness":** Doyle, "Americans, Their Physicians Should Take Sleep Seriously."

166 **"Baby steps":** Daniel Coyle, *The Talent Code: Greatness Isn't Born, It's Grown. Here's How* (New York: Bantam Dell, 2009), 94.

166 **"When a little child":** Louise L. Hay, *You Can Heal Your Life* (Carlsbad, CA: Hay House, 1984), Kindle edition.

166 **As Marcus Aurelius put it:** Marcus Aurelius, *Meditations*, trans. Maxwell Staniforth (New York: Penguin, 2005), Kindle edition.

167 **"When we wake up":** Alan Watts, *The Philosophies of Asia* (Clarendon, VT: Tuttle Publishing, 1999), 105.

167 **"Calling up the stress response":** Neil A. Fiore, *Awaken Your Strongest Self: Break Free of Stress, Inner Conflict, and Self-Sabotage* (New York: McGraw-Hill Professional, 2006), 68.

168 **"We need to rethink sleep":** Rath, *Eat Move Sleep.*

168 **Agapi modeled her sleep:** Agapi Stassinopoulos, conversation with the author, June 23, 2015.

170 **a *minimum* of seven hours:** Nathaniel F. Watson, M. Safwan Badr, Gregory Belenky, Donald L. Bliwise, Orfeu M. Buxton, Daniel Buysse, David F. Dinges, James Gangwisch, Michael A. Grandner, Clete Kushida, Raman K. Malhotra, Jennifer L. Martin, Sanjay R. Patel, Stuart F. Quan, and Esra Tasali, "Joint Consensus Statement of the American Academy of Sleep Medicine and Sleep Research Statement on the Recommended Amount of Sleep for a Healthy Adult: Methodology and Discussion," *SLEEP* 38 (2015): 1161–83.

170 **broken it down accordingly:** "National Sleep Foundation Recommends New Sleep Times," National Sleep Foundation press release, February 2, 2015, www.sleepfoundation.org.

170 **Dr. Harvey Karp:** Harvey Karp, email to the author, September 6, 2015.

171 **researchers in Norway:** Børge Sivertsen, Allison G. Harvey, Ted Reichborn-Kjennerud, Leila Torgersen, Eivind Ystrom, and Mari Hysing, "Later Emotional and Behavioral Problems Associated with Sleep Problems in Toddlers: A Longitudinal Study," *JAMA Pediatrics* 169 (2015): 575–82.

171 **parents' education:** Laura McDonald, Jane Wardle, Clare H. Llewellyn, Cornelia H. M. van Jaarsveld, and Abigail Fisher, "Predictors of Shorter Sleep in Early Childhood," *Sleep Medicine* 15 (2014): 536–40.

171 **"Sleep in the Modern Family":** "National Sleep Foundation 2014

Sleep in America Poll Finds Children Sleep Better When Parents Establish Rules, Limit Technology and Set a Good Example," National Sleep Foundation press release, March 3, 2014, www.sleepfoundation.org.

172 **"attachment parenting":** William Sears and Martha Sears, "The Benefits of Attachment Parenting," in *The Attachment Parenting Book: A Commonsense Guide to Understanding and Nurturing Your Child* (New York: Hachette Book Group, 2001), Kindle edition.

172 **Angelina Jolie and Brad Pitt:** Rich Cohen, "Angelina the Conqueror," *Vanity Fair*, August 2010, www.vanityfair.com.

173 **Beyond the emotional bond:** James McKenna, email to the author, April 16, 2015.

173 **"Sweet dreams, form a shade":** William Blake, "A Cradle Song," in *The Book of Georgian Verse*, ed. William Stanley Braithwaite (New York: Brentano's, 1909), 313.

173 **The American Academy of Pediatrics:** "AAP Expands Guidelines for Infant Sleep Safety and SIDS Risk Reduction," American Academy of Pediatrics press release, October 18, 2011, www.aap.org.

174 **tips from Dr. Karp:** Harvey Karp, "Ask Dr. Karp: Should We Consider Co-sleeping?," BabyCenter, https://blogs.babycenter.com.

174 ***I Love Lucy:*** "Lucy Hires a Maid," *I Love Lucy*, CBS (April 27, 1953).

174 **"Parenthood has worn me down":** Stuart Heritage, "I've Hit a Sleep Wall and I'm Seeing Double," *The Guardian*, June 13, 2015, www.theguardian.com.

174 **A 2014 *Today* show survey:** A. Pawlowski, "Does Mommy Brain Really Exist? Help for Sleep-Deprived Parents," *TODAY*, November 11, 2014, www.today.com.

174 **"drunk parenting":** Karp, email to the author.

175 **Mika Brzezinski:** Mika Brzezinski, *All Things at Once* (New York: Weinstein Books, 2009), Kindle edition.

175 **"How could I":** Ibid.

175 **lasting effect on Mika:** Ibid.

176 **A *New York Times* article:** Aimee Molloy, "Sleep Training At 8 Weeks: 'Do You Have the Guts?'" *The New York Times*, March 26, 2015, www.nytimes.com.

176 **call it heart-wrenching:** Zach Johnson, "Zoe Saldana Is Having a Hard Time Sleep Training Her Twins (Although Vodka Makes It a Little Easier)—Watch Now!," *E! Online*, June 12, 2015, www.eonline.com.

176 **"It's important that you pick":** Rachel Grumman Bender, "Sleep Training: What Is the Perfect Age?," *Yahoo Parenting*, May 11, 2015, www.yahoo.com.

177 **Swedish author Carl-Johan:** Sarah Knapton, "Bedtime Phenomenon: Scientist Develops Book to Send Children to Sleep in Minutes," *The Telegraph*, August 15, 2015, www.telegraph.co.uk.

177 **"I thought I'd listen to it":** Tinman Mom, August 17, 2015, review of *The Rabbit Who Wants to Fall Asleep: A New Way of Getting Children to Sleep*, Amazon.com, www.amazon.com.

177 **According to one study:** Ariel Kalil, Rachel Dunifon, Danielle Crosby,

and Jessica Houston Su, "Working Hours, Schedules, and Insufficient Sleep Among Mothers and Their Young Children," *Journal of Marriage and Family* 76 (2014): 891–904.

177 **In the United States:** "Employment Characteristics of Families Summary," Bureau of Labor Statistics economic news release, April 23, 2015, www.bls.gov.

177 **Only three states:** Nadja Popovich, "Only Three US States Have Paid Family Leave Policies—Will New York Be Next?," *The Guardian*, March 17, 2015, www.theguardian.com.

177 **Sweden and Norway:** Rebecca Ray, Janet C. Gornick, and John Schmitt, "Who Cares? Assessing Generosity and Gender Equality in Parental Leave Policy Designs in 21 Countries," *Journal of European Social Policy* 20 (2010): 196-216; "Working Mother Statistics," Statistic Brain Research Institute, www.statisticbrain.com.

177 **The Family and Medical Leave Act:** "Fact Sheet #28: The Family and Medical Leave Act," U.S. Department of Labor Wage and Hour Division, www.dol.gov.

178 **40 percent of the American workforce:** "A Look at the U.S. Department of Labor's 2012 Family and Medical Leave Act Employee and Worksite Surveys," National Partnership for Women & Families, www.nationalpartnership.org.

178 **Netflix announced in 2015:** Tawni Cranz, "Starting Now at Netflix: Unlimited Maternity and Paternity Leave," *Netflix US & Canada Blog*, August 4, 2015, www.blog.netflix.com; Emily Peck, "Not All Netflix Workers Will Get 'Unlimited' Parental Leave," *The Huffington Post*, August 6, 2015, www.huffingtonpost.com.

178 **British telecommunications company Vodafone:** "Vodafone Pioneers Global Maternity Policy Across 30 Countries," Vodafone press release, March 6, 2015, www.vodafone.com.

178 **"There is an epidemic of obesity":** Clifford Saper, email to the author, April 3, 2015.

178 **Researchers from the University of Illinois:** Katherine E. Speirs, Janet M. Liechty, Chi-Fang Wu, and Strong Kids Research Team, "Sleep, but Not Other Daily Routines, Mediates the Association Between Maternal Employment and BMI for Preschool Children," *Sleep Medicine* 15 (2014): 1590–93.

179 **average start time for public high schools:** "Schools and Staffing Survey (SASS)," National Center for Education Statistics, www.nces.ed.gov.

179 **American Academy of Pediatrics recommended:** "Let Them Sleep: AAP Recommends Delaying Start Times of Middle and High Schools to Combat Teen Sleep Deprivation," American Academy of Pediatrics press release, October 25, 2014, www.aap.org.

180 **only 14 percent of schools:** "Schools and Staffing Survey (SASS)."

180 **A 2011 study:** Dubi Lufi, Orna Tzischinsky, and Stav Hadar, "Delaying School Start Times by One Hour: Some Effects on Attention Levels in Adolescents," *Journal of Clinical Sleep Medicine* 7 (2011): 137–43.

180 **in the United Kingdom:** Hannah Richardson, "Later School Start Time 'May Boost GSCE Results,'" *BBC News*, October 9, 2014, www.bbc.com.

180 **"Teensleep":** "Teensleep," University of Oxford Nuffield Department of Clinical Neurosciences Medical Sciences Division, www.ndcn.ox.ac.uk.

180 **Japan's education ministry:** Jun Hongo, "5 Facts from Survey on Sleep Habits of Students in Japan," *The Wall Street Journal*, May 1, 2015, www.blogs.wsj.com.

180 **Brown University professor Mary Carskadon:** Carskadon, email to the author.

181 **In August 2015, New Jersey:** Adam Clark, "Christie Agrees to Study Later School Start Times," August 10, 2015, *NJ.com*, www.nj.com.

181 **In Singapore:** Adrian Lim, "Less Travel Time, More Sleep for Pupils," *AsiaOne*, April 19, 2015, www.news.asiaone.com.

181 **Deerfield Academy:** Justin Pope, "Colleges Wake Up to Notion That Better Sleep Means Better Grades," *The Associated Press*, September 3, 2012, www.washingtontimes.com.

181 **Eighty-two percent of British teens:** Lisa Artis, "Revision Robs Teens of Sleep," The Sleep Council press release, March 27, 2015, www.sleepcouncil.org.uk.

182 **"This is not just about teens":** Maanvi Singh, "Teens Who Skimp on Sleep Now Have More Drinking Problems Later," *NPR Shots*, January 16, 2015, www.npr.org.

183 **"Sleep Week":** Tyler Kingkade, "College Students Aren't Getting Enough Sleep. These Universities Are Trying to Change That," *The Huffington Post*, April 19, 2015, www.huffingtonpost.com.

183 **Duke University eliminated 8 a.m. classes:** Francie Grace, "Help for Sleep-Deprived Students," *CBS News*, April 19, 2004, www.cbsnews.com.

183 **Penn State followed suit:** Alex Muller, "University Departments Reduce the Amount of 8 a.m. Course Offerings," *The Daily Collegian*, April 27, 2005, www.collegian.psu.edu.

183 **At Stanford:** "PSYC 235: Sleep and Dreams (PSYC 135)," Stanford University, www.explorecourses.stanford.edu.

183 **launching its "Refresh" initiative:** Mickey Trockel, Rachel Manber, Vickie Chang, Alexandra Thurston, and Craig Barr Tailor, "An E-mail Delivered CBT for Sleep-Health Program for College Students: Effects on Sleep Quality and Depression Symptoms," *Journal of Clinical Sleep Medicine* 7 (2011): 276–81.

184 **At Dartmouth:** Priya Ramaiah, "Refresh Pilot Tracks Student Sleep Habits," *The Dartmouth*, October 7, 2014, thedartmouth.com.

184 **its own version of Stanford's Refresh:** Ibid.

184 **health service actively screens:** Caitlin Barthelmes (director of student health promotion and wellness, Dartmouth College), email to the author, August 14, 2015.

184 **Refresh is also being replicated:** Mickey Trockel (clinical assistant

professor, Stanford University School of Medicine), email to the author, July 23, 2015.

184 **Hastings College:** Justin Pope, "Enough Zzzzzs Can Help You Get A's," *The Associated Press*, September 4, 2012, www.thechronicleherald.ca.

184 **University of Georgia:** "Let the Bulldawg Sleep!," University of Georgia University Health Center, www.uhs.uga.edu.

185 **At the University of Michigan:** Olivia B. Waxman, "Napping Around: Colleges Provide Campus Snooze Rooms," *TIME*, August 29, 2014, www.time.com.

185 **at Berkeley, Melissa Hsu campaigned:** "Melissa Hsu #123 for ASUC Senate," Facebook, www.facebook.com.

185 **At the University of Arizona:** UA Campus Health Service, "CHTV 5.2: Get in Bed with Campus Health," YouTube video, December 5, 2014, www.youtube.com.

185 **"zombie campaign":** "My Transformation into a George Romero Zombie," J. Farrell Studio, October 30, 2011, www.farrellstudio.wordpress.com.

185 **James Madison University has the "Nap Nook":** Waxman, "Napping Around."

186 **University of East Anglia:** Natasha Preskey, "Nap Time for University Students," *The Telegraph*, February 3, 2015, www.telegraph.co.uk.

186 **Institute of Advanced Media Arts and Sciences:** "Outline," Institute of Advanced Media Arts and Sciences, www.iamas.ac.jp.

186 **"nap maps":** "Napping," University of Texas at Austin University Health Services, healthyhorns.utexas.edu.

186 **Christina Kyriakos:** Nikolas Markantonatos, "Holy Cross Senior Brings Sleep Education Program to Worcester," *College of the Holy Cross*, March 1, 2011, https://news.holycross.edu.

187 **The program's motto:** "Simply Profound," Sweet Dreamzzz, www.sweetdreamzzz.org; "Sweet Dreamzzz at a Glance," Sweet Dreamzzz, www.sweetdreamzzz.org.

187 **"We delivered the REM":** Christina Kyriakos, email to the author, July 22, 2015.

8. SLEEPING TOGETHER

189 **"Among the lower classes":** Jon Methven, "Why We Sleep Together," *The Atlantic*, June 11, 2014, www.theatlantic.com.

189 **"Never did families feel more vulnerable":** Ibid.

189 **"Often a bedmate became":** Ibid.

190 **"No man prefers":** Herman Melville, *Moby-Dick, Or The Whale*, eds. Harrison Hayford, Hershel Parker, and G. Thomas Tanselle (Evanston: Northwestern University Press, 1988), 17.

191 **A study from the University of Vienna:** John Dittami, Marietta

Keckeis, Ivo Machatschke, Stanislav Katina, Josef Zeitlhofer, and Gerhard Kloesch, "Sex Differences in the Reactions to Sleeping in Pairs Versus Sleeping Alone in Humans," *Sleep and Biological Rhythms* 5 (2007): 271–76.

191 **Lee Crespi:** Methven, "Why We Sleep Together."

191 **University of Hertfordshire:** Alexandra Sifferlin, "What Your Sleeping Position Says About Your Relationship," *TIME*, April 16, 2014, www.time.com.

191 **the farther apart a couple slept:** *Richard Wiseman's Night School*, presented by Richard Wiseman (Edinburgh: Edinburgh International Science Festival, 2014), www.youtube.com.

192 **these couples "have more conflict":** Elizabeth Bernstein, "Couples on Different Sleep Schedules Can Expect Conflict—and Adapt," *The Wall Street Journal*, September 9, 2014, www.wsj.com.

192 **found that women slept better:** Brant P. Hasler and Wendy M. Troxel, "Couples' Nighttime Sleep Efficiency and Concordance: Evidence for Bidirectional Associations with Daytime Relationship Functioning," *Psychosomatic Medicine* 72 (2010): 794–801.

192 **"Women are more sensitive":** Bernstein, "Couples on Different Sleep Schedules Can Expect Conflict—and Adapt."

192 **Another study of Troxel's:** Ibid.

192 **"Some couples end up sleeping apart":** Ibid.

192 **"If one partner is not sleeping well":** Jillian Kramer, "Should Married Couples Always Sleep in the Same Bed?," *Brides*, March 11, 2015, www.brides.com.

193 **2015 study:** David A. Kalmbach, J. Todd Arnedt, Vivek Pillai, and Jeffrey A. Ciesla, "The Impact of Sleep on Female Sexual Response and Behavior: A Pilot Study," *The Journal of Sexual Medicine* 12 (2015): 1221–32.

193 **In terms of men:** Judith L. Reishtein, Greg Maislin, and Terri E. Weaver, "Outcome of CPAP Treatment on Intimate and Sexual Relationships in Men with Obstructive Sleep Apnea," *Journal of Clinical Sleep Medicine* 6 (2010): 221–26.

194 **one-third of adults snore:** "Snoring and Sleep," National Sleep Foundation, www.sleepfoundation.org.

194 **American Academy of Dental Sleep Medicine:** "A 'Snore-fire' Way to Hurt Your Relationship," American Academy of Dental Sleep Medicine press release, February 12, 2015, www.aadsm.org.

194 **"Hope suddenly cries out":** David Foster Wallace, *Oblivion: Stories* (New York: Little, Brown and Company, 2004), Kindle edition.

195 **Snoring happens when your airways:** "Snoring and Sleep."

195 **"When you are snoring":** Sarah Klein, "Want to Stop Snoring? Here's What Works (and What Doesn't)," *The Huffington Post*, April 27, 2015, www.huffingtonpost.com.

195 **half of America's 90 million snorers:** Dennis Hwang, "Is It Snoring or Sleep Apnea?," American Sleep Apnea Association, www.sleepapnea.org.

195 **Badr finds that:** Klein, "Want to Stop Snoring?"
195 **"Most people like sleeping":** Judy McGuire, "Sawing Logs: 7 Ways to Get More Sleep with a Snorer," *TODAY Health & Wellness*, November 13, 2014, www.today.com.
196 ***Huffington Post* reporter Yagana Shah:** Yagana Shah, "How Separate Beds Are the Key to a Happy Relationship for Many Couples," *The Huffington Post*, October 20, 2014, www.huffingtonpost.com.

9. WHAT TO DO, WHAT NOT TO DO

198 **The National Sleep Foundation advises:** "See," National Sleep Foundation, www.sleepfoundation.org.
198 **"Turn off the lights":** Mathias Basner, email to the author, March 26, 2015.
198 **Lighting Science Group Corporation:** Jen Christensen, "Warning Labels on Your Light Bulbs," *CNN*, June 9, 2015, www.cnn.com.
198 **"an alert stimulus":** Laura Beil, "In Eyes, a Clock Calibrated by Wavelengths of Light," *The New York Times*, July 4, 2011, www.nytimes.com.
199 **"People are exposing their eyes":** Justin Gmoser and Alana Kakoyiannis, "This Is What Happens to Your Brain and Body When You Check Your Phone Before Bed," *Business Insider*, February 17, 2015, www.businessinsider.com.
199 **71 percent of Americans sleep:** "Trends in Consumer Mobility Report."
199 **Heather Cleland Woods:** Alexis Sobel Fitts, "Teens Obsessed with Facebook May Struggle with Anxiety, Sleep Problems," *The Huffington Post*, September 14, 2015, www.huffingtonpost.com.
200 **highest emotional investment:** Ibid.
200 **the ideal sleeping temperature:** S. H. Onen, F. Onen, D. Bailly, and P. Parquet, "Prevention and Treatment of Sleep Disorders Through Regulation of Sleeping Habits," *La Presse Médicale* 23 (1994): 485–89.
200 **The National Sleep Foundation recommends:** "Touch," National Sleep Foundation, www.sleepfoundation.org; "How to Sleep Comfortably Through Hot Summer Nights," National Sleep Foundation, www.sleepfoundation.org.
200 **our bodies have a temperature cycle:** Onen et al., "Prevention and Treatment of Sleep Disorders Through Regulation of Sleeping Habits."
200 **As Natalie Dautovich:** Lindsay Holmes, "Why We Sleep Better in Cooler Climates," *The Huffington Post*, March 30, 2015, www.huffingtonpost.com.
201 **2014 study from the University of Georgia:** Rodney K. Dishman, Xuemei Sui, Timothy S. Church, Christopher E. Kline, Shawn D. Youngstedt, and Steven N. Blair, "Decline in Cardiorespiratory Fitness and Odds of Incident Sleep Complaints," *Medicine & Science in Sports & Exercise* 47 (2015): 960–66.

201 **"Staying active won't cure":** Molly Berg, "UGA Study Links Declining Fitness, Sleep Complaints," University of Georgia press release, October 6, 2014, www.news.uga.edu.

201 **"regular physical activity":** "Study: Physical Activity Impacts Overall Quality of Sleep," Oregon State University News & Research Communications press release, November 22, 2011, www.oregonstate.edu.

201 **Michael Grandner:** "Yoga, Running, Weight Lifting, and Gardening: Penn Study Maps the Types of Physical Activity Associated with Better Sleep Habits," Penn Medicine press release, June 4, 2015, www.uphs.upenn.edu.

202 **"The real danger":** Markham Heid, "You Asked: Is It Better to Sleep In or Work Out?," *TIME*, June 10, 2015, www.time.com.

202 **A 2013 study from Northwestern University:** Kelly Glazer Baron, Kathryn J. Reid, and Phyllis C. Zee, "Exercise to Improve Sleep in Insomnia: Exploration of the Bidirectional Effects," *Journal of Clinical Sleep Medicine* 9 (2013): 819–24.

202 **"The timing of exercise":** Kim Painter, "Exercising Close to Bedtime is OK, Sleep Experts Say," *USA TODAY*, March 4, 2013, www.usatoday.com.

203 **caffeine can decrease sleep:** Christopher Drake, Timothy Roehrs, John Shambroom, and Thomas Roth, "Caffeine Effects on Sleep Taken 0, 3, or 6 Hours Before Going to Bed," *Journal of Clinical Sleep Medicine* 9 (2013): 1195–200.

204 **involved in sleep regulation:** "Insomnia: Studies Suggest Calcium and Magnesium Effective," *Medical News Today*, September 8, 2009, www.medicalnewstoday.com; Deborah Enos, "3 Nutrients Linked with a Better Night's Sleep," *Live Science*, July 24, 2013, www.livescience.com; Jessica Lewis, "Vitamins That Help You Sleep," *Livestrong*, June 22, 2015, www.livestrong.com.

204 **2014 study from Louisiana State University:** Ann Liu, Russell Tipton, Weihong Pan, John Finley, Alfredo Prudente, Namrata Karki, Jack Losso, and Frank Greenway, "Tart Cherry Juice Increases Sleep Time in Older Adults with Insomnia," *The Journal of the Federation of American Societies for Experimental Biology* 28 (2014): Supplement 830.9.

204 **40 percent of Americans:** Jamie A. Koufman, "The Dangers of Eating Late at Night," *The New York Times*, October 25, 2014, www.nytimes.com.

204 **"Over the past two decades":** Ibid.

204 **"We have this illusion":** A. Pawlowski, "Why Eating Late at Night May Be Bad for Your Brain," *TODAY*, February 22, 2015, www.today.com.

205 **Australian researchers found:** S. J. Edwards, I. M. Montgomery, E. Q. Colquhoun, J. E. Jordan, and M. G. Clark, "Spicy Meal Disturbs Sleep: An Effect of Thermoregulation," *International Journal of Psychophysiology* 13 (1992): 97–100.

205 **rats put on a high-fat diet:** "Weight Gain Induced by High-Fat Diet Increases Active-Period Sleep and Sleep Fragmentation," Society

for the Study of Ingestive Behavior press release, July 10, 2012, www.eurekalert.org.

206 **"The number one weakness":** Patricia Fitzgerald, email to the author, July 27, 2015.

206 **Winston Churchill to James Bond:** Warren F. Kimball, "'Like Goldfish in a Bowl': The Alcohol Quotient," *Finest Hour,* Spring 2007, www.winstonchurchill.org; *The Spy Who Loved Me,* directed by Lewis Gilbert (1977; London: Eon Productions, 2002), DVD.

207 **study from the University of Melbourne:** Julia K. M. Chan, John Trinder, Ian M. Colrain, and Christian L. Nicholas, "The Acute Effects of Alcohol on Sleep Electroencephalogram Power Spectra in Late Adolescence," *Alcoholism: Clinical and Experimental Research* 39 (2015): 291–99.

207 **"The take-home message here":** "Pre-Sleep Drinking Disrupts Sleep," *Alcoholism: Clinical and Experimental Research* press release, January 16, 2015, www.eurekalert.com.

207 **"at all dosages":** I. O. Ebrahim, C. M. Shapiro, A. J. Williams, and P. B. Fenwick, "Alcohol and Sleep I: Effects on Normal Sleep," *Alcoholism: Clinical and Experimental Research* 37 (2013): 539–49.

207 **acupuncture had positive effects:** Wei Huang, Nancy Kutner, and Donald L. Bliwise, "A Systematic Review of the Effects of Acupuncture in Treating Insomnia," *Sleep Medicine Reviews* 13 (2009): 73–104.

207 **auricular acupuncture:** H. Y. Chen, Y. Shi, C. S. Ng, S. M. Chan, K. K. Yung, and Q. L. Zhang, "Auricular Acupuncture Treatment for Insomnia," *Journal of Alternative and Complementary Medicine* 13 (2007): 669–76.

207 **acupuncture was just as effective:** Huijuan Cao, Xingfang Pan, Hua Li, and Jianping Liu, "Acupuncture for Treatment of Insomnia: A Systematic Review of Randomized Controlled Trials," *Journal of Alternative and Complementary Medicine* 15 (2009): 1171–86.

207 **how acupuncture reduces insomnia:** D. W. Spence, L. Kayumov, A. Chen, A. Lowe, U. Jain, M. A. Katzman, J. Shen, B. Perelman, and C. M. Shapiro, "Acupuncture Increases Nocturnal Melatonin Secretion and Reduces Insomnia and Anxiety: A Preliminary Report," *The Journal of Neuropsychiatry & Clinical Neurosciences* 16 (2004): 19–28.

208 **"in Traditional Chinese Medicine":** Janet Zand, email to the author, September 23, 2015.

208 **Patricia Fitzgerald has found:** Fitzgerald, email to the author.

208 **lavender:** Joe-Ann McCoy, "Lavender: History, Taxonomy, and Production," NC Herb, 1999, www.ces.ncsu.edu.

208 **Other studies have found:** George T. Lewith, Anthony D. Godfrey, and Philip Prescott, "A Single-Blinded, Randomized Pilot Study Evaluating the Aroma of Lavandula Augustifolia as a Treatment for Mild Insomnia," *Journal of Alternative and Complementary Medicine* 11 (2005): 631–37; C. Alford, L. Austin, T. Bachel, E. Bulbrooke, E. Taylor, and G. Lewith, "Preliminary Investigations of the Use of Aromatherapy for Treating Mild to Moderate Insomnia," *Abstracts: European Sleep Research Society Annual Meeting* (Glasgow: 2009).

208 **And in Germany:** James A. Duke and Michael Castleman, *The Green*

Pharmacy Anti-Aging Prescriptions: Herbs, Foods, and Natural Formulas to Keep You Young (Emmaus: Rodale, 2000), 459.

209 **Valerian root:** "Valerian," National Center for Complementary and Integrative Health, www.nccih.nih.gov.

209 **effectiveness has been supported:** Teruhisa Komori, Takuya Matsumoto, Eishi Motomura, and Takashi Shiroyama, "The Sleep-Enhancing Effect of Valerian Inhalation and Sleep-Shortening Effect of Lemon Inhalation," *Chemical Senses* 31 (2006): 731–37.

209 **Dr. Frank Lipman also recommends:** Frank Lipman, email to the author, July 22, 2015.

209 **Interior designer Michael Smith:** Michael Smith, conversation with the author, September 26, 2015.

209 **"Sleep is the best meditation":** Pearl Marshall and Margaret Studer, "Enthroned at 4, Exiled at 23, Tibet's Dalai Lama Visits the U.S., but Can He Go Home Again?," *People*, September 10, 1979, www.people.com.

210 **"They generally tend to handle":** Maria Basta, George P. Chrousos, Antonio Vela-Bueno, and Alexandros N. Vgontzas, "Chronic Insomnia and Stress System," *Sleep Medicine Clinics* 2 (2007): 279–91.

210 **"If you are having a lot of trouble sleeping":** Jon Kabat-Zinn, *Full Catastrophe Living* (New York: Bantam Dell, 1990), 363.

211 **"I would stress three words":** Jennifer Ailshire, email to the author, May 16, 2015.

211 **So is qigong:** Fitzgerald, email to the author.

211 **"Finish every day":** Ralph Waldo Emerson, *The Letters of Ralph Waldo Emerson in Six Volumes, Volume Four*, ed. Ralph L. Rusk (New York: Columbia University Press, 1939), 439.

211 **"mind dump":** Joey Hubbard, conversation with the author, October 18, 2015.

212 **"People look for retreats":** Christopher Gill, trans., *Marcus Aurelius: Meditations, Books 1–6* (New York: Oxford University Press, 2013), 20.

213 **Jim Gordon:** Jim Gordon, conversation with the author, September 29, 2015.

214 **A 2009 Stanford study:** Jason C. Ong, Shauna L. Shapiro, and Rachel Manber, "Mindfulness Meditation and Cognitive Behavioral Therapy for Insomnia: A Naturalistic 12-Month Follow-up," *EXPLORE: The Journal of Science & Healing* 5 (2009): 30–36.

214 **kindness and gratitude help us sleep:** Richard Davidson, email to the author, June 22, 2015.

214 **Matthieu Ricard:** Matthieu Ricard, email to the author, July 12, 2015.

215 **"Like dropping through a hole":** Clark Strand, *Meditation Without Gurus: A Guide to the Heart of Practice* (Woodstock: Skylight Paths Publishing, 1998), 3–5.

215 ***The Mary Tyler Moore Show:*** "Mary's Insomnia," *The Mary Tyler Moore Show*, MTM Enterprises (December 4, 1976).

215 **4-7-8 method:** Lizette Borreli, "A Life Hack for Sleep: The 4-7-8 Breathing Exercise Will Supposedly Put You to Sleep in Just 60 Seconds," *Medical Daily*, May 5, 2015, www.medicaldaily.com.

216 **"Visualize images that evoke":** Brent Menninger, "Half-Smile and Serenity," *DBT Self Help*, www.dbtselfhelp.com.

216 **researchers at the University of Glasgow:** Niall M. Broomfield and Colin A. Espie, "Initial Insomnia and Paradoxical Intention: An Experimental Investigation of Putative Mechanisms Using Subjective and Actigraphic Measurement of Sleep," *Behavioural and Cognitive Psychotherapy* 31 (2003): 313–24.

216 **"Patients realize when they try":** Anna Magee, "Want Better Sleep? Worry Less About How Much You're Getting," *Healthista*, June 16, 2014, www.healthista.com.

217 **"Stay awake, don't rest your head":** *Mary Poppins*, directed by Robert Stevenson (1964; Burbank, CA: Walt Disney Productions, 2004), DVD.

217 **"We need more stillness":** Christine Carter, "Starved for Time? Here's a Surprising—and Easy—Solution," *Greater Good*, November 4, 2014, www.greatergood.berkeley.edu.

218 **"It changes what time we get up":** Steven Pressfield, *Turning Pro: Tap Your Inner Power and Create Your Life's Work* (New York: Black Irish Entertainment, 2012), 72.

220 **Steve Jobs:** Steve Jobs, "'You've Got to Find What You Love,' Jobs Says," *Stanford News*, June 14, 2005, http://news.stanford.edu.

220 **"Military and economic command":** Lewis H. Lapham, "Memento Mori," *Lapham's Quarterly*, Fall 2013, www.laphamsquarterly.com.

220 **"I would lie awake at night":** Ira Glass, "361: Fear of Sleep," *This American Life*, WBEZ, August 8, 2008, www.thisamericanlife.org.

221 **"Unresting death":** Philip Larkin, *Philip Larkin Poems Selected by Martin Amis* (London: Faber and Faber, 2011), Kindle edition.

221 **"To practice death":** Michel Montaigne, *The Complete Essays*, trans. M. A. Screech (New York: Penguin, 2004), Kindle edition.

222 **Clare Sauro:** Clare Sauro, email to the author, September 25, 2015.

223 **74 percent of Americans:** "National Sleep Survey Pulls Back the Covers on How We Doze and Dream," Anna's Linens press release, December 26, 2012, www.prnewswire.com.

223 **In another poll, 57 percent:** Lizette Borreli, "Sleeping Naked Helps Couples Have Healthy Relationships with More Intimacy," *Medical Daily*, July 2, 2014, www.medicaldaily.com.

223 **"When you and your partner both sleep":** Ibid.

10. CATNAPS, JET LAG, AND TIME ZONES

225 **"a pleasant luxury":** "Napping," The National Sleep Foundation, www.sleepfoundation.org.

225 **"primes our brains":** David K. Randall, "Rethinking Sleep," *The New York Times*, September 22, 2012, www.nytimes.com.

225 **Sorbonne University:** "Napping Reverses Health Effects of Poor Sleep," Endocrine Society press society, February 10, 2013, www.eurekalert.org.

226 **a study by Allegheny College:** Ryan Brindle and Sarah Conklin, "Daytime Sleep Accelerates Cardiovascular Recovery after Psychological Stress," *International Journal of Behavioral Medicine* 19 (2012): 111–14.

226 **5 percent decrease in blood pressure:** "Midday Naps Associated with Reduced Blood Pressure and Fewer Medications," European Society of Cardiology press release, August 29, 2015, www.escardio.org.

226 **a NASA report:** Mark R. Rosekind, Roy M. Smith, Donna L. Miller, Elizabeth L. Co, Kevin B. Gregory, Lissa L. Webbon, Philippa H. Gander, and J. Victor Lebacqz, "Alertness Management: Strategic Naps in Operational Settings," *Journal of Sleep Research* 4 (1995): 62–66.

226 **"Let me tell you about the nap":** Philip Roth, interview with Scott Simon, "At 80, Philip Roth Reflects on Life, Literature and the Beauty of Naps," *Weekend Edition*, NPR, March 23, 2013, www.npr.com.

227 **"a five-fold improvement":** "Neuropsychology: Power Naps Produce a Significant Improvement in Memory Performance," *Science Daily*, March 29, 2015, www.sciencedaily.com.

227 **Georgetown University Medical Center:** "Might Lefties and Righties Benefit Differently from a Power Nap?," Georgetown University press release, October 17, 2012, https://explore.georgetown.edu.

227 **Yo-Yo Ma told me:** Yo-Yo Ma, conversation with the author, October 4, 2015.

227 **A study of older adults:** Hideki Tanaka, Kazuhiko Taira, Masashi Arakawa, Hiroki Toguti, Chisae Urasaki, Yukari Yamamoto, Eiko Uezu, Tadao Hori, and Shuichiro Shirakawa, "Effects of Short Nap and Exercise on Elderly People Having Difficulty in Sleeping," *Psychiatry and Clinical Neurosciences* 55 (2001): 173–74.

227 **the best "circadian timing":** Nicole Lovato and Leon Lack, "The Effects of Napping on Cognitive Functioning," *Progress in Brain Research* 185 (2010): 155–66.

228 **if you're deciding between the two:** Sara Mednick, Denise J. Cai, Jennifer Kanady, and Sean P. A. Drummond, "Comparing the Benefits of Caffeine, Naps and Placebo on Verbal, Motor and Perceptual Memory," *Behavioural Brain Research* 193 (2008): 79–86.

228 **Margaret Thatcher:** Alena Hall, "The Energy Secret These 15 Successful People Swear By," *The Huffington Post*, May 6, 2014, www.huffingtonpost.com.

228 **John F. Kennedy:** Michael O'Brien, *John F. Kennedy: A Biography* (New York: St. Martin's Griffin, 2006), 743.

229 **Charlie Rose:** Charlie Rose, email to the author, September 28, 2015.

229 **Night owl Bill Clinton:** Laura Barnett, "An Afternoon Nap Is Good for Your Health," *The Guardian*, March 2, 2011, www.theguardian.com.

229 **"You must sleep sometime":** Jane E. Brody, "New Respect for the Nap, a Pause That Refreshes," *The New York Times*, January 4, 2000, www.nytimes.com.

229 **Pope Francis:** Jaweed Kaleem, "The Secret to How Pope Francis Keeps His Hectic Travel Schedule," *The Huffington Post*, September 25, 2015, www.huffingtonpost.com.

229 **spiritual leader, the Dalai Lama:** "The Dalai Lama, Arianna Huffington Interview: His Holiness Discusses Compassion, Science, Religion and Sleep," *The Huffington Post*, May 14, 2015, www.huffingtonpost.com.

230 **disrupt sleep like travel:** "Jet Lag and Sleep," National Sleep Foundation, www.sleepfoundation.org.

230 **the term "jet lag":** Rebecca Maksel, "When Did the Term 'Jet Lag' Come into Use?," *Air & Space Magazine*, June, 17, 2008, www.airspacemag.com.

230 **researchers from Rush University Medical Center:** Charmane I. Eastman and Helen J. Burgess, "How to Travel the World Without Jet Lag," *Sleep Medicine Clinics* 4 (2009): 241–55.

231 **"Weary with toil":** William Shakespeare, *Sonnets*, ed. Thomas Tyler, (London: David Nutt, 1890), Kindle edition.

231 **the term "social jet lag":** McGrath, "Unlocking the Science of Social Jet Lag and Sleep."

231 **clock genes:** Sally Pobojewski, "The Rhythm of Life," *Michigan Today*, Spring 2007, www.deepblue.lib.umich.edu.

231 **"When food is plentiful":** Patrick M. Fuller, Jun Lu, and Clifford B. Saper, "Differential Rescue of Light- and Food-Entrainable Circadian Rhythms," *Science* Magazine 320 (2008): 1074–77.

232 **"A period of fasting":** Jeanna Bryner, "How to Beat Jet Lag: Don't Eat," *Live Science*, May 22, 2008, www.livescience.com.

232 **for a fourteen-hour flight:** "Avoiding Food 'May Beat Jet Lag,'" *BBC News*, May 22, 2008, www.bbc.com.

233 **Argonne Anti-Jet-Lag Diet:** Jane E. Brody, "The Jet Lag Diet," *The New York Times*, May 22, 1983, www.nytimes.com.

233 **The diet was tested in 2002:** Steve Hendricks, "The Empty Stomach: Fasting to Beat Jet Lag," *Harper's Magazine*, March 5, 2012, www.harpers.org.

233 **another common travel misstep:** Amy Capetta, "6 Ways to Fight Jet Lag (and Not Be Too Tired to Enjoy Your Trip!)," *TODAY*, September 13, 2014, www.today.com.

233 **Entrain:** "Entrain Yourself," University of Michigan, entrain.math.lsa.umich.edu.

234 **Re-Timer:** "Re-Timer Light Therapy 'Sunglasses' May Help Regulate Circadian Rhythms," *Sleep Review*, July 28, 2014, www.sleepreviewmag.com.

234 **"For a quick trip":** Chris Winter, email to the author, June 5, 2015.

234 **"If you're on vacation":** Capetta, "6 Ways to Fight Jet Lag."

235 **As Betty Thesky:** Sid Lipsey, "Flight Attendants' Tips for Sleeping Well on a Plane," *Yahoo! Travel*, September 17, 2015, www.yahoo.com.

11. SLEEP AND THE WORKPLACE

236 **George Costanza:** "The Nap," *Seinfeld*, NBC (April 10, 1997).

237 **work burnout and bad sleep:** Torbjörn Åkerstedt, Johanna Garefelt,

Anne Richter, Hugo Westerlund, Linda Magnusson Hanson, and Magnus Sverke, "Work and Sleep—A Prospective Study of Psychosocial Work Factors, Physical Work Factors, and Work Scheduling," *SLEEP* 38 (2015): 1129–36.

237 **work is the number-one reason:** Mathias Basner, Andrea M. Spaeth, and David F. Dinges, "Sociodemographic Characteristics and Waking Activities and Their Role in the Timing and Duration of Sleep," *SLEEP* 37 (2014): 1889–906.

238 **For each hour later that we start work:** Ibid.

238 **simply training managers:** Ryan Olson, Tori L. Crain, Todd E. Bodner, Rosalind King, Leslie B. Hammer, Laura Cousino Klein, Leslie Erickson, Phyllis Moen, Lisa F. Berkman, and Orfeu M. Buxton, "A Workplace Intervention Improves Sleep: Results from the Randomized Controlled Work, Family, and Health Study," *Sleep Health* 1 (2015): 55–65.

238 **Dr. Carol Ash:** Carol Ash, interview with Gayle King, Charlie Rose, and Norah O'Donnell, "Resting Easier," *CBS This Morning*, January 26, 2015, www.cbsnews.com.

238 **study of Chinese workers:** Nicholas Bloom, James Liang, John Roberts, and Zhichun Jenny Ying, "Does Working from Home Work? Evidence from a Chinese Experiment," *The Quarterly Journal of Economics* 130 (2015), 165–218.

238 **"Our advice":** Nicholas Bloom and John Roberts, "A Working from Home Experiment Shows High Performers Like It Better," *Harvard Business Review*, January 23, 2015, www.hbr.org.

238 **more than 13 million people:** Peter J. Mateyka, Melanie A. Rapino, and Liana Christin Landivar, "Home-Based Workers in the United States: 2010," United States Census Bureau, October 2012, www.census.gov.

238 **13.9 percent of all workers:** "Characteristics of Home Workers, 2014," Office for National Statistics, June 2014, www.ons.gov.uk.

238 **whose offices had windows:** Mohamed Boubekri, Ivy N. Cheung, Kathryn J. Reid, Chia-Hui Wang, and Phyllis C. Zee, "Impact of Windows and Daylight Exposure on Overall Health and Sleep Quality of Office Workers: A Case-Control Pilot Study," *Journal of Clinical Sleep Medicine* 10 (2014): 603–11.

238 **"There is increasing evidence that exposure to light":** Marla Paul, "Natural Light in the Office Boosts Health," *Northwestern University News*, August 4, 2014, www.northwestern.edu.

239 **more and more companies:** "Sleeping at Work: Companies with Nap Rooms and Snooze-Friendly Policies," *Sleep*, www.sleep.org.

239 **Karen May:** Karen May, "Getting More Sleep, and Sticking With It," *The Huffington Post*, September 2, 2015, www.huffingtonpost.com.

239 **tips she's developed:** Ibid.

240 **Brian Halligan:** Adam Bryant, "Brian Halligan, Chief of HubSpot, on the Value of Naps," *The New York Times*, December 5, 2013, www.nytimes.com.

240 **philosophy shared by Ryan Holmes:** Alyssa Kritsch, "5 Secrets for a

Better Work-Life Balance: Inside Hootsuite Culture," *Hootsuite*, October 18, 2013, www.blog.hootsuite.com.

241 **"Many of the same tech start-ups":** Ryan Holmes, "Why I Want My Employees to Sleep on the Job," *LinkedIn*, September 11, 2014, www.linkedin.com.

241 **Shampa Bagchi:** Shampa Bagchi, "My 'Arianna Huffington Wakeup Call,'" *The Huffington Post*, November 15, 2014, www.huffingtonpost.com.

242 **Alicia Hansen:** Alicia Hansen, "My Wake-Up Call Came in the Form of a Broken Face," *The Huffington Post*, March 27, 2015, www.huffingtonpost.com.

242 **Hans Ulrich Obrist:** Hans Ulrich Obrist, email to the author, November 6, 2015.

243 **Aleen Keshishian:** Aleen Keshishian, conversation with the author, January 6, 2015.

243 **"When forced to choose":** "2008 Annual Report," Berkshire Hathaway Inc., www.berkshirehathaway.com.

244 **Microsoft CEO Satya Nadella:** Satya Nadella, interview with Rebecca Jarvis, "What Time Does This Tech Titan Wake Up in the Morning?," *ABC News*, February 4, 2015, www.abcnews.go.com.

244 **Goldman Sachs has banned summer interns:** Jackie Wattles, "Goldman Sachs Bans Interns from Staying Overnight at the Office," *CNN Money*, June 17, 2015, www.money.cnn.com.

244 **help the bankers sleep more:** Jena McGregor, "The Average Worker Loses 11 Days of Productivity Each Year Due to Insomnia, and Companies Are Taking Notice," *The Washington Post*, July 30, 2015, www.washingtonpost.com.

244 **recognizing the need for change:** Emily Peck, "Goldman Tells Interns: You Can't Work All Night Anymore," *The Huffington Post*, July 17, 2015, www.huffingtonpost.com.

244 **Pat Wadors:** Pat Wadors, "I Got My 8 Hours in—Did You?," *The Huffington Post*, October 7, 2015, www.huffingtonpost.com.

244 **"Without a good night's rest":** Ibid.

245 **Amazon CEO Jeff Bezos:** Nancy Jeffrey, "Sleep Is the New Status Symbol for Successful Entrepreneurs," *The Wall Street Journal*, April 2, 1999, www.wsj.com.

245 **Marc Andreessen:** Ibid.

245 **Campbell's Soup CEO Denise Morrison:** Denise Morrison, email to the author, November 3, 2015.

245 **Google Chairman Eric Schmidt:** Rebecca Jarvis and Nicole Sawyer, "C-Suite Insider: A Day in the Life of Google's Eric Schmidt," *ABC News*, September 23, 2014, www.abcnews.go.com.

245 **licensed pilot:** Matt Rosoff, "Eric Schmidt Has a Need for Speed," *Business Insider*, March 22, 2012, www.businessinsider.com.

245 **Mark Bertolini:** David Gelles, "At Aetna, a C.E.O.'s Management by Mantra," *The New York Times*, February 27, 2015, www.nytimes.com.

246 **Ursula von der Leyen:** Jeevan Vasagar, "Out of Hours Working

Banned by German Labour Ministry," *The Telegraph*, August 30, 2013, www.telegraph.co.uk.

246 **Andrea Nahles:** Philip Oltermann, "Germany Ponders Ground-Breaking Law to Combat Work-Related Stress," *The Guardian*, September 18, 2014, www.theguardian.com.

246 **Nahles has declared her support:** "Anti-Stress Law Moves Step Closer in Germany," *The Local*, August 26, 2014, www.thelocal.de.

246 **Volkswagen:** Tom de Castella, "Could Work Emails Be Banned After 6pm?," *BBC News*, April 10, 2014, www.bbc.com.

246 **other German companies:** David Meyer, "Germany Mulls Ban on After-Hours Work Emails and Calls," *Gigaom*, August 27, 2014, www.gigaom.com.

247 **France has established rules:** de Castella, "Could Work Emails Be Banned After 6pm?"

12. FROM HOLLYWOOD AND WASHINGTON TO HOSPITALS AND HOTELS: DISCOVERING THE POWER OF SLEEP

248 **Bobbi Brown:** "Secrets of the Most Productive People," *Fast Company*, November 18, 2014, www.fastcompany.com.

248 **"Sleep and rest and happiness":** Bobbi Brown and Annemarie Iverson, *Bobbi Brown Teenage Beauty: Everything You Need to Look Pretty, Natural, Sexy, and Awesome* (New York: William Morrow and Co., 2001), 11.

249 **Supermodel Karlie Kloss agrees:** "Karlie Kloss 'Spoils' Herself with Sleep," *The Washington Post*, May 26, 2015, www.washingtonpost.com.

249 **Cindy Crawford:** Sasha Bronner, "8 Surprisingly Down-to-Earth Wellness Tips from Cindy Crawford," *The Huffington Post*, February 13, 2015, www.huffingtonpost.com.

249 **Christina Aguilera:** "How Much Beauty Sleep Do You Get?," *People*, April 25, 2011, www.people.com.

249 **Lauren Conrad:** Lauren Conrad, "Inspirations: Beauty Sleep," *The Beauty Department*, May 18, 2011, www.thebeautydepartment.com.

249 **Gwyneth Paltrow:** Kate Hogan, "Gwyneth Paltrow's Biggest Beauty Secret? Sleep!," *People*, October 20, 2011, www.peoplestylewatch.com.

249 **"And if tonight my soul":** D. H. Lawrence, *Complete Works of D. H. Lawrence* (Hasting: Delphi Classics, 2015), www.books.google.com.

249 **"Sleep is my weapon":** "Lopez' Beauty Tip," *Contactmusic*, February 15, 2006, www.contactmusic.com.

249 **"I think sometimes":** Rebecca Ascher-Walsh, "Jennifer Lopez and Her New Leading Role to Help Kids," *WebMD Magazine*, February 1, 2012, www.webmd.com.

249 **Beyoncé's "definition of beauty":** "How Much Beauty Sleep Do You Get?"

249 **Jane Fonda:** Rod McPhee and Veronica Parker, "Jane Fonda from Sex Symbol to Pensioner and How She Keeps Her Youthful Spirit," *The Mirror*, July 5, 2015, www.mirror.co.uk.

250 **Cameron Diaz:** Cameron Diaz, *The Body Book: The Law of Hunger, the Science of Strength, and Other Ways to Love Your Amazing Body* (New York: HarperCollins, 2014), 188–94.

250 **"Sleep can completely":** Poehler, *Yes Please*, 1850–52.

250 **President Franklin D. Roosevelt:** Doris Kearns Goodwin, *No Ordinary Time: Franklin & Eleanor Roosevelt: The Home Front in World War II* (New York: Simon & Schuster, 1994), 191–92.

250 **Harry Hopkins later said:** Ibid., 193.

251 **Robert Sherwood:** Ibid.

251 **when Hillary Clinton stepped down:** Gail Collins, "Hillary's Next Move," *The New York Times*, November 10, 2012, www.nytimes.com.

251 **"I do believe sleep deprivation":** Mark Leibovich, "Fatigue Factor Gives Equal Time to Candidates," *The New York Times*, January 3, 2008, www.nytimes.com.

252 **World Health Organization:** Birgitta Berglund, Thomas Lindvall, and Dietrich H. Schwela, eds., "Guidelines for Community Noise," *World Health Organization Institutional Repository for Information Sharing*, April 1999, www.who.int.

252 **In 2014, researchers from Oxford:** Julie L. Darbyshire and J. Duncan Young, "An Investigation of Sound Levels on Intensive Care Units with Reference to the WHO Guidelines," *Critical Care* 17 (2013): doi: 10.1186/cc12870.

253 **hospital noise peaked:** Jordan C. Yoder, Paul G. Staisiunas, David O. Meltzer, Kristen L. Knutson, and Vineet M. Arora, "Noise and Sleep Among Adult Medical Inpatients: Far from a Quiet Night," *Archives of Internal Medicine* 172 (2012): 68–70.

253 **2013 study by researchers at Johns Hopkins University:** Biren B. Kamdar, Lauren M. King, Nancy A. Collop, Sruthi Sakamuri, Elizabeth Colantuoni, Karin J. Neufeld, O. Joseph Bienvenu, Annette M. Rowden, Pegah Touradji, Roy G. Brower, and Dale M. Needham, "The Effect of a Quality Improvement Intervention on Perceived Sleep Quality and Cognition in a Medical ICU," *Critical Care Medicine* 41 (2013): 800–9.

253 **sleep lost due to high noise:** Pauline W. Chen, "The Clatter of the Hospital Room," *The New York Times*, August 2, 2012, www.well.blogs.nytimes.com.

253 **St. Luke's Hospital in New York City:** Alison Connor and Elizabeth Ortiz, "Staff Solutions for Noise Reduction in the Workplace," *The Permanente Journal* 13 (2009): 23–27.

253 **reduce nighttime noise in the ICU:** "Simple Measures to Promote Sleep Can Reduce Delirium in Intensive Care Patients," Johns Hopkins Medicine press release, February 20, 2013, www.hopkinsmedicine.org.

254 **the "SHHH" system:** Diane Rogers, "Shhhhh: Stanford Hospital Team Works to Keep Things Quiet in Patient Units," *Stanford Medicine News*, May 27, 2009, www.med.stanford.edu.

254 **"Too Loud" initiative:** "Too Loud Program at Newark Beth Helps Reduce Noise," *Local Talk News*, January 4, 2010, www.localtalknews.com.

254 **Department of Veterans Affairs:** Chen, "The Clatter of the Hospital Room."

254 **"Sleep is such a powerful source":** Ibid.

254 **a hospital in Mexico:** Gabriela Torres, "Should Doctors Be Allowed to Nap on the Job?," *BBC News*, May 16, 2015, www.bbc.com.

255 **"Awake at the Wheel":** Timothy Morgenthaler, "Awake at the Wheel: Healthy Sleep Project Launches Campaign to Decrease Avoidable Drowsy Driving-Related Motor Vehicle Accidents," *The Huffington Post*, November 11, 2014, www.huffingtonpost.com.

255 **"Tiredness Can Kill, Take a Break":** Lockley and Foster, *Sleep*, 104.

255 **using GPS technology to detect car deviations:** Drew M. Morris, June J. Pilcher, and Fred S. Switzer III, "Lane Heading Difference: An Innovative Model for Drowsy Driving Detection Using Retrospective Analysis Around Curves," *Accident Analysis & Prevention* 80 (2015): 117–24.

255 **Ford Fusion sounds an alarm:** "All-New 2013 Ford Fusion to Offer Lane Keeping Assist," *Kelley Blue Book*, December 30, 2011, www.kbb.com.

255 **Mercedes' "Attention Assist":** "Safety," Mercedes-Benz, www.mbusa.com.

255 **"Drowsy driving is deadly":** "Healthy Sleep Project Urges Parents to Teach Teens to Avoid Drowsy Driving," American Academy of Sleep Medicine, April 7, 2015, www.aasmnet.org.

256 **John Timmerman:** John Timmerman, email to the author, September 25, 2015.

256 **Benjamin Hotel in New York City:** Rebecca Robbins, phone call with the author, July 31, 2015.

256 **array of sleep-inducing amenities:** Ibid.

257 **"I opened the bed fastidiously":** Flann O'Brien, *The Complete Novels* (New York: Everyman's Library, 2008), 324.

258 **Four Seasons:** "Disconnect to Reconnect," Four Seasons, www.fourseasons.com.

258 **InterContinental:** "Discover the Difference of Crowne Plaza Sleep Advantage," Crowne Plaza Hotels & Resorts, https://ihg.com.

258 **Marriott:** John Wolf (consumer PR, Marriott), email to Suzy Strutner (associate lifestyle editor, *The Huffington Post*), September 10, 2015.

13. THE SPORTS WORLD'S ULTIMATE PERFORMANCE ENHANCER

259 **Equinox:** Ciara Bryne, "A Fitness Giant Eyes the Next Frontier of Personal Training: Sleeping," *Fast Company*, February 26, 2015, www.fastcompany.com.

259 **Liz Miersch:** Liz Miersch, email to the author, November 6, 2015.

259 **"The body is super busy":** Kym Perfetto, email to the author, July 12, 2015.

260 **"It is everything":** Sue Molnar, email to the author, July 12, 2015.

260 **"Eating well and working well":** Joey Gonzalez, email to the author, July 16, 2015.

261 **"Just as athletes need more calories":** R. Morgan Griffin, "Can Sleep Improve Your Athletic Performance?," *WebMD*, August 13, 2014, www.webmd.com.

261 **the cheetah:** "Cheetah," *National Geographic*, animals.nationalgeographic.com; Laura Walters, "Walking with the Cheetahs," *Stuff*, October 24, 2014, www.stuff.co.nz.

261 **"actually one of the older coaches":** Jon Gruden and Vic Carucci, *Do You Love Football?!: Winning with Heart, Passion, and Not Much Sleep* (New York: HarperCollins, 2004), 232–41.

261 **George Allen of the Washington Redskins:** Derickson, *Dangerously Sleepy;* Deacon Jones, "George Allen's Enshrinement Speech," Pro Football Hall of Fame, August 3, 2002, www.profootballhof.com.

262 **"Several collegiate swimmers":** Cheri Mah, email to the author, March 15, 2015.

262 **Mah's focus began to shift:** Ibid.

263 **"multiple weeks of sleep extension":** Ibid.

263 **her most widely cited studies:** Cheri D. Mah, Kenneth E. Mah, Eric J. Kezirian, and William C. Dement, "The Effects of Sleep Extension on the Athletic Performance of Collegiate Basketball Players," *SLEEP* 34 (2011): 943–50.

263 **Mah conducted another study:** "Getting Extra Sleep Improves the Athletic Performance of Collegiate Football Players," American Academy of Sleep Medicine, May 27, 2010, www.aasmnet.org.

263 **"Some sports teams":** Mah, email to the author.

264 **"if I can get a pro athlete":** Winter, email to the author.

264 **"Teams view what I do":** Ibid.

264 **"When it comes to the precision":** Pete Carroll, email to the author, June 12, 2015.

265 **"Fatigue and performance":** Michael Gervais and Sam Ramsden, email to the author, June 12, 2015.

265 **quarterback Tom Brady:** Tom Brady, interview with John Dennis and Gerry Callahan, "Tom Brady on the Bye Week," *The Dennis & Callahan Morning Show*, WEEI 93.7 FM, November 10, 2014, www.media.weei.com.

265 **The Chicago Bears are employing:** Rich Campbell, "Bears' Eyes Are Wide Open to the Advantages of Proper Sleep Habits," *Chicago Tribune*, August 17, 2015, www.chicagotribune.com.

265 **former NBA All-Star Grant Hill:** "Grant Hill–NBA FIT Team Member," *NBA FIT*, December 1, 2009, fit.nba.com.

265 **LeBron James:** Zach McCann, "Sleep Tracking Brings New Info to Athletes," *ESPN*, June 1, 2012, www.espn.go.com.

265 **NBA MVP Steve Nash:** "Training Tips from NBA Superstar Steve Nash," *Canada.com*, www.canada.com.

266 **triathlete Jarrod Shoemaker:** Ben Greenfield, *Beyond Training: Mastering Endurance, Health, and Life* (Las Vegas: Victory Belt Publishing, 2014), 231.

266 **Usain Bolt:** "Sleep to Be an All-Star: Winners Sleep, Losers Weep," *Speed Endurance*, November 2013, www.speedendurance.com.

266 **Kerri Walsh Jennings:** Ibid.

266 **Roger Federer:** Ru-an, "Awesome Federer Interview," *The Ultimate Tennis Blog*, January 15, 2010, www.theultimatetennisblog.com.

266 **Before Wimbledon in 2015:** Thomas Burrows, "Roger Federer's Formula for Final? Renting TWO Houses to Avoid Being Disturbed by His Young Family," *Daily Mail*, July 11, 2015, www.dailymail.co.uk.

266 **the Southampton soccer club:** Alec Fenn, "How Gareth Bale and Real Madrid Sleep Their Way to the Top," *BBC Sport*, April 21, 2015, www.bbc.com.

266 **Manchester City soccer club:** Jack Crone, "Manchester City Players Given Wallpaper with Special Sleep-Inducing Patterns in Their Bedrooms at Club's £200m Training Base," *Mail Online*, January 3, 2015, www.dailymail.co.uk.

266 **Nick Littlehales:** "Testimonials," Sport Sleep Coach, www.sportsleepcoach.com.

266 **"I have been preparing":** Nick Littlehales, email to the author, September 30, 2015.

267 **A 2015 *Wall Street Journal* headline:** Jonathan Clegg, "College Football Wakes Up to a New Statistic: Sleep," *The Wall Street Journal*, August 20, 2015, www.wsj.com.

267 **Pat Fitzgerald:** Ibid.

267 **Tyler Scott:** Ibid.

267 **University of Tennessee:** Brian Rice, "Sleeping to Better Performance," *UT Sports*, August 16, 2015, www.utsports.com.

267 **players also wear orange-tinted glasses:** Clegg, "College Football Wakes Up to a New Statistic."

267 **"It was very powerful to see":** Leon Sasson (founder, Rise Science), email to the author, November 7, 2015.

268 **coach Pat Narduzzi makes sure his players:** Clegg, "College Football Wakes Up to a New Statistic."

268 **one of the focal points of Chris Winter's work:** Christopher Winter, William R. Hammond, Noah H. Green, Zhiyong Zhang, and Donald L. Bliwise, "Measuring Circadian Advantage in Major League Baseball: A 10-Year Retrospective Study," *International Journal of Sports Physiology & Performance* 4 (2009): 394–401.

268 **"Basically, we proved what hardcore gamblers":** Winter, email to the author.

269 **Researchers studied thirty Major League Baseball teams:** Jason Koebler, "Study: MLB Players' Plate Discipline Degrades Over Season," *USA TODAY*, May 31, 2013, www.usatoday.com.

269 **Winter has been working with the San Francisco Giants:** Janie McCauley, "Sweet Dreams: Sleep Expert Helps Giants in October," *USA TODAY*, October, 25, 2014, www.usatoday.com.

269 **Peak physical performance:** Sue Shellenbarger, "The Peak Time for Everything," *The Wall Street Journal*, September 26, 2012, www.wsj.com.

269 **Since Winter started consulting:** McCauley, "Sweet Dreams."

270 **Seattle Mariners baseball team:** Mark McClusky, *Faster, Higher, Stronger: How Sports Science Is Creating a New Generation of Superathletes—and What We Can Learn from Them* (New York: Penguin, 2014), Kindle edition.

270 **In 2014, the Mariners began wearing:** Dan Hughes, "Seattle Mariners Use Technology and Stuff to Fight Travel Fatigue," *SODO MOJO*, November 3, 2014, www.sodomojo.com.

270 **Readibands monitor:** "What Impact Is a Lack of Sleep Having on Your Athletes' Performance?," Fatigue Science, www.fatiguescience.com.

270 **researchers from the University of Birmingham:** Elise Facer-Childs and Roland Brandstaetter, "The Impact of Circadian Phenotype and Time Since Awakening on Diurnal Performance in Athletes," *Current Biology* 25 (2015), 518–22.

270 **"If you're an early type":** James Gallagher, "Bedtime 'Has Huge Impact on Sport,'" *BBC News*, January 30, 2015, www.bbc.com.

270 **Major League Baseball players:** Winter, email to the author.

270 **"For players who want":** Ibid.

272 **Jason Smith:** Ian Begley, "The Science of Sleep: For New Dad Jason Smith, It's Hard to Beat a Good Night's Rest," *ESPN*, January 30, 2015, www.espn.go.com.

272 **his job performance suffered:** Nakia Hogan, "New Orleans Pelicans Center/Forward Jason Smith's Season Plagued by Injuries Again," *The Times-Picayune*, May 1, 2014, www.nola.com.

272 **the sleep-deprived first half of the season:** Begley, "The Science of Sleep."

272 **And as her sleep time increased:** Ibid.

273 **Iguodala also makes sleep a priority:** Pablo S. Torre and Tom Haberstroh, "New Biometric Tests Invade the NBA," *ESPN*, October 10, 2014, www.espn.com.

273 **The pattern went on for years:** Ibid.

273 **"Sleep good, feel good, play good":** Juliet Spies-Gans, "Andre Iguodala Attributes Strong Play to Better Sleep Cycles," *The Huffington Post*, October 6, 2015, www.huffingtonpost.com.

273 **When Iguodala adjusted:** Sweetser, "How MVP Andre Iguodala Improved His Game with UP."

273 **he Instagrammed a picture:** Nick Schwartz, "Andre Iguodala's Perfect Instagram Photo with His Finals MVP Trophy," *For the Win*, July 17, 2015, ftw.usatoday.com.

273 **"I've grown":** Philip Galanes, "For Arianna Huffington and Kobe Bryant: First, Success. Then Sleep.," *The New York Times*, September 26, 2015, www.nytimes.com.

14. PUTTING TECHNOLOGY IN ITS PLACE (NOT ON YOUR NIGHTSTAND)

275 **global wearables market is predicted:** BI Intelligence, "The Wearables Report: Growth Trends, Consumer Attitudes, and Why Smartwatches Will Dominate," *Business Insider*, May 21, 2015, www.businessinsider.com.

275 **One in five Americans:** "Consumer Intelligence Series: The Wearable Technology Future," PricewaterhouseCoopers, www.pwc.com.

275 **A big percentage of these are fitness trackers:** Ananya Bhattacharya, "Fitbit Is Now Worth $4.1 Billion After IPO," *CNN Money*, June 25, 2015, www.money.cnn.com.

276 **Lumoid:** "Wearable Gear," LUMOID, www.lumoid.com.

276 **2015 study by Sleep Number:** "National Survey Shows 75 Percent of Americans Don't Get Enough Sleep; 58 Percent Wish They Knew More About Improving Sleep Quality, Yet Only 16 Percent Track Sleep," Sleep Number, community.sleepnumber.com.

276 **It's a nonwearable sleep tracker:** "Meet Sense," hello, www.hello.is.

276 **Proud told me:** James Proud, email to the author, June 15, 2015.

276 **The data come from a bedside orb:** Ibid.

277 **Chrona, created by Ultradia:** "Chrona," Chrona, www.chronasleep.com.

277 **Ultradia cofounder Ben Bronsther:** Ben Bronsther, email to the author, May 25, 2015.

277 **The Samsung Gear S:** "S Health: Sleep Monitor," Samsung, www.samsung.com.

277 **Jawbone's UP3 band:** "UP3," Jawbone, www.jawbone.com.

277 **"The app's Smart Coach":** Hosain Rahman, email to the author, September 14, 2015.

277 **Fitbit:** "Sleep Tracking FAQs," Fitbit, https://help.fitbit.com.

277 **"There's a saying":** James Park, email to the author, September 14, 2015.

277 **In 2014, Withings:** "Aura Connected Alarm Clock + Sleep Sensor Accessory," Withings, www.withings.com.

278 **light can suppress the body's production:** "Blue Light Has a Dark Side," *Harvard Health Publications*, May 1, 2012, www.health.harvard.edu.

278 **f.lux:** "f.lux," f.lux, www.justgetflux.com.

278 **As Michael Herf told me:** Michael Herf, email to the author, August 20, 2015.

EPILOGUE

283 **Japanese tea ceremony:** Andrea L. Stanton, Edward Ramsamy, Peter J. Seybolt, and Carolyn M. Elliott, eds., *Cultural Sociology of the Middle East, Asia, and Africa: An Encyclopedia* (Thousand Oaks, CA: SAGE Publications, 2012), 137; Pradyumna Karan, *Japan in the 21st Century: Environment, Economy, and Society* (Lexington: University of Kentucky Press, 2010), 97.

APPENDIX C: THE HOTEL SLEEP REVOLUTION

298 **"Light levels":** Paul Scialla, email to the author, April 13, 2015.

APPENDIX D: GOING TO THE MATTRESSES

305 **"The market for beds":** Charlie Wells, "The New Mattress Professionals," *The Wall Street Journal*, September 30, 2015, www.wsj.com.

305 **"We noticed that everyone":** "Interview with Philip Krim, cofounder and CEO of Casper Sleep," *Slumber Sage*, www.slumbersage.com.

306 **"When you buy a car":** Mike Efmorfidis, conversation with the author, June 5, 2015.

INDEX